# Genes and Proteins Underlying Microbial Urinary Tract Virulence

## Basic Aspects and Applications

# ADVANCES IN EXPERIMENTAL MEDICINE AND BIOLOGY

A Continuation Order Plan is available for this series. A continuation order will bring delivery of each new volume immediately upon publication. Volumes are billed only upon actual shipment. For further information please contact the publisher.

# Genes and Proteins Underlying Microbial Urinary Tract Virulence

## Basic Aspects and Applications

Edited by

**Levente Emődy**
**Tibor Pál**
*University of Pécs*
*Pécs, Hungary*

and

**Jörg Hacker**
**Gabriele Blum-Oehler**
*University of Würzburg*
*Würzburg, Germany*

Kluwer Academic / Plenum Publishers
New York, Boston, Dordrecht, London, Moscow

Library of Congress Cataloging-in-Publication Data

Genes and proteins underlying microbial urinary tract virulence: basic aspects and applications/edited by Levente Emődy ... [et al.].
    p.   ; cm.—(Advances in experimental medicine and biology: v. 485)
    "Proceedings of the FEMS Symposium on Genes and Proteins Underlying Microbial Urinary Tract Virulence: Basic Aspects and Applications, held September 16–19, 1999, in Pécs, Hungary"—T.p. verso
    Includes bibliographical references and index.
    ISBN 0-306-46455-1
        1. Urinary tract infections—Congresses.   2. Virulence (Microbiology)—Molecular aspects—Congresses.   3. Escherichia coli infections—Congresses.   I. Emődy, Levente.   II. FEMS Symposium on Genes and Proteins Underlying Microbial Urinary Tract Virulence: Basic Aspects and Applications (1999: Pécs, Hungary)   III. Series.
        [DNLM:   1. Urinary tract infections—genetics—Congresses.   2. Enterobacteriaceae—pathogenicity—Congresses.   3. Virulence—genetics—Congresses.   WJ 15I G327 2000]
    RC901.8 .G46 2000
    616.6′01—dc21

                                                                                          00-042249

Proceedings of the FEMS Symposium on Genes and Proteins Underlying Microbial Urinary Tract Virulence: Basic Aspects and Applications, held September 16–19, 1999, in Pécs, Hungary

ISBN 0-306-46455-1

©2000 Kluwer Academic / Plenum Publishers, New York
233 Spring Street, New York, N.Y. 10013

http://www.wkap.nl/

10  9  8  7  6  5  4  3  2  1

A C.I.P. record for this book is available from the Library of Congress

# PREFACE

Urinary tract infections are among the most frequent diseases caused by microbial pathogens. Their clinical manifestations range from uncomplicated episodes to life threatening conditions like urosepsis with septic shock. The molecular basis of bacterial mechanisms and host-parasite interactions underlying the pathogenesis of these infections as well as the modern approaches to the diagnosis, therapy and preventive measures have attracted the attention of a wide range of experts. A FEMS supported symposium was held on this subject September 16-19, 1999, at Pécs, Hungary. The aim of the meeting was to bring together basic researchers, clinical microbiologists and clinicians to exchange the latest ideas covering four major aspects of the main topic, namely:

- genetic information, synthesis, and assembly of virulence factors in urinary pathogens
- regulation of genes involved in the phenotypic appearence of virulence
- host-parasite interactions determining the process and outcome of the infection
- possible applications of the above aspects in diagnosis, therapy, and prevention

The presentations delivered at this symposium provided the basis for the chapters of this volume.

The organisers of the conference wish to express their special thanks to the following organisations for their financial support and contribution to the realisation of the symposium: Federation of the European Microbiological Societies (FEMS), German Society for Hygiene and Microbiology (DGHM) and Hungarian Society for Microbiology.

Levente Emődy      Jörg Hacker
Tibor Pál      Gabriele Blum-Oehler

Pécs      Würzburg

# CONTENTS

## SESSION III. HOST-PARASITE INTERACTIONS

## SESSION IV. APPLICATIONS: DIAGNOSIS, THERAPY AND PREVENTION

# URINARY TRACT INFECTION: FROM BASIC SCIENCE TO CLINICAL APPLICATION

Jörg Hacker

*Institut für Molekulare Infektionsbiologie der Universität Würzburg, Röntgenring 11, D-97070 Würzburg, Tel. 0931/31-2575, Fax 0931/ 31-2578*

## 1.     INTRODUCTION

Urinary tract infections (UTIs) represent one of the most important infectious syndroms in countries of the industrialized world. In addition to the main uropathogen, *Escherichia coli*, more and more non-*E. coli* pathogens have been detected as causative agents of UTI. Thus, gram-positive bacteria (Staphylococci, Enterococci) as well as fungal pathogens (*Candida albicans, Candida glabrata*) are able to cause urinary tract infections especially in elderly persons and hospitalized patients. However, for many years, urinary pathogens have been chosen as model organisms to study issues of molecular pathogenesis. The genome structure of pathogens, the concept of virulence factors, important features of gene regulation, host-parasite interactions and the role of host factors in infectious diseases have been studied with urinary pathogens. This article describes recent developments in the analysis of UTI and future trends, presented during the FEMS Symposium on UTI, held in Pecs (Hungary) in summer 1999.

## 2.     UROPATHOGENIC ORGANISM

Urinary tract infections can be divided into complicated and non-complicated infectious diseases. The main pathogen of non-complicated urinary tract infections is *Escherichia coli*. *E. coli* is not only detected in

*Genes and Proteins Underlying Microbial Urinary Tract Virulence*
Edited by L. Emődy *et al.*, Kluwer Academic/Plenum Publishers, 2000

1

urinary tract infections in humans but also plays an important role in UTI of certain animals, especially dogs. It is interesting to note that also intestinal pathogens of porcine origin exhibit features of uropathogenic *E. coli*[1].

Over the last few years several non-E. coli bacteria were identified to be uropathogenic. Those bacteria were often found in patients suffering from complicated urinary tract infections, including patients with either catheters or suffering from stone formation or in immunocompromized patients. Thus, multiresistant *Klebsiella pneumoniae* and *Pseudomonas aeruginosa* as well as certain Proteus species are important of non-*E. coli* uropathogens. One has to take in mind that especially the newly established species *Proteus penneri* seems to be a newly emerging uropathogen[2]. In addition, gram-positive bacteria also play an increasing role as nosocomial pathogens in UTI. Thus, the biofilm forming *S. aureus* and *S. epidermidis* species are of particular importance. Moreover, *Chlamydia trachomatis*, *Mycoplasma hominis* and *Ureaplasma urealyticum* represent important uropathogens. Anaerobic bacteria play an important role especially during prostatitis. Fungi (*Candida albicans*, *Candida glabrata*) also represent an emerging group of uropathogens, especially in patients following organ transplantation and chemotherapy.

## 3.       GENE STRUCTURE OF UROPATHOGENS

Studies on the genome structure of uropathogens were performed especially with uropathogenic *E. coli*[3]. It is of interest that the complete genome sequence of the non-pathogenic *E. coli* K-12 isolate was established two years ago on the basis of this sequence. It became obvious that pathogenic *E. coli*, including uropathogenic organisms, contain additional pieces of DNA, which can be part of plasmids, bacteriophages or may represent particular fragments of the genome, termed pathogenicity islands[4]. Enterohemorrhagic *E. coli*, another group of intestinal pathogenic *E. coli* bacteria, contain at least one megabase additional DNA compared to *E. coli* K-12. It is suggested that uropathogenic *E. coli* may also carry additional 300 to 400 kb of DNA. The analysis of the genome of the uropathogenic *E. coli* strain 536 exhibited four additional pieces of DNA forming pathogenicity islands with a size range from 25 - 190 kb. In the future, the application of new techniques, including the representative difference analysis (RDA) and the two-dimensional (2D) protein gel electrophoresis will be of great advantage in the discovery and characterization of additional virulence factors which may be part of pathogenicity islands in uropathogenic bacteria.

## 4.     VIRULENCE FACTORS

Pathogenicity islands carry genes, which encode important virulence factors (see Fig 1), including iron uptake systems[5].

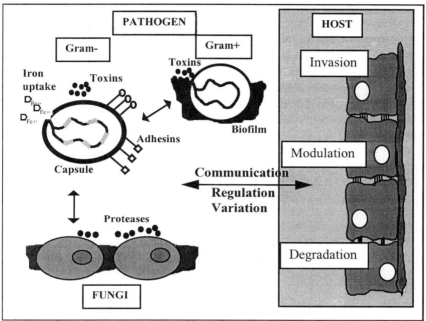

*Figure1.* Schematic diagram on the interaction between uropathogenic organism and host cell structures (for details see text).

It is of particular importance that yersiniabactin, an iron uptake system, first described for pathogenic *Yersinia*, is also encoded by the majority of uropathogenic *E. coli*[6]. This iron uptake system is located on a conserved pathogenicity island which is present in many enterobacteria. In addition, yersiniabactin and the seven iron uptake systems described for the non-pathogenic *E. coli* K-12 organisms, aerobactin is also produced by uropathogenic *E. coli* strains. Toxins are important for the pathogenesis of urinary tract infections[7]. In uropathogenic *E. coli*, the $\alpha$-hemolysin toxin was described many years ago. Recently, an accumulating amount of data concerning the maturation of the $\alpha$-hemolysin toxin in UPEC, its secretion and the regulation of the corresponding genes appeared. In addition, the cytotoxic necrotizing factor I, which is responsible for Rho modification and subsequent activation of small host GTPases has been analyzed. A newly identified toxin, the cytolethal destending toxin (CDT), was also found to be produced by uropathogenic *E. coli*, its role in the pathogenesis, however, remains to be elucidated.

Another import feature of pathogenic bacteria are adherence factors. The fimbriae from uropathogenic *E. coli* are well described[3]. It was shown that P-fimbriae, which are able to bind to Gal α1-4 Gal-receptors carry receptor binding molecules, termed PapG, exhibiting the receptor binding domain in their N-terminal parts. Recently, the importance of sequence alterations of the major subunit FimA and the minor subunit FimH of mannose-specific type I fimbriae were illustrated by the finding that pathoadaptive mutations are important for the binding capacity of the type I adherence factors. S-fimbriae and type I C-fimbriae are also important adherence factors of uropathogenic *E. coli*. These adherence factors have the capacity to bind to an asialo GM2 receptor structure. It is of great interest whether additional binding factors, especially thin aggregative fimbriae are of importance for the pathogenesis of UTI. Other non *E. coli* uropathogenic bacteria also produce important binding molecules. This is especially true for the capacity of biofilm formation, which is exhibited by Enterococci and Staphylococci[8]. In Enterococci the aggregative slime substance is identical to the clumping factor, which plays an important role in DNA transfer via conjugation. *In S. epidermidis* and as described recently, also in *S. aureus*, the so-called PIA antigen, a β 1,6 N-Acetyl Glucosamine polymer is important for biofilm formation.

However, capsules are also important virulence factors of gram-negative uropathogens. The flagella seem to play a role in the virulence of *Proteus* strains[9]. Proteases are necessary for full virulence of *Candida albicans*. The analysis of the newly established *Proteus penneri* strains exhibit an array of new important virulence factors, such as IgA proteases and ureases[2]. With the help of the newly established techniques in molecular biology and on the basis of the emerging genome sequences, new virulence factors will be identified and analyzed within the next few years.

## 5.      HOST-PARASITE INTERACTIONS

The different virulence factors identified, play a key-role in the interaction of uropathogens with host cell structures (see Fig 1). It is of particular importance that the adherence factors do not simply bind to uroepithelial cells, but that the majority of these factors play a role in these interaction of the pathogens with extracellular matrix molecules. Thus, the FimH-adhesin has the capacity to interact with laminin. In addition, FimA may act as a receptor for plasminogen, which in turn leads to plasmin activation and fibrinolysis. G-fimbriae bind to type IV collagen and P (Pap)-pili have the capacity to interact with fibronectin. These interactions, of course, have important consequences for the penetration of the bacteria through the extracellular matrix. Therefore, the penetration process has also been termed as „bacterial metastasis".

Fimbriae, however, may also be involved in triggering the invasion capacity of uropathogens into eukaryotic cells. A gene cluster, similar to type I fimbriae of *Salmonella* is responsible for the production of proteins, which act as invasion factors of *Citrobacter freundii*. Also other uropathogens, including uropathogenic E. coli, have the capacity to invade eukaryotic cells. Furthermore, fimbriae are able to trigger the cytokine response of epithelial cells. As shown by C. Svanborg and co-workers[10], P-fimbriae have the capacity to induce the IL-6 response of infected loot cells. A particular variant of type I fimbriae is involved in IL-8 expression. The expression of the IL-8 receptor molecule is important for the penetration of neutrophiles through the tissue layer. It is interesting to note that epithelial cells from patients, suffering from diabetes mellitus show a low level response with respect to cytokine production, compared to cells isolated from healthy persons.

Also patients with a reconstituted bladder show a different cytokine response to uropathogens compared to a control group. The analysis of host factors is extremely important to understand the development of urinary tract infections. Thus, the blood group antigen is involved in the binding capacity of uropathogens to host cells via P-fimbriae. Future studies, which will include the microarray chip technology will certainly lead to new observations regarding the host response on urinary pathogens. Using the chip technology it will be possible to analyse the expression of various host genes, including cytokine specific gene clusters, genetic determinants encoding receptor molecules and gene loci, whose products are involved in cell signalling. These data will broaden our knowledge on the host response to urinary tract infections.

## 6.     GENE REGULATION AND PHASE VARIATION

Uropathogens, especially uropathogenic *E. coli* were used in the last years as model organism to study the regulation of virulence associated genes[11]. Fimbriae, flagella, capsules as well as hemolysin determinants were described with respect to the acting gene regulators. Activators as well as repressors were found to play a role in the regulation of these gene clusters. The regulators Lrp, H-NS, Hha as well as PapI and PapB belong to these regulating molecules.

These regulators also play a role in the response of virulence gene expression in response to environmental signals. In addition, two component systems, such as the AirS (BarA) systems, are involved in environmental regulation. The AirS system seems to be activated by the binding of P-fimbriae through their eukaryotic receptor molecules. In addition, quorum sensing seems to play a role in the expression of virulence genes of uropathogens. This is also true for the biofilm gene cluster of pathogenic Staphylococci. Stress response is also involved in regulatory cascades which involve alternativ σ-factors, such as RpoS. In addition to these regulatory factors which act on the transcriptional level, translational regulation seems to be of importance (2, 5). Recently, the CNF1-gene cluster was shown to be regulated on the translation level involving the 5′ region of the molecule. Antitermination plays a role in the regulation of the hly-operon. Here, the regulator RfaH is important. Messenger (m) RNA processing is involved in the regulation of the Pap- and Sfa-fimbriae as well as in capsule synthesis.

In addition to gene regulation, phase variation on the basis of genetical alterations plays a role in adaptation of uropathogens in their environment. The expression of Pap-fimbriae is based on the methylation status of promoter regions due to the action of the Dam methylase. In addition, the inversion of a promotor carrying element directs the phase variation of type I fimbriae of enterobacteria. On the other hand, biofilm formation *of S. epidermidis* is modulated by the integration and precise excision of an IS-element. It will be interesting to determine, whether antimicrobial substances, which may act on the basis of gene regulation represent a new class of antimicrobial drugs. Such new antimicrobial drugs, however, will require a deep analysis until they will appear as real antimicrobial agents in clinical trials.

## 7.        DIAGNOSTICS, THERAPY, PREVENTION

Clinical diagnostics of uropathogens is based on classical microbiological methods (see Table 1). In addition, nucleic acid-based systems became more and more of importance. The detection of *Chlamydia trachomatis* and *Mycoplasma species* occured due to the employment of gene probes, PCR and LCR (ligase chain reaction) methods. The application of the Chip technology will allow the establishment of arrays covering a large number of factors important for virulence (e. g. adherence factors) and therapy (e. g. resistance factors) of UTI. In therapy, certain antibiotics are essential. A simple cystitis should be treated three days, pyelonephritis 10 to 14 days and a prostatitis over three months. Trimethoprim and other substances are well established in therapy of urinary tract infections. It will be certainly possible to use new drugs in the near future. For prevention antibiotics and oestrogens are used for certain groups of patients. It is doubtful, whether vaccination against uropathogens will play a major role in the future. Newly developed display systems, such as the FimH-molecule or the Flagella-protein, however, will certainly lead to new dead and live vaccine strains of potential importance for prevention of UTI. In addition, immue stimulation may also play a role in prevention of this infectious disease.

*Table 1.* Present and future methods of diagnosis, therapy and prevention of urinary tract infections

| Method / Treatment | Presently available |
|---|:---:|
| Diagnostics | |
| Classical microbial methods | + |
| PCR reactions | + |
| Gene probes | + |
| Chip technology | - |
| | |
| Therapy | |
| Traditional antibiotics | + |
| Pathogenicity blocker | - |
| | |
| Prevention | |
| Antibiotics/Oestrogen | + |
| Immune stimulation | + |
| Dead vaccine | + |
| Live vaccine | - |

# 8.    CONCLUSIONS

It is obvious that in the future urinary tract infections will play an important role in basic science and in practical medicine. In my opinion, the number of non-*E. coli* uropathogens will emerge. Especially nosocomial urinary tract infections will play a major role, because the number of eldery persons, persons receiving organ transplantation and chemotherapy and patients with other medical devices will increase. The analysis of urinary tract infections will benefit from the area of genomics and proteomics. DNA chips will be available for the analysis of uropathogens. The integrated activity of molecular biologists and physicians will be necessary to solve the future problems of urinary tract infections.

## ACKNOWLEDGEMENTS

Our own work regarding these topic was supported by the „Deutsche Forschungsgemeinschaft" (SFB 379) and the „Fond der Chemischen Industrie". I thank B. Janke (Würzburg), I. Mühldorfer (Konstanz) and C. Borde (Würzburg) for help and advise in preparing the manuscript.

## REFERENCES

1. Toth, I., Oswald, E., Mainil, J., Awad-Masalmeh, M., and Nagy, B., 2000, Porcine postweaning diarrhea isolates of *Escherichia coli* with uropathogenic characters. In *Adv. Exper. Med. Biol.*, in press.

2. Kustos, I., Toth, V., Kilar, F., Kocsis, B., and Emödy, L., 2000, Effect of spontaneous and induced mutations on outer membrane proteins and lipopolysaccharides of *Proteus penneri* strain 357. In *Adv. Exper. Med. Biol.*, in press.

3. Hacker, J., Blum-Oehler, G., Janke, B., Nagy, G., and Goebel, W., 1999, Pathogenicity islands of extraintestinal *Escherichia coli*. In *Pathogenicity islands and other mobile virulence elements* (J. Kaper, and J. Hacker, eds.), ASM-Press, Washington D.C., pp. 59 - 76.

4. Hacker, J., and Kaper, J., 1999, The concept of pathogenicity islands. In *Pathogenicity islands and other mobile virulence elements* (J. Kaper, and J. Hacker, eds.), ASM-Press, Washington D.C., pp. 1 - 11.

5. Braun, M., Killmann, H., and Braun, V., 1999, The ß-barrel domain of FhuAdelta5-160 is sufficient for TonB-dependent FhuA activities of *Escherichia coli. Mol. Microbiol.*, in press.

6. Rakin, A., Schubert, S., Pelludat C., Brem, D., and Heesemann, J., 1999, The High Pathogenicity Islands of *Yersinia*. In Kaper, J.B., Hacker, J. (ed): *Pathogenicity Islands and Other Mobile Virulence Elements* (J. Kaper and J. Hacker, eds.), ASM-Press, Washington, D.C., pp. 77 – 90.

7. Fabbri, A, Gauthier, M and Boquet, P., 1999, The 5' region of CNF1 harbours a translational regulatory mechanism for CNF1 synthesis and encodes the cell-binding domain of the toxin. *Mol. Microbiol.* **33**: 108-118.

8. Heilmann, C., Schweitzer, O., Gerke, C., Nonguch, V., Mack, D., and Götz, F., 1996, Molecular basis of intercellular adhesion in the biofilm-forming *Staphylococcus epidermidis. Mol. Microbiol.* **20**: 1083-1091.

9. Fraser, G.M., Bennett, J.C.Q., and Hughes, C., 1999, Substrate specific binding of hook-associated proteins by FlgN and FliT, putative chaperones for flagellum assembly. *Mol. Microbiol* **32**: 569-580

10. Godaly, G., Bergsten, G., Frendéus B., Long, H., Hedlund, M., Karpman, D., Samuelsson, P., Svensson, M., Otto, G., Wullt, B., and Svanborg, C., 2000, Epithelial cytokine responses elicited by bacterial adherence in the urinary tract. In: *Adv. Exper. Med. Biol.*, in press.

11. Foley, I., Marsch, P. Wellington, E. M. H., Smith, A. W. and Brown, M.R.W., 1999, General stress response master regulator *rpo* is expressed in human infection: a possible role in chronicity. *J. Antimicrob. Chemother.* **43**: 164-165.

# INNATE DEFENCES AND RESISTANCE TO GRAM NEGATIVE MUCOSAL INFECTION

Gabriela Godaly, Göran Bergsten, Björn Frendéus, Long Hang, Maria Hedlund, Diana Karpman, Patrik Samuelsson, Majlis Svensson, Gisela Otto, Björn Wullt and Catharina Svanborg
*Institute of Laboratory Medicine, Department of MIG, Lund University, Lund, Sweden*

## 1.     INTRODUCTION

Mucosal surfaces are continuously exposed to a diverse environmental microflora. Yet, infections are fairly rare and health is maintained. So, how is this achieved? Many and diverse effectors of the host defense have converged at mucosal sites and cooperate to resist the onslaught of pathogens. These are commonly assigned to two categories; the specific or the ''innate'' defenses. Specific immunity is executed by different lymphocyte populations in response to specific microbial antigens. The term ''innate'' immunity is used to denote the defenses, which lack antigen specificity, but execute their defense functions through effector molecules with highly specialized anti-microbial activity. While many aspects of specific and ''innate'' defense mechanisms have been worked out *in vitro*, we understand relatively little about their contribution to host resistance *in vivo* at a given infection site.

Specific and innate defenses cooperate to achieve the efficient anti-microbial defense at mucosal surfaces. The epithelium provides an efficient barrier that prevents the microbes from invading the tissues, and different secreted and cellbound defenses have converged at these sites. For example,

*Genes and Proteins Underlying Microbial Urinary Tract Virulence*
Edited by L. Emödy *et al.*, Kluwer Academic/Plenum Publishers, 2000

more than half of the B lymphocytes in the human body are localized along the intestinal mucosa, emphasizing the importance of specific immunity for the mucosal defense. There is a wealth of ''innate'' effectors, ranging from secreted bactericidal defensins, to mucins and receptor analogs preventing adhesion, NO production, complement activation and the influx of different cellular elements like neutrophils, mast cells and macrophages.

How should a successful outcome of the mucosal defense be described? At normally sterile sites like the lungs, upper intestinal tract or kidney, the host defense is designed to maintain sterility by destroying all invading microbes. Yet, at other sites, which normally are colonized by an indigenous microflora, the defense has to counteract the pathogens, while permitting the indigenous flora to persist. Clearly, very different host defense strategies are needed to achieve these two end points.

By the same token, pathogens and commensals use quite different strategies to overcome the defense and infect their hosts. Pathogens that cause symptomatic infections have evolved mechanisms to first establish at the mucosal site of infection and to survive the defense at this site. They then act as a ''danger signal'' and trigger the first wave of host response mediators that later get amplified through a variety of pathways, to cause symptoms and tissue damage. Indeed, we normally define virulence according to the severity of the host response. Consequently, the virulence of mucosal pathogens can be regarded as a direct read out of their ability to trigger a host response. The molecular basis of individual virulence factors should be analyzed in cellular systems involving responsive host cells. The commensals on the other hand, have evolved mechanisms of persisting without causing overt host responses. They may share with the pathogens the properties required for the initial establishment and for persistence but lack pathogenicity islands and genes that encode the molecular determinants required for host response induction.

## 2.  URINARY TRACT INFECTION AS A MODEL FOR STUDIES OF MICROBIAL VIRULENCE AND HOST RESISTANCE TO MUCOSAL INFECTION

The urinary tract infection model is suitable to study virulence mechanisms of mucosal pathogens and the antimicrobial mucosal defense. The kidney and bladder mucosa is normally sterile, due to an efficient defense that purges invading microbes and maintains sterility.

Uropathogenic *E. coli* causes symptomatic infections involving the kidneys (acute pyelonephritis) or bladders (acute cystitis). These infections are accompanied by strong host responses that cause symptoms and tissue pathology, but eventually most individuals clear the infection. Asymptomatic bacteriuria is quite frequent, occuring in about 1 % of girls, 2 % of pregnant women and up to 20% of elderly men and women[1]. In this case, bacteria are present in the urinary tract, but the patients appear totally healthy, and do not suffer long-term effects of the infection.

Urinary tract infections may thus be used as a model to study the molecular basis of virulence or commensalism, the key elements of the acute anti-microbial defense that maintains sterility of the mucosa, and the mechanisms that allow long-term symptomatic carriage of bacteria at mucosal sites.

## 2.1     Kinetics of the Host Defense

Hypotheses about the key defense mechanisms that maintain urinary tract sterility, should be based on kinetics of bacterial clearance from the urinary tract of resistant hosts. Following injection of $10^8$ cfu/ml of *E.coli* into the urinary bladder, there was an initial reduction in bacterial counts to about $10^4$ cfu/ml during the first two hours (phase I). Subsequently, bacterial numbers decrease even further until about 24 hours (phase II), and are completely eliminated by two to seven days depending on virulence and host background (phase III).

The reduction in bacterial numbers during the first two hours probably depends largely on mechanic factors, like the urine flow. Even phase II is too short to allow for a specific immune response. There is little or no pre-existing mucosal immunity against a specific pathogen in the uninfected urinary tract, and the induction of a primary specific immune response in the urinary tract takes at least 7 days. Infection is cleared before the specific immune response needs to be activated. We have therefore sought to explain host resistance as a function of innate immunity.

Two approaches were used:

1 To characterize host responses to bacteria during the short time period when infection is cleared, and attempts to identify response pathways that might be involved in bacterial clearance.

2 Identification of host defects that upset the specific or innate defenses.

## 3.    THE EARLY HOST RESPONSE TO URINARY TRACT INFECTION

In view of the rapid clearance kinetics following intravesical instillation of bacteria, we have investigated the molecular mechanisms used by the bacteria to elicit the early host response to urinary tract infection.

### 3.1    Attachment, Trans-membrane Signalling and Epithelial Cell Activation

The different cell populations in the mucosal barrier are equipped to sense and respond to the molecular contents in the lumen and to translate this molecular information into signals that can reach local or distant tissue sites. Inflammatory mediators provide a direct link between the microbe and the host in disease pathogenesis[2]. Inflammatory cascades are often the first to be activated by bacteria or viruses, and explain many aspects of acute disease. It is not the presence of microbes in the tissues that makes us sick. Vast numbers of bacteria may colonise different sites in the body, and viruses may persist for long periods of time, while the individual remains perfectly healthy. It is the host response to the infecting agents that causes the symptoms and tissue damage.

It is commonly accepted that the most virulent bacteria cause the most severe acute symptoms and long-term effects, but we know relatively little about the mechanisms used by specific bacterial components to trigger acute disease manifestations. Both virulent bacteria and members of the indigenous microflora contain molecules that can trigger inflammation, but only the pathogens elicit a strong host response. This is quite puzzling, but at least two factors may explain the difference. First, pathogens have a broader repertoire of host activating molecules than the commensals or express molecular variants with a better specificity for the host response pathways. Second, the pathogens present host activating molecules more efficiently to the responding cells in the mucosa[3].

The process starts with attachment to the urinary tract mucosa. Uropathogenic *E. coli* elaborate specific adherence factors which bind to receptor epitopes in the epithelial cells or cellular elements of the mucosal barrier. While epithelial cells serve to maintain the border between the lumen and internal tissues, they are also highly responsive cells that can be triggered by pathogens to secrete host response molecules. Epithelial cells respond to external danger and produce an array of mediators that transmit signals across the barrier to adjacent cells or underlying tissues[4,5,6]. Our group was the first to study mucosal cytokine responses to infection[4] and to demonstrate that human urinary tract epithelial cells produce inflammatory mediators in response to bacterial stimulation[6]. Our continued studies concern the molecular and cellular determinants of these responses and their role in disease pathogenesis.

Bacterial adherence enhances epithelial cell cytokine responses[5,7,8]. P fimbriated and type 1-fimbriated *E. coli* strains elicit higher cytokine responses *in vivo* and *in vitro* than isogenic, non-fimbriated strains[8,9,10]. Inhibition of epithelial cells glycolipid expression reduced the cytokine response to P-fimbriated *E. coli*, but had no effect on the cytokine response to type 1-fimbriated *E. coli,* that bind different glycoconjugate receptors[8]. Furthermore, inhibition of binding by receptor analogues inhibited epithelial cell cytokine responses to whole bacteria[11].

### 3.1.1     P Fimbriae and Trans-membrane Signalling through Ceramide

Membrane sphingolipids play an important role in signal transduction. Earlier studies of sphingolipid structure and function focused on the carbohydrate headgroups of the glycosphingolipids and their role in cell-cell or cell-microbial recognition. After sphingosine was found to inhibit protein kinase C[12,13,14], sphingomyelin cycle was elucidated, and ceramide was identified as a second messenger[3].

The P fimbriae bind to glycosphingolipid receptors[15]. The recognition sites are Galα1-4Galβ epitopes in oligosaccharide sequences bound to ceramide in the outer leaflet of the epithelial cell lipid bilayer. We have shown that the receptors are altered as a consequence of ligand binding and that ceramide release is important for cell activation by P fimbriated *E. coli*[16,17]. Free ceramide was detected by *in vitro* phosphorylation after approximately 20 min. Phosphorylation of ceramide to ceramide-1-phosphate was detected around 20 minutes after stimulation with P fimbriated *E. coli.* Type 1 fimbriated or non-fimbriated isogens did not release ceramide in the A498 cells, and increases in ceramide-1-phosphate levels were not detected.

Ceramide activates Ser/Thr kinases with specificity for proline[18]. Inhibitors of Ser/Thr kinases blocked the IL-6 response to P-fimbriated *E.coli* but had no effect on the IL-6 response to the non-fimbriated *E.coli* control. Inhibitors of tyrosine kinases had no effect on the response to P-fimbriae, but reduced the cytokine response to the type 1 fimbriated isogen.

So which mechanisms explain the P fimbriae specific ceramide response? Activation of the sphingomyelin cycle by exogenous ligands like vitamin D3, IL-1, TNF or gamma interferon[19], involves sphingomyelinase activation. Sphingomyelin is hydrolysed and released ceramide activates CAPP, a subtype of heterotrimeric protein phosphatase and of Ser/Thr specific protein kinases. Downstream cellular targets include c-myc, NF-kB and MAP kinases. Ceramide has been proposed to modulate cell growth and differentiation, cell death and secretion of proteins including cytokines[12,13,14].

In contrast to the previously described ligands, P fimbriated *E. coli* trigger the release of ceramide in a sphingomyelinase independent manner[16]. We have shown that the sphingomyelinase cycle is fully functional in our cells, and that exogenous sphingomyelinases cleave sphingomyelin and activate the cells. P fimbriated *E. coli* produced low amounts of this enzyme, but there was no evidence of sphingomyelin break-down in the cells, suggesting that P fimbriated *E. coli* release ceramide from previously unrecognized precursors. P fimbriae differ from other activators of the ceramide-signaling pathway in that it binds directly to a ceramide anchored receptor. It is possible that enzymes of bacteria or cellular origin are activated and cleave the receptor glycolipid. Preliminary experiments showed the release of Gal and a reduction in the amount of receptor glycosphingolipid following stimulation with P frimbriated bacteria[16].

Receptor fragmentation into ceramide and free oligosaccharide may represent a highly efficient strategy of the host defence. Release of the carbohydrate receptor makes the bacteria "lose their grip" until novel receptors are expressed. Soluble receptors may competitively inhibit further attachment and prevent experimental urinary tract infection *in vivo*[20]. In addition, the ceramide signalling pathway triggers chemokines that recruit inflammatory cells which clear bacteria from the local site (see below)[21,22].

### 3.1.2    Cell Activation by P Fimbriated *E. coli* is LPS Independent

LPS is an integral component of the outer membrane of Gram negative bacteria and a potent activator of inflammation in the systemic compartment, but these effects can not be generalised to mucosal sites. Epithelial cells differ from macrophages and inflammatory cells, in that they do not express surface CD14, and are refractory to purified LPS regardless of the polysaccharide structure. Inactivation of LPS in virulent isolates by BPI and PolymyxinB or mutational inactivation of Lipid A, had no effect on epithelial cytokine responses to whole bacteria[23].

Some studies have suggested that LPS is a structural analogue of ceramide that can bypass ceramide as an activator of Ser/Thr specific signalling mechanisms in CD14 positive cells[24]. So could LPS be a second signal and a costimulatory molecule in cell activation by P fimbriated *E. coli*[21]? This would be consistent with the observed *in vivo* synergy between LPS and fimbriae[7,23,24].

We compared the cellular responses to P fimbriated isogens with intact LPS or with dysfunctional LPS resulting from mutational inactivation of the *msb* gene that determines myristoylation of lipid A[24]. This lipid A is inactive in other cellular assays. The results clearly demonstrated that epithelial cell activation by P fimbriated *E. coli* is lipidA independent. These findings make sense, since mucosal surfaces are under constant bombardment by LPS and still do not appear to be in a state of constant inflammation.

## 3.2 Epithelial Cells as Arbitrators of Neutrophil Recruitment to Mucosal Sites

Cytokines have local and systemic effects. Local inflammation causes changes in vascular permeability, recruitment of inflammatory cells, and disruption of tissue function. Systemic effects include fever, and the symptoms and signs of sepsis. We detected an IL-6 response in urine and blood of children with acute pyelonephritis[25,26]. The urine IL-6 response was specific for febrile UTI; it was not found in children with other febrile infections. We also found positive correlations between fever, CRP and local or circulating IL-6 concentrations in adults with febrile UTI[27,28].

Chemokines are commonly assigned to two groups, depending on the position of the first two cysteins and disulphide bridges[29,30]. The ELR-motif containing C-X-C chemokines are involved in neutrophil recruitment and activation[29]. The C-C chemokines are mainly active in interactions with monocytes and macrophages[31]. Mucosal infections trigger a broad chemokine response. After our initial observation that epithelial cells secrete chemokines in response to *E. coli*, different epithelial cells have been shown to express a broad range of chemokines, including IL-8, GRO-α, GRO-β, GRO-γ, ENA78, MCP-1 and RANTES[32]. The chemokine responses provide a basis for differential recruitment of reactive cell populations to mucosal sites.

The different steps involved in neutrophil migration to mucosal sites are outlined in Fig 1. Similar results have been obtained by several groups using the Transwell model system pioneered by Madara *et al.*[33] and most aspects of the model have been confirmed in human patients or experimental animal models[21,34,35]. Bacteria first stimulate the epithelial cells to secrete chemokines, and a gradient is established. Neutrophils leave the blood stream, migrate through the tissues and cross the epithelial barrier into the lumen. While human uroepithelial cells secrete several chemokines, IL-8 is the main force that drives neutrophil migration across epithelial cell layers. Inhibition with Mab to IL-8 was shown to completely inhibit neutrophil transmigration *in vitro*[35]. Urine IL-8 concentrations increased rapidly and the concentrations correlated with the urine neutrophil numbers after urinary tract colonisation of human volunteers[21].

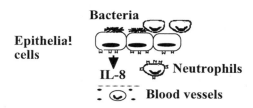

*Figure 1.* Bacterial activation of epithelial cells induces increased cytokine production and the recruitment of neutrophils from the blood vessels to the infected site.

The role of epithelial chemokine production for neutrophil recruitment to mucosal site was studied *in vivo,* using the mouse UTI model. Following intravesical *Escherichia coli* infection, several C-X-C chemokines were secreted into the urine, but only MIP-2 concentrations correlated to neutrophil numbers[36]. Immunohistochemistry identified the kidney epithelium as a main source of MIP-2. MIP-2 antibody treatment of the mice caused the neutrophils to aggregate under the pelvic epithelium, but in control mice the neutrophils crossed the urothelium into the urine. The results demonstrate that MIP-2 directs neutrophil migration through the lamina propria and across the epithelium. Neutrophils cross the epithelial cell barriers in a highly regulated manner, in response to chemokines elaborated at this site. This is yet another mechanism that defines the mucosal compartment and differentiates the local from the systemic host resistance.

# 4. IDENTIFICATION OF HOST DEFECTS THAT UPSET THE SPECIFIC OR INNATE DEFENSES

## 4.1    Specific Immunity

Early studies in the UTI model indicated that specific immunity was of minor importance for the mucosal host defense. *Nude, xid,* and *scid* mice with defective T lymphocyte, immunoglobulin, and B and T lymphocyte function, respectively, were shown to be fully resistant to infection[37]. Since the defects in these mice are vaguely defined and in some cases incomplete we wanted to re-evaluate the role of specific immunity, using mutant mice that lack specific lymphocyte populations.

Experimental UTI was thus established in βT cell receptor (TCR) mutant[38,39], δTCR mutant[40], RAG-1 mutant[41], and control mice. TCR αβ mutant mice lack cytotoxic and helper T cells and have defective humoral and cellular responses to T-cell dependent antigens[42] TCR δ mutant mice have a normal peripheral αβ T cell repertoire[39] and intact humoral and cellular responses to T-cell dependent antigens[42], but low levels of mucosal IgA[43]. γδ T cells have been implicated in the antimicrobial defense against *Staphylococci, Streptococci, Mycobacteria* and *E.coli*[44,45]. RAG-1 mutant mice are deficient in the V(D)J recombination activating gene (RAG-1) responsible for the recombinatorial events during B and T cell development and consequently lack B and T cells altogether[41]. RAG-1 mutant mice also lack mature thymus independent αβ and γδ intraepithelial lymphocytes[46].

There was no difference in resistance to infection between the lymphocyte mutant mice and their immunocompetent controls as determined by bacterial counts 24 hours after inoculation (Table 1). The results prove that specific lymphocyte populations are of marginal importance for the early defense against UTI in the mouse.

*Table 1.* Host resistance to E.coli urinary tract infection is lymphocyte independent

|  | genotype | Log no. of bacteria[a] (Mean ± SEM) | | | |
|---|---|---|---|---|---|
|  |  | Kidneys | p | Bladders | p |
| B10.Q | TCRB (-/-) | 0.27 ± 0.27 | n.s. | 2.44 ± 0.142 | n.s. |
| B10.Q | TCRB (+/+) | 0.986 ± 0.566 |  | 2.69 ± 0.139 |  |
| B10.Q | TCRD (-/-) | 1.04 ± 1.04 | n.s. | 3.86 ± 0.04 | n.s. |
| B10.Q | TCRD (+/+) | 1.76 ± 0.69 |  | 4.37 ± 0.38 |  |
| B6 | RAG-1 (-/-) | 1.68 ± 0.72 | n.s. | 4.24 ± 0.76 | n.s. |
| B6 | RAG-1 (+/+) | 1.88 ± 0.66 |  | 3.69 ± 0.55 |  |

[a] Bacterial persistence was determined by viable counts of kidney and bladder homogenates 24h after intravesical inoculation.

## 4.2    Innate Immunity

We have shown that innate immune mechanisms provide the most potent defence of the mucosal barrier against UTI, and have identified neutrophils as important local effectors of the mucosal defence[36]. The work was based on earlier observation in C3H/HeJ (*lps^d*, *lps^d*) mice that lack the neutrophil response to UTI, and fail to clear bacteria from the tissues[47,48]. More recently, studies directly addressing the role of neutrophils have been performed.

Peripheral neutrophil depletion in C3H/HeN mice was achieved by pretreatment with the granulocyte specific antibody RB6-8C5. As a consequence, bacterial clearance from kidneys and bladders was drastically impaired[49]. Antibody treatment of C3H/HeJ mice had only a marginal effect. The results demonstrate that neutrophils are essential for bacterial clearance from the urinary tract, and that the neutrophil recruitment deficiency in C3H/HeJ mice explains their susceptibility to Gram negative mucosal infection.

## 4.3    The IL-8R Deficiency Confers Susceptibility to Acute Pyelonephritis.

IL-8R mutant mice were used to disrupt neutrophil recruitment to the mucosa and to study the effect on resistance to infection. This approach was preferred over the more complex procedure of eliminating all potential IL-8 homologues in the mouse[9,50,51,52]. IL-8R mutant mice were raised from a single breeder pair. The genotypes were confirmed by PCR on DNA extracted from tail clippings, using validated primers specific for the murine IL-8R gene or the inserted neomycine gene[9]. The phenotype was confirmed by staining of kidney and bladder tissue sections from control and IL-8R mutant mice with monoclonal antibodies to the IL-8R. The IL-8R mutant mice had an intact mucosal chemokine response to infection as shown by staining of tissue sections obtained 6 hours after infection. An epithelial cell MIP-2 response was detected in both IL-8R mutant and control mice with no evidence of a decrease in the receptor mutant mice.

A marked loss of resistance to infection was noted in the IL-8R mutant mice. IL-8R mutant mice were unable to clear the bacteria from kidney and bladder tissue and showed abnormal neutrophil recruitment to the mucosa. They eventually developed bacteremia and symptoms of systemic disease. These results emphasize the role of innate immunity and IL-8 receptor function for the resistance to urinary tract infection in the mouse. The findings in neutrophil depleted and IL-8R mutant mice prove that neutrophils are essential defense elements in the urinary tract.

Many aspects of these finding need to be explored further

1. Is it the neutrophil receptor deficiency or the epithelial cell that determines the susceptibility to UTI?
2. Where are the bacteria killed? It is unclear if uropathogens are eradicated by the host response as they attach to the mucosal lining or in the tissues.
3. The IL-8 mutant mice show tissue changes that resemble renal scarring in humans. The long-term effects of infection should be explored in these mice.

## 5.    FIMBRIAE-MEDIATED ADHERENCE, CYTOKINE RESPONSES AND DISEASE IN THE HUMAN URINARY TRACT

### 5.1    Influence of P Fimbrial Expression on the Mucosal Cytokine Response

Biopsies from the human urinary tract mucosa showed that the prerequisites for IL-8 and IL-8 receptor responses are in place at this site. Immuno-histochemical staining of tissue biopsies with specific antibodies showed that the epithelium contains IL-8 and that the kidney and bladder epithelial cells express the CXCR1 and CXCR2 receptors.

The response to UPEC was examined by injection of bacteria into the urinary tract of patients. Colonization with non-virulent bacteria was performed in an attempt to protect special patient groups from recurrent, symptomatic UTI. This strategy was based on clinical observations that ABU in children protected against symptomatic UTI. Those who were left untreated were shown to have a lower frequency of symptomatic recurrences than the patients who were given antibiotics in order to eliminate the bacteriuria, and there were no adverse effects on renal function.

This study examined the role of P fimbriae for the establishment and persistence of bacteria in the human urinary tract[53]. Eleven patients with recurrent symptomatic urinary tract infections (UTI) were subjected to urinary tract colonization with an asymptomatic bacteriuria (ABU) strain or P fimbriated transformants of this strain. P fimbriae were shown to facilitate the initial establishment but not the long-term persistence of bacteriuria. Fimbrial expression was rapidly lost *in vivo*, but the *pap* sequences remained intact and P-fimbriae were re-expressed after *in vitro* culture. The loss of P fimbrial expression may be just as important as the initial P-fimbriae mediated enhancement of colonization, and may be a prerequisite for a non-virulent strain to persist in the urinary tract. The results are consistent with earlier observations that ABU strains carry the *pap* sequences, but rarely express the phenotype.

The cytokine response coincided in time with the expression of the P fimbriae but waned when the strains switched to a non-fimbriated phenotype. In a subsequent colonization, with a P-fimbriae negative variant of *E.coli* 83972, low cytokine responses were observed. These findings suggest that it is sufficient to transform a non-virulent strain with P fimbriae in order to make it a host response inducer in the urinary tract.

## 5.2    The IL-8 Receptor Deficiency and Susceptibility to Recurrent Pyelonephritis

The findings in the mutant mice demonstrated that IL-8R expression influences the susceptibility to E.coli UTI through an effect on neutrophil recruitment. So, could abnormal IL-8R expression be a cause of susceptibility to UTI also in man? To address this question we examined the expression of the two high affinity IL-8 receptors, CXCR1 and CXCR2, on cells from patients and controls. Children with recurrent UTI and episodes of acute pyelonephritis were enrolled in a prospective study of IL-8 receptor expression and were compared to healthy age-matched controls.

CXCR1 receptor expression was low in the pyelonephritis group compared to the healthy age-matched controls as determined by flow cytometry and confocal microscopy. In contrast, there was no difference in CXCR2 expression between patients and controls. The results demonstrate heterogeneity in CXCR1 expression among children with acute pyelonephritis, and show that patients with recurrent pyelonephritis have a large fraction of neutrophils with low surface CXCR1, but unchanged CXCR2 expression.

# REFERENCES

1. Andersen, H., 1966, Studies of urinary tract infections in infancy and childhood. VII. The relation of E.coli antibody in pyelonephritis as measured by homologous and common (Kunin) antigens. J. Pediatr. 68: 542-550.
2. Hedges, S., Agace, W., and Svanborg, C., 1995, Epithelial cytokine responses and mucosal cytokine networks. Trends in Microbiol. 3: 266-270.
3. Sansonetti, P. J., 1998, Molecular and cellular mechanisms of the intestinal barrier by enteric pathogens. The paradigm of Shigella. Folia Microbiol. (Praha). 43: 239-246.
4. de Man, P., Van Kooten, C., Aarden, L., Engberg, I., and Svanborg-Edén, C., 1989, Interleukin-6 induced by Gram-negative bacterial infection at mucosal surfaces. *Infect. Immun.* 57: 3383-3388.
5. Hedges, S., de Man, P., Linder, H., van Kooten, C., and Svanborg-Edén, **C.,** 1990, Interleukin-6 is secreted by epithelial cells in response to Gram-negative bacterial challenge. In *Advances in mucosal immunology*. International Conference of Mucosal Immunity (T. Macdonald, ed.), Kluwer, London, pp. 144-148.
6. Hedges, S., Svensson, M.,and Svanborg, C., 1992, Interleukin-6 response of epithelial cell lines to bacterial stimulation *in vitro. Infect. Immun.* 60: 1295-1301.
7. Linder, H., Engberg, I., Hoschützky, H., Mattsby Baltzer, I.,and Svanborg-Edén, C., 1991, Adhesion dependant activation of mucosal IL-6 production. *Infect. Immun.* 59: 4357-4362.
8. Svensson, M., Lindstedt, R., Radin, N., and Svanborg, C., 1994, Epithelial glycosphingolipid expression as a determinant of bacterial adherence and cytokine production. *Infect. Immun.* 62: 4404-4410.
9. Cacalano, G., Le, J., Kikly, K., Ryan, A.M., Pitts-Meek, S., Hultgren, B., Wood, W.I., and Moore, M.W., 1994, Neutrophil and B cell expansion in mice that lack the murine IL-8 receptor homolog. *Science* 265: 682-684.
10. Hedges, S., Anderson, P., Lidin-Janson, G., de Man, P.,and Svanborg. C., 1991, Interleukin-6 response to deliberate colonization of the human urinary tract with gram-negative bacteria. *Infect. Immun.* 59: 421-427.
11. Godaly, G., Frendéus, B., Prodfoot, A., Svensson, M., Klemm, P., and Svanborg, C., 1998, Role of fimbriae-mediated adherence for neutrophil migration across *Escherichia coli* -infected epithelial cell layers. *Mol. Microbiol.* 30: 725-735.
12. Hannun, Y., and Bell, R., 1989, Functions of sphingolipids and sphingolipid break-down products in cellular regulation. *Science* 247: 500-507.
13. Obeid, L. M., Linardic, C.M., Karolak, L.A., and Hannun, Y.A., 1993, Programmed cell death induced by ceramide. *Science* 259: 1769-1771.
14. Okazaki, T., Bell, R.M., and Hannun, Y.A., 1989, Sphingomyelin turnover induced by vitamin D3 in HL-60 cells. Role in cell differentiation. *J. Biol. Chem.* 264: 19076-19080.
15. Leffler, H., and Svanborg-Edén, C., 1980, Chemical identification of a glycosphingolipid receptor for *Escherichia coli* attaching to human urinary tract epithelial cells and agglutinating human erythrocytes. *FEMS Microbiol. Lett.* 8: 127-134.
16. Hedlund, M., Nilsson, Å., Duan, R.D., and Svanborg, C., 1998, Sphingomyelin, glycosphimgolipids and ceramide signalling in cells exposed to P fimbriated *Escherichia coli. Mol. Microbiol.* 29: 1297-1306.
17. Hedlund, M., Svensson, M.,. Nilsson, Å., Duan, R., and Svanborg, C., 1996, Role of the ceramide signalling pathway in cytokine responses to P fimbriated *Escherichia coli. J. Exp. Med.* 183: 1-8.

18. Schütze, S., Potthoff, K., Machleidt, T., Berkovic, C., Weigman, K., and Krönke, M., 1992, TNF activates NF-κB by phosphatidylcholine-specific phospholipase C-induced "acidic" sphingomyelin breakdown. *Cell* **71**: 765-776.

19. Kim, M.-Y., Linardic, C., Obeid, L., and Hannun Z.A., 1991, Identification of sphingomyelin turn-over as an effector mechanism for the activation of TNFa and IFNγ. Specific role in celldifferentiation. *J. Biol. Chem.* **266**: 484-489.

20. Svanborg-Edén, C., Freter, R., Hagberg, L., Hull, R., Hull, S., Leffler, H., and Schoolnik, G., 1982, Inhibition of experimental ascending urinary tract infection by an epithelial cell-surface receptor analogue. *Nature (London).* **298**: 560-562.

21. Agace, W., Hedges, S., Ceska, M.,and Svanborg, C., 1993, IL-8 and the neutrophil response to mucosal Gram negative infection . *J. Clin. Invest.* **92**: 780-785.

22. Svanborg, C., Hedlund, M., Connell, H., Agace, W., Duan, R.-D., Nilsson, Å., and Wullt, B., 1996, Bacterial adherence and mucosal cytokine responses. Receptors and transmembrane signaling. *Ann. NY Acad. Sci.* **797**: 177-198.

23. Hedlund, M., Wachtler, M., Johansson, E., Hang, L., Somerville, J.E., Darveau, R.P., and Svanborg, C., 1999, P fimbriae dependent, LPS independent activation of epithelial cytokine responses. *Mol. Microbiol.* **33**: 693-703.

24. Joseph, C., Wright, S., Bornmann, W., Randolph, J., Kumar, E., Bittman, R., Liu, J., and Kolesnick, R., 1994, Bacterial lipopolysaccharide has structural similarity to ceramide and stimulates ceramide-activated protein kinase in myeloid cells. *J. Biol. Chem.* **269**: 17606-17610.

25. Benson, M., Jodal, U., Agace, W., Andreasson, A., Mårild, S., Stokland, E., Wettergren, B., and Svanborg, C., 1996, Interleukin-6 and interleukin-8 in children with febrile urinary tract infection and asymptomatic bacteriuria. *J. Infect. Dis.* **174**: 1080-1084.

26. Benson, M., Jodal, U., Andreasson, A., Karlsson, Å., Rydberg, J., and Svanborg, C., 1994, The interleukin-6 response to urinary tract infection to urinary tract infection in childhood. *Ped. Infect. Dis. J.* **13**: 612-616.

27. Hedges, S., Stenquist, K., Lidin-Janson, G., Martinell, J., Sandberg, T.,and Svanborg, C., 1992, Comparison of urine and serum concentrations of interleukin-6 in women with acute pyelonephritis or asymptomatic bacteriuria. *J. Infect. Dis.* **166**: 653-6.

28. Otto, G., Branconier, J., Andreasson, A.,and Svanborg, C., 1998, Interleukin-6 responses and disease severity in bacteremic and non bacteremic febrile urinary tract infection. *J. Infect. Dis.* **179**: 172-179.

29. Baggiolini, M., Dewald, B., and Moser, B., 1994, Interleukin-8 and related chemotactic cytokines-CXC and CC chemokines. *Adv. Immunol.* **55**: 97-179.

30. Schall, T., and Bacon, K., 1994, Chemokines, leukocyte trafficking, and inflammation. *Curr. Opin. Immunol.* **6**: 865-873.

31. Moser, B., Loetscher, M., Piali, L.,and Loetscher, P., 1998, Lymphocyte responses to chemokines. *Intern. Rev. Immunol.* **16**: 323-344.

32. Kagnoff, M. F., Eckmann, L., Yang, S.-K., Huang, G., Jung, H.C., and Reed, S.L., 1996, Intestinal epithelial cells: an integral component of the mucosal immune system., In *Mucosal Immunology* (M. F. Kagnoff and H. Kiyono, eds). Academic Press, San Diego, pp. 63-71.

33. Parkos, C., Delp, C., Armin Arnout, M.,and Madara, J., 1991, Neutrophil migration across cultured intestinal epithelium. *J. Clin. Invest.* **88**: 1605-1612.

34. Godaly, G., Proudfoot, A.E.I., Offord, R.E., Svanborg, C., and Agace, W.,. 1997, Role of epithelial interleukin-8 and neutrophil IL-8 receptor A in *Escherichia coli* -induced transuroepithelial neutrophil migration. *Infect. Immun.* **65**: 3451-3456.

35. McCormick, B., Colgan, S., Delp-Archer, C., Miller, S., and Madara, J., 1993, *Salmonella typhimurium* attachment to human intestinal epithelial monolayers: Transcellular signalling to subepithelial neutrophils. *J. Cell. Biol.* **123**: 895-907.

36. Hang, L., Haraoka, M., Agace, W.W., Burdick, M., Strieter, R., and Svanborg, C., 1998, MIP-2 is required for neutrophil passage across the epithelial barrier of the infected urinary tract. *J. Immunol.* **162**: 3037-3044.

37. Svanborg-Edén, C., Hagberg, L., Briles, D., McGhee, J., and Michalek, S., 1985, Suspectibility of *Escherichia coli* urinary tract infection and LPS responsiveness. In *Genetic Control of Host Resistance to Infection and Malignancy.* (E. Skamene, (ed.), Alan R Liss Inc. pp. 385-391.

38. Mombaerts, P., Clarke, A.R., Hooper, M.L., and Tonegawa, S., 1991, Creation of a large genomic deletion at the T-cell antigen receptor β-subunit locus in mouse embryonic stem cells by gene targeting. *Proc. Natl. Acad. Sci.* **88**: 3084-3087.

39. Mombaerts, P., Clarke, A.R., Rudnicki, M.A., Lacomini, J., Itohara, S., Lafaille, J.J., Wang, L., Ichikawa, Y., Jaenisch, R., Hooper, M.L., and Tonegawa, S., 1992, Mutations in T-cell antigen receptor genes α and β block thymocyte development at different stages. *Nature* **360**: 225-231.

40. Itohar.a, S., Mombaerts, P., Lafaille, J., Iacomini, J., Nelson, A., Clarke, A.R., Hooper, M.L., Farr, A., and Tonegawa, S., 1993, T cell receptor delta gene mutant mice: independent generation of alpha beta T cells and programmed rearrangements of gamma delta TCR genes. *Cell* **72**: 337-348.

41. Mombaerts, P., Lacomini, J., Johnson, R.S., Herrup, K.,Tonegawa, S., and Papaioannou, V.E., 1992, RAG-1 deficient mice have no mature B and T lymphocytes. *Cell* **68**: 869-877.

42. Mombaerts, P., Mizoguchi, E., Ljunggren, H.-G., Lacomini, J., Ishikawa, H., Wang, L., Grusby, M.J., Glimcher, L.H., Winn, H.J., Bhan, A.K., and Tonegawa, S., 1994, Peripheral lymphoid development and function in TCR mutant mice. *International Immunology* **6**: 1061-1070.

43. Fujihashi, K., McGhee, J.R., Kweon, M.N., Cooper, M.D., Tonegawa, S., Takahashi, I., Hiroi, T., Mestecky, j., and Kiyono, H., 1996, γ/δ T cell-deficient mice have impaired mucosal immunoglobulin A responses. *J. Exp. Med.* **183**: 1929-1935.

44. Haas, W., Pereira, P., and Tonegawa., S., 1993, Gamma/delta T cells. *Ann.. Rev. Immunol.* .637-685.

45. Jones-Carson, J., Balish, E., and Uehling, D.T., 1999, Susceptibility of immunodeficient gene-knockout mice to urinary tract infection. *J. Urol.* **161**: 338-341.

46. Page, S. T., van Oers, N.S., Perlmutter, R.M., Weiss, A., and Pullen, A.M., 1997, Differential contribution of Lck and Fyn protein tyrosine kinases to intraepithelial lymphocyte development. *Eur. J. Immunol.* **27**: 554-62.

47. Shahin, R. D., Engberg, I., Hagberg, L., and Svanborg-Eden, C., 1987, Neutrophil recruitment and bacterial clearance correlated with LPS responsiveness in local gram-negative infection. *J. Immunol.* **138**: 3475-80.

58. Svanborg-Edén, C., Shahin, R., and Briles, D., 1987, Host resistance to mucosal Gram-negative infection. Suspectibility of LPS non-responder mice. *J. Immunol.* **140**: 3180-3185.

49. Haraoka, M., Hang, L., Frendéus, B., Godaly, G., Burdick, M., Strieter, R.,and Svanborg, C., 1999, Neutrophil recruitment and resistance to Urinary Tract Infection. *J. Infect. Dis.* **180**: 1220-1229.

50. Bozic, C. R., Gerard, N.P., von Uexkull-Guldenband, C., Kolakowski, L.F., Conklyn, M.J., Breslow, R., Showell, H.J., and Gerard, C., 1994, The murine interleukin 8 type b receptor homologue and its ligands. *J. Biol. Chem.* **269**: 29355-29358.

51. Lee, J., Cacalano, G., Camerato, T., Toy, K., Moore, M.W., and Wood, W.I., 1995, Chemokine binding and activities mediated by the mouse IL-8 receptor. *J. Immunol.* **155**: 2158-2164.

52. Schuster, D. E., Kehrli, M.E.J., and Ackermann, M.R., 1995, Neutrophilia in mice that lack the murine IL-8 receptor homolog. *Science* **269:** 1590-1591.
53. Wullt, B., Bergsten, G., Connell, H., Röllano, P., Gebretsadik, N., Hull, R., and Svanborg, C., 1999, P fimbriae enhance the establishment but not the long term persistence of *Escherichia coli* in the human urinary tract. Manuscript.

# PATHOGENICITY ISLANDS OF UROPATHOGENIC *E. COLI* AND EVOLUTION OF VIRULENCE

Gabriele Blum-Oehler, Ulrich Dobrindt, Britta Janke, Gábor Nagy, Katharine Piechaczek and Jörg Hacker
*Institut für Molekulare Infektionsbiologie der Universität Würzburg, Röntgenring 11, D-97070 Würzburg*

## 1. INTRODUCTION

*E. coli* bacteria are able to cause a large range of infectious diseases in humans. Among these are infections of the gastrointestinal tract as well as extraintestinal infections of great importance. Intestinal *E. coli* can be grouped in at least six different pathotypes including enterotoxigenic (ETEC), enteropathogenic (EPEC), enterohemorrhagic (EHEC) and enteroaggregative (EaggEC) *E. coli*. Extraintestinal *E. coli* fall into three groups: meningitis (MENEC), septicemia (SEPEC) and uropathogenic (UPEC) *E. coli*. UPECs are by far the most common cause of uncomplicated bacterial urinary tract infections (UTIs)[1,2]. About 80 % of all UTIs are due to *E. coli*. UPECs differ from non-pathogenic *E. coli* variants by the presence of certain virulence factors which contribute to their ability to cause disease. These are two different types of toxins, α-hemolysin (Hly) and the cytotoxic necrotizing factor 1 (CNF1), fimbrial adhesins e. g. P-, type 1 and S-fimbriae and iron-uptake systems like aerobactin, enterobactin or yersiniabactin. Furthermore, UPECs belong to certain serotypes and have the capacity to survive in human serum.

About ten years ago it was detected that UPECs contain distinct blocks of DNA carrying closely linked virulence genes[3]. Later on these structures were

*Genes and Proteins Underlying Microbial Urinary Tract Virulence*
Edited by L. Emödy *et al.*, Kluwer Academic/Plenum Publishers, 2000

renamed pathogenicity islands (PAIs)[4]. Since then UPECs have been intensively used as model system for structural and evolutionary studies on pathogenic *E. coli* bacteria.

α-hemolysin and P fimbrial adhesin gene clusters were the first determinants which were shown to be closely linked on PAIs [3]. The presence of at least one virulence gene cluster is one of the main features of PAIs. In addition they may be characterised as follows:

    i)      they occupy large, genomic DNA regions,

    ii)    they are inserted near or within tRNA genes

    iii)   they contain direct repeats and mobility sequences

    iv)   they have a G+C content different from that of the host bacterium[5].

## 2.  THE PATHOGENICITY ISLANDS OF THE UROPATHOGENIC *E. COLI* STRAIN 536

The first PAIs have been described for the UPEC strains 536 and J96[4, 6.] Strain 536 was isolated from a patient with acute pyelonephritis. The genome of this strain contains several virulence gene clusters encoding two α-hemolysins, P-related-, S- and type 1 fimbriae, enterobactin and yersiniabactin and it exhibits serumresistance properties. Strain 536 contains four PAIs varying significantly in size between about 25 and 190 kb [7]. PAI I$_{536}$ is 70 kb in size and carries the *hly*I genes, PAI II$_{536}$ is about 190 kb in size and carries a P-related fimbrial gene cluster (*prf*) in addition to the *hly* genes. PAI III$_{536}$ is about 25 kb in size and is characterised by the presence of an S fimbrial gene cluster (*sfa*), PAI IV$_{536}$ is 40 kb in size and is characterised by the presence of the ferric yersiniabactin uptake (*fyuA*) gene and the iron-repressible protein (*irp1-5*) genes (Table 1).

*Table 1.* Main characteristics of PAIs of the uropathogenic *E. coli* strain 536

| Designation of PAI | Virulence genes encoded on PAI | Size (kb) | Associated tRNA | Location (min) | Boundary |
|---|---|---|---|---|---|
| PAI I$_{536}$ | α-hemolysin | 70 kb | *selC* | 82 | direct repeats |
| PAI II$_{536}$ | α-hemolysin, P-related fimbriae | 190 kb | *leuX* | 97 | direct repeats |
| PAI III$_{536}$ | S-fimbrial adhesin | ~25 kb | *thrW* | 5,6 | ? |
| PAI IV$_{536}$ | Yersiniabactin, iron-repressible proteins | 40 kb | *asnT* | 44 | - |

Originally PAI IV$_{536}$ has been found in the genome of different *Yersinia*, where it has been called "high-pathogenicity island" (HPI). The four PAIs of strain 536 differ in their ability to delete spontaneously from the chromosome. The deletion process of PAI I$_{536}$ and II$_{536}$ is due to two short direct repeats (repeat I and II) which flank the islands and are involved in a homologous recombination process. In *Yersinia* the HPI is flanked by 17 bp direct repeats but in the *E. coli* genome only one repeat is left[8,9]. For PAI III$_{536}$ and also PAI IV$_{536}$ deletion has not been detected yet.

## 2.1 tRNA Genes as Parts of Pathogenicity Islands of the Uropathogenic *E. coli* Strain 536

One copy each of repeat I of PAI I$_{536}$ and repeat II of PAI II$_{536}$ belong to a tRNA gene. Repeat I is part of the tRNA gene *sel*C which is responsible for the incorporation of the amino acid selenocysteine in the formate dehydrogenase protein. This protein is essential for the mixed acid fermentation of strain 536[10]. Repeat II is part of the tRNA gene *leuX*. It transfers leucine and seems to be an important regulator of the virulence properties of strain 536. The deletion of PAI II$_{536}$ leads to the truncation of the *leuX* gene which is no longer transcriptionally active. PAI II$_{536}$ as well as *leuX* deletion mutants show a reduced production of type 1 fimbriae, flagellae and the iron uptake system enterobactin[11]. Furthermore, they show delayed hemolysin production and are reduced in their *in vivo* pathogenicity. Especially regulatory proteins have been shown to contain more *leuX* specific codons than structural genes arguing for a regulation on the translational level[12]. PAI III$_{536}$ and IV$_{536}$ are also flanked by tRNA genes. While PAI III$_{536}$ is associated with the tRNA gene *thrW*, PAI IV$_{536}$ is flanked by the tRNA gene *asnT*.

## 2.2 Genome and Proteome Analysis of the Uropathogenic *E. coli* Strain 536

As already mentioned, UPECs are considered as a model system to study the genomic structure of pathogenic microorganisms. Therefore, the decoding of the genome sequence of the non-pathogenic *E. coli* K-12 strain MG1655 was extremely useful to analyse pathogenic *E. coli* variants[13]. From the *E. coli* K-12 sequence it can be estimated that about 17,6% of the genome represent horizontally transferred DNA[14]. Horizontal gene transfer must have played a major role in the development of pathogenic enteric bacteria.

With regard to this question sequence analysis was performed on the entire sequences of PAIs of UPECs. Overlapping PAI specific cosmid clones of a cosmid library of strain 536 have been used. Although strain 536 is not known to have an integrated prophage limited sequence similarity to bacteriophages was found. For PAI $I_{536}$ the homology search revealed the presence of a cryptic integrase gene next to the tRNA gene *selC*. This integrase gene shows striking homology to the $\Phi R73int$, the integrase gene of the retronphage $\Phi R73$[15]. Interestingly, homologous sequences specific for bacteriophage integrase genes were found on all PAIs of strain 536. DNA sequences corresponding to the P4 integrase gene occur immediately downstream of the *leuX* tRNA gene of PAI $II_{536}$, an additional copy was found on PAI $IV_{536}$. PAI $III_{536}$ carries a DLP12*int* next to the tRNA gene *thrW*. The DNA sequence analysis also revealed the presence of other mobility genes on PAIs of strain 536 i. e. ORFs typical for insertion elements (IS) and transposases. These genes do not necessarily originate from *E. coli* or other enterobacteriae but they have been found e. g. in *Yersinia, Shigella,* and also outside the enterobacteriae e. g. in *Agrobacteria*. Another example for mobility genes on PAIs is a stretch of sequence exhibiting sequence similarity to an intron-like structure originally identified in eukaryotes. It is a so-called group II intron which was first described for the organellar genomes of fungi and plants but it was also found in bacteria in the plasmid sequence of an enterotoxigenic *E. coli* strain[16]. The intron specific sequences described for PAI $I_{536}$ show homologies to the intron sequences of ETEC strains.

Another interesting result of the DNA sequence analysis of PAI $I_{536}$ was the detection of *cnf1* specific sequences downstream of *hlyI*. The coding region of the *cnf1* gene is missing but the up- and downstream sequences are still present. The *cnf1* gene is known to be closely linked to the *hly* genes in uropathogenic *E. coli*[17]. The coding region of the *cnf1* gene in strain 536 seems to be replaced by a 6.5 kb DNA fragment.

*Table 2.* Genes/ORFs located on PAIs I-IV$_{536}$ of the uropathogenic *E. coli* strain 536

| Genes | Functional genes | Pseudogenes |
|---|---|---|
| Toxins | 2 | - |
| Putative virulence genes | 3 | - |
| Iron uptake | 1 | - |
| Mobility genes | 4 | 9 |
| Regulatory genes | 1 | 1 |
| Genes/ORFs with unknown function | 5 | 20 |

In conclusion it can be summarised that the DNA sequence analysis of PAI specific sequences of strain 536 revealed the presence of different types of virulence, mobility and regulatory genes as well as the presence of genes/ORFs with unknown functions (see Table 2).

## 3. SUBTRACTIVE HYBRIDIZATION AND PROTEOME ANALYSIS - NEW TECHNIQUES FOR THE CHARACTERISATION OF PAIS

With more sequence information available, it becomes more and more obvious that there is a correlation between the so far identified PAIs of *E. coli* and PAIs of other species. PAI I$_{536}$ e. g. contains sequences which were also found in enterohemorrhagic *E. coli* and the intron group II structure which was also described for ETEC and *Shigella* strains [16,18].

The application of techniques such as signature tagged mutagenesis, subtractive hybridization, representational difference analysis, differential display of mRNA, proteome analysis and the already described cosmid cloning combined with sample sequencing offers the possibility to identify further virulence genes or new PAIs. The approach taken in our laboratory was the PCR based subtractive hybridization technique. This method allows the identification of genetic differences between two different strains, e. g. a pathogenic and a non-pathogenic strain. The genomic DNA of the *E. coli* strain 536 was compared to the genomic DNA of the *E. coli* K-12 strain MG1655. In total, 22 different PCR fragments could be detected which were specific for strain 536. Eleven fragments map on PAI I and II$_{536}$ including fragments exhibiting significant similarity to the already known virulence gene clusters *hly* and *prf* but also fragments with no homology at either a nucleotide nor amino acid level to sequences of the database. The other 11 identified fragments map elsewhere in the genome of strain 536 including fragments with similarity to lipopolysaccharide and capsule biosynthesis and iron receptors. Further investigation is necessary to show the location of these fragments in the genome of strain 536 and their possible function.

The second approach taken in our laboratory was the proteome analysis. 2-D-polyacrylamide gels of the wild-type strain 536 and PAI deletion as well as *leuX* mutants showed that the expression of several gene products appear to be PAI-dependent and may possibly be *leuX*-regulated. Proteins were identified which showed different expression patterns in the wild-type strain and the mutant strains. Some of these proteins were further analysed by mass fingerprinting using matrix-assisted laser desorption/ionization-time of flight (MALDI-TOF) mass spectrometry and by partial peptide sequencing. Most of the identified proteins are involved in biochemical and amino acid biosynthesis pathways and in iron uptake.

# 4.    PAIS OF UROPATHOGENIC *E. COLI* - IMPLICATIONS FOR EVOLUTION

DNA sequence analysis of PAIs from uropathogenic *E. coli* showed that they represent heterogenous pieces of DNA. The PAI regions are characterised by an unusual genetic organisation, comprising virulence genes, mobility and regulatory genes or pseudogenes as well as genes/ORFs with unknown function. The occurrence of such diverse sequences in PAIs of UPEC strongly argues for a stepwise acquisition of these DNA fragments from very heterogeneous sources, leading to the mosaic-like structure of the islands. Usually, PAIs are characterised by a different G+C content compared to the host bacterium. Therefore, the genomes of prokaryotic organisms seem to be composed of a core genome, which is stable for long periods of time, and newly acquired sequences [19]. These new sequences may be acquired by different mechanisms. Point mutations, genomic rearrangements and horizontal gene transfer are driving forces in microbial evolution [20]. Horizontal gene transfer processes involving bacteriophages, plasmids and pathogenicity islands quickly generate new variants of strains.

PAIs are not restricted to UPEC strains, they were also found in other bacterial species[5]. Although PAIs can vary significantly in size and function they have some features in common, e. g. the association with tRNA genes. tRNA genes seem to play a key role in the development and function of PAIs. Thus, the 3' ends of tRNAs may generally act as sites for the integration of foreign DNA into bacterial genomes[21]. Some tRNA genes seem to be hot spots for the integration of PAIs or bacteriophages. The *selC* gene serves as integration site for various mobile elements not only in uropathogenic *E. coli* but also in enterotoxigenic, enterohemorrhagic and enteropathogenic *E. coli* and in *Salmonella*. In addition, *selC* carries the attachment site for the bacteriophage ΦR73[19].

PAIs of uropathogenic *E. coli* are excellent examples for the evolution of prokaryotic genomes in pathogenic and non-pathogenic microbes. Since the discovery of PAIs in UPEC, several other examples of pathogenic and genomic islands have been described. The principal mechanisms underlying these genetic processes resemble the basic mechanisms of UPECs to a striking extent.

## ACKNOWLEDGEMENTS

Part of the work from our laboratory was supported by grants from the DFG Sonderforschungsbereich 479 "Erregervariabilität und Wirtsreaktionen bei infektiösen Krankheitsprozessen".

# REFERENCES

1. Mühldorfer, I., and Hacker, J., 1994, Genetic aspects of *Escherichia coli* virulence. *Microb. Pathogen.* **16:** 171-181.
2. Sussman, M., 1997, *Escherichia coli* and human disease, In *Escherichia coli: mechanisms of virulence.* (M. Sussman, ed.), Cambridge University Press, Cambridge, pp. 3-48.
3. High, N.J., Hales, B.A., Jann, K., and Boulnois, G. J., 1988, A block of urovirulence genes encoding multiple fimbriae and hemolysin in *Escherichia coli* O4:K12:H⁻. *Infect. Immun.* **56:** 513-517.
4. Hacker, J., Bender, L., Ott, M., Wingender, J., Lund, B., Marre, R., and Goebel, W., 1990, Deletions of chromosomal regions coding for fimbriae and hemolysins occur *in vivo* and *in vitro* in various extraintestinal *Escherichia coli* isolates. *Microb. Pathogen.* **8:** 213-225.
5. Hacker, J., Blum-Oehler, G., Mühldorfer, I., and Tschäpe, H., 1997, Pathogenicity islands of virulent bacteria: structure, function and impact on microbial evolution. *Mol. Microbiol.* **23:** 1089-1097.
6. Hull, R.A., Gill, R.E., Hsu, P., Minshew, B.H., and Falkow, S., 1981, Construction and expression of recombinant plasmids encoding type 1 or D-mannose-resistant pili from a urinary tract infection *Escherichia coli* isolate. *Infect. Immun.* **33:** 933-938.
7. Blum-Oehler, G., Dobrindt, U., Weiß, N., Janke, B., Schubert, S., Rakin, A., Heesemann, J., Marre, R., and Hacker, J., 1998, Pathogenicity islands of uropathogenic *Escherichia coli*: Implications for the evolution of virulence, In *Bacterial Protein Toxins* (Hacker et al., eds.), *Zent.bl. Bakteriol. Suppl.* **29:** pp. 380-386.
8. Buchrieser, C., Brosch, R., Bach, S., Guiyoule, A., and Carniel, E., 1998, The high-pathogenicity island of *Yersinia pseudotuberculosis* can be inserted into any of the three chromosomal *asn* tRNA genes. *Mol. Microbiol.* **30:** 965-978.
9. Schubert, S., Rakin, A., Karch, H., Carniel, E., and Heesemann, J., 1998, Prevalence of the "high-pathogenicity island" of *Yersinia* species among *Escherichia coli* strains that are pathogenic to humans. *Infect. Immun.* **66:** 480-485.
10. Blum, G., Ott, M., Lischewski, A., Ritter, A., Imrich, H., Tschäpe, H., and Hacker, H., 1994, Excision of large DNA regions termed pathogenicity islands from tRNA-specific loci in the chromosome of an *Escherichia coli* wild-type pathogen. *Infect. Immun.* **62:** 606-614.
11. Ritter, A., Blum, G., Emödy, L., Kerenyi, M., Böck, A., Neuhierl, B., Rabsch, W., Scheutz, F., and Hacker, J., 1995, tRNA genes and pathogenicity islands: influence on virulence and metabolic properties of uropathogenic *Escherichia coli. Mol. Microbiol.* **17:** 109-121.
12. Ritter A., Gally, D.L., Olsen, P.B., Dobrindt, U., Friedrich, A., Klemm, P., and Hacker, J., 1997, The PAI-associated *leu*X specific tRNA5(Leu) affects type 1 fimbriation in pathogenic *Escherichia coli* by control of FimB recombinase expression. *Mol. Microbiol.* **25:** 871-882.
13. Blattner, F.R., Plunkett III, G., Bloch, C.A., Perna, N.T., Burland, V., Riley, M., Collado-Vides, J., Glasner, J.D., Rode, C.K., Mayhew, G.F., Gregor, J., Davis, N.W., Kirkpatrick, H.A., Goeden, M.A., Rose, D.J., Mau, B., and Shao, Y., 1997, The complete genome sequence of *Escherichia coli* K-12. *Science* **277:** 1453-1474.
14. Lawrence, J.G., and Ochman, H., 1998, Molecular archaeology of the *Escherichia coli* genome. *Proc. Natl. Acad. Sci. USA* **95:** 9513-9417.

15. Pierson III, L.S., and Kahn, M.L., 1987, Integration of satellite bacteriophage P4 in *Escherichia coli*. DNA sequences of the phage and host regions involved in site-specific recombination. *J. Mol. Biol.* **196:** 487-496.

16. Knoop, V., and Brennicke, A., 1994, Evidence for a group II intron in *Escherichia coli* inserted into a highly conserved reading frame associated with mobile DNA sequences. *Nucleic Acids Res.* **22:** 1167-1171.

17. Falbo, V., Famiglietti, M., and Caprioli, A., 1992, Gene block encoding production of cytotoxic necrotizing factor 1 and hemolysin in *Escherichia coli* isolates from extraintestinal infections. *Infect. Immun.* **60:** 2182-2187.

18. Rajakumar, K., Sasakawa, C., and Adler, B., 1997, Use of a novel approach, termed island probing, identifies the *Shigella flexneri she* pathogenicity island which encodes a homolog of the immunoglobulin A protease-like family of proteins. *Infect. Immun.* **65:** 4606-4614.

19. Hacker, J., Blum-Oehler, G., Janke, B., Nagy, G., and Goebel, W., 1999, Pathogenicity islands of extraintestinal *Escherichia coli*. In *Pathogenicity Islands and Other Mobile Virulence Elements* (J.B. Kaper and J. Hacker, eds.), American Society for Microbiology, Washington D.C., pp. 59-76.

20. Arber, W., 1993 Evolution of prokaryotic genomes. *Gene* **135:** 49-56.

21. Reiter, W.-D., Palm, P., and Yeats, S., 1989, Transfer RNA genes frequently serve as integration sites for prokaryotic genetic elements. *Nucleic Acids Res.* **17:** 1907-1914.

# IRON TRANSPORT IN *ESCHERICHIA COLI*
*Crystal Structure of FhuA, an Outer Membrane Iron and Antibiotic Transporter*

Volkmar Braun, Michael Braun and Helmut Killmann
*Mikrobiologie/Membranphysiologie, Universität Tübingen, Auf der Morgenstelle 28, D-72076 Tübingen, Germany*

## 1.    INTRODUCTION

*Escherichia coli* is the most frequent cause of bacterial disease in the human urinary tract. *E. coli* strains isolated from the urine without further cultivation contain large amounts of outer membrane proteins with molecular masses of approximately 80 kDa; these proteins are transporters of $Fe^{3+}$–siderophores and heme[1,2]. Under sufficient iron supply, several thousand copies of these proteins are synthesized per cell and can increase to 30,000 copies under iron-limiting growth conditions. The outer membrane transporters are the most abundant iron-transport proteins and can be detected by staining after SDS-PAGE, whereas the proteins involved in transport across the cytoplasmic membrane are made in amounts below the detection limit of protein staining and can be visualized by radiolabeling after cloning the encoding genes on multicopy plasmids. The $Fe^{3+}$–siderophores and heme transporters in the cytoplasmic membrane belong to the group of the ABC transporters, which are the most frequently occurring transport systems in bacteria. They consist of a periplasmic binding protein, one or two integral cytoplasmic membrane transport proteins, and a cytoplasmic ATPase that is associated with the inner side of the cytoplasmic membrane (Fig 1). During transport, ATP is consumed; ATP hydrolysis is initiated by binding of the substrate-loaded periplasmic protein to the inner membrane transporters[3]. Evidence has been found that the periplasmic protein interacts with transmembrane domains and a cytoplasmically

*Genes and Proteins Underlying Microbial Urinary Tract Virulence*
Edited by L. Emödy *et al.*, Kluwer Academic/Plenum Publishers, 2000

33

exposed region of an integral cytoplasmic membrane protein that is close to the binding site of the ATPase and suggests that the periplasmic protein may directly interact with the ATPase[4,5].

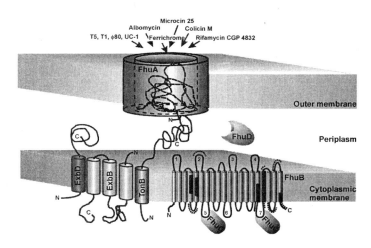

*Figure 1.* Subcellular location of the FhuABCD proteins, which transport ferrichrome and albomycin across the outer membrane and cytoplasmic membrane of *E. coli* (see text for details). The actual structure of FhuA is shown in Fig. 3. The TonB-ExbB-ExbD protein complex is thought to transmit the energy of the proton-motive force across the cytoplasmic membrane via a conformational change of TonB to FhuA. The stoichiometry of the complex is not known, but it has been shown that ExbB binds to TonB and ExbD[1].

All transport proteins are subject to iron regulation exerted by the Fur protein, which acts as a repressor when loaded with $Fe^{2+}$. $Fe^{2+}$–Fur recognizes a consensus sequence in the promoter of iron-regulated genes, termed the Fur box. Fur regulation has been found in all gram-negative bacteria and in some gram-positive bacteria with a low G+C content. In contrast, iron regulation in the gram-positive, high G+C bacterium *Corynebacterium diphtheriae* is mediated by the DtxR protein, which represses diphtheria toxin synthesis when loaded with $Fe^{2+}$. Diphtheria toxin production documents iron-restricted growth conditions of *C. diphtheriae* in humans. Fur and DtxR seem to function similarly although they share little sequence similarity[1].

## 2. THE MULTIFUNTIONAL FhuA PROTEIN AS A PARADIGMATIC OUTER MEMBRANE IRON TRANSPORTER

The FhuA protein is considered as a typical example of a gram-negative outer membrane transport protein for which the most advanced knowledge has been gained. FhuA serves as transporter for ferrichrome, a $Fe^{3+}$–hydroxamate (Fig 2) synthesized by the fungus *Ustilago sphaerogena* and released into the growth medium. $Fe^{3+}$–ferrichrome can be used by *E. coli* and many other gram-negative and gram-positive bacteria as an iron source. FhuA also transports the antibiotic albomycin, a structural analogue of ferrichrome (Fig 2), and the antibiotic rifamycin CGP 4832, which has no structural similarity to ferrichrome (Fig 2).

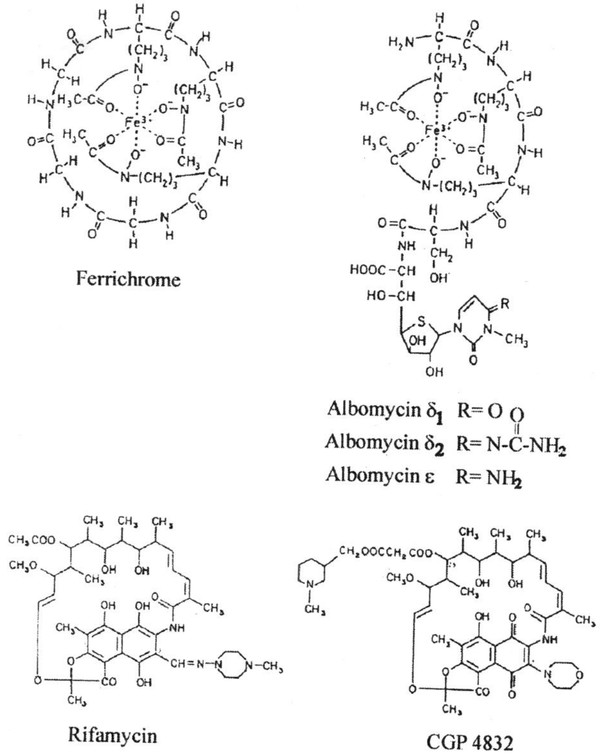

Ferrichrome

Albomycin $\delta_1$ R= O

Albomycin $\delta_2$ R= N-C-NH$_2$

Albomycin ε R= NH$_2$

Rifamycin

CGP 4832

*Figure 2.* Comparison of the chemical structures of ferrichrome, albomycin, and rifamycin CGP 4832.

FhuA also mediates the transport of two toxins, the 21-residue microcin J25 peptide and the 271-residue colicin M protein, both of which are plasmid-encoded and synthesized by certain clinically isolated *E. coli* strains and kill other *E. coli* strains. Furthermore, FhuA serves as receptor for the infection of *E. coli* by the phages T1, T5, φ80, and UC-1 (Fig. 1). FhuA deletion mutants are resistant to the antibiotics, toxins, and phages. These multifunctional properties makes FhuA an attractive model protein to study energy-driven transport, which contrasts the diffusion of most substrates through protein pores in the outer membrane.

## 2.1    Crystal Structure of the FhuA Protein

In December 1998, two groups independently published the crystal structure of FhuA with and without bound ferrichrome at atomic resolution[6,7]. FhuA consists of 22 antiparallel β-strands that form a β-barrel (Fig 3), similar to the porins that form β-barrels of 16 or 18 strands. In contrast to the porins, the β-barrel of FhuA is completely closed by residues 19 to 159, which form a globular structure that enters the β-barrel from the periplasmic side and is for this reason designated the cork[6] or plug[7]. Loop 4, which forms the principal phage binding site[8], is located at the cell surface.

Ferrichrome binds in a pocket exposed to the cell surface above the external outer membrane interface (Fig 3). Binding of ferrichrome causes movement of the cork by 1.7 Å towards ferrichrome and a large structural transition in the periplasmically exposed portion where a short α-helix unwinds and Glu-19 moves 17.3 Å from its former α-carbon position. The ferrichrome-induced structural transition through the FhuA molecule and across the entire outer membrane does not open the channel of the β-barrel. The opening of the channel is thought to occur by input of energy from the cytoplasmic membrane, mediated by the Ton complex composed of the proteins TonB, ExbB, and ExbD[9].

Energization of transport across the outer membrane by the proton-motive force of the cytoplasmic membrane differs entirely from energization of transport across the cytoplasmic membrane by ATP hydrolysis. The crystal structure does not elucidate the active transport mechanism since it represents a static state and cannot reveal the dynamics of ferrichrome transport. However, the portion of FhuA that has been shown to interact with the TonB protein[10], termed the TonB box (residues 7–11), is exposed to the periplasm, but has not been identified in the ferrichrome-loaded or unloaded crystal structure since it is disordered.

It is tentative to assume that the ferrichrome-induced large structural change in the periplasmic pocket of FhuA exposes the TonB box and facilitates its interaction with the TonB protein. Energy input from the cytoplasmic membrane may release ferrichrome from the FhuA binding site and open the channel in the FhuA β-barrel, resulting in translocation of ferrichrome through FhuA into the periplasm where it binds to the FhuD protein. The dissociation constant of FhuA for ferrichrome is below 0.1 μM, that of the FhuD protein is 1 μM[11].

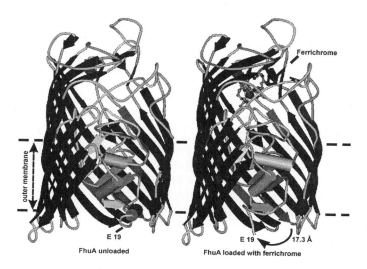

*Figure 3.* Structure of FhuA loaded with ferrichrome and in the unloaded form. In the ribbon representations, residues 621 to 723 are left out to allow a better view of the cork domain (shown in gray). The horizontal lines indicate the two boundaries of the outer membrane, with the cell surface on top.

## 3.    FhuA AS AN ACTIVE ANTIBIOTIC TRANSPORTER

Most antibiotics diffuse into bacteria. Their efficiency, as measured by the minimal inhibitory concentration (MIC), is determined by the diffusion rate and the activity at the target sites. Gram-negative bacteria are usually less sensitive to antibiotics than gram-positive bacteria because they contain an outer membrane that functions as a permeability barrier. However, if antibiotics are actively transported across the outer membrane, their MIC may be lower in gram-negative bacteria than in gram-positive bacteria because the antibiotic is accumulated in the periplasm, forming a steep concentration gradient across the cytoplasmic membrane and thereby enhancing the diffusion rate into the cytoplasm, or the antibiotic may even be actively transported across the cytoplasmic membrane. Examples for both uptake routes will be given.

## 3.1     The Crystal Structure of FhuA–Albomycin, the First Example of an Antibiotic Protein Transporter

Albomycin is a broad-spectrum antibiotic with an excellent inhibitory activity toward gram-positive and gram-negative bacteria. It belongs to the class of sideromycins that contain $Fe^{3+}$. The chemical structure of albomycin has been determined by $^1$H and $^{13}$C nuclear magnetic resonance spectroscopy, UV spectroscopy, and mass spectroscopy of chemical degradation products[12]. The albomycin-producing strain *Streptomyces* specWS116 synthesizes three derivatives that differ in the pyrimidine side chains (Fig 2).

The high specific activity of albomycin comes from the active transport into bacteria via the transport system of the structural analogue ferrichrome. Albomycin, like ferrichrome, is transported across the outer membrane by the FhuA protein. In the periplasm albomycin binds to the FhuD protein, which then donates albomycin to the FhuB protein in the cytoplasmic membrane. Transport across the cytoplasmic membrane is energized by ATP hydrolysis catalyzed by the FhuC protein, which is associated with FhuB at the cytoplasmic side of the cytoplasmic membrane (Fig 1). The moiety of albomycin that is analogous to ferrichrome (Fig 2) serves as carrier of the antibiotically active thioribosyl pyrimidine group[13]. After transport into the cytoplasm, iron is released from albomycin, and the thioribosyl pyrimidine group has to be cleaved from the carrier to be inhibitory; in *E. coli*, this cleavage is mainly achieved by peptidase N[14]. Mutants devoid of peptidase N activity are resistant to albomycin, and albomycin then serves only as an iron carrier. Most of the thioribosyl pyrimidine moiety remains inside the cells, whereas the carrier is released into the culture medium[13]. Albomycin is one of the very few antibiotics for which transport and intracellular activation have been characterized. The intracellular target has not been identified. The lack of albomycin-resistant target mutants suggests several targets and/or essential functions of the targets. It is likely that albomycin interferes with nucleic acid metabolism and/or nucleic-acid-dependent functions.

Albomycin has been co-crystallized with FhuA to determine whether it binds to the ferrichrome binding site of FhuA, how it fits into the binding site, and whether the thioribosyl pyrimidine moiety sterically hinders access to the ferrichrome binding site (Fig 2). Extra binding sites for albomycin on FhuA could result in a stronger binding to FhuA and a transport rate of albomycin lower than that of ferrichrome.

The crystal structure reveals[15] that the $Fe^{3+}$–hydroxamate portion of albomycin occupies the same site on FhuA and is bound by the same amino acid chains as ferrichrome. The predominant binding sites of albomycin on FhuA are aromatic residues (69%). Binding of the thioribosyl pyrimidine moiety occurs in the external pocket and involves five residues. These additional binding sites as compared to ferrichrome do not prevent release of albomycin from FhuA and transport through FhuA. The albomycin transport rate is 50% lower than the transport rate of ferrichrome, but it is not clear whether the lower rate is caused by transport across the outer membrane or across the cytoplasmic membrane.

The structure of the FhuA–albomycin co-crystal also has revealed the hitherto unknown conformation of albomycin and the conformation in the transport-competent form. The most unexpected result was the existence of two albomycin conformations in the crystal, an extended and a compact conformation. Both conformations fit into the external cavity of FhuA and occupy different amino acid ligands. The solvent-exposed external cavity of FhuA is sufficiently large to accommodate the voluminous side chain bound to the $Fe^{3+}$–hydroxamate moiety of albomycin.

With the modular composition of albomycin, in which the iron carrier is linked by a peptide linker to the antibiotically active thioribosyl pyrimidine, nature provides a clue of how to design highly efficient antibiotics that are actively transported into bacteria. Such antibiotics could be synthetically assembled from $Fe^{3+}$–hydroxamates, which fit into the active center of the transporters, and from an antibiotic that diffuses too slowly into cells to be useful by itself as a drug. The FhuA–albomycin structure demonstrates that the water-filled cavities in transporters can tolerate rather large antibiotics that are structurally unrelated to the carrier. The tolerance toward the antibiotic structure is not confined to FhuA since albomycin is also transported across the cytoplasmic membrane very well and is recognized by the FhuD and the FhuB proteins during this process.

## 3.2    Crystal Structure of FhuA with Bound Rifamycin CGP 4832

In 1987 a group from Ciba-Geigy reported on a semisynthetic rifamycin derivative, rifamycin CGP 4832, with an activity against many gram-negative bacteria 200-fold higher than that of unmodified rifamycin[16]. It was then shown with our mutants[17] that CGP 4832 is transported by FhuA across the outer membrane of *E. coli* and that the TonB activity is required[18]. Mutants in the *fhuBCD* genes, which encode the proteins required for active transport of ferrichrome across the cytoplasmic membrane, display unaltered CGP 4832 sensitivity. Our attempts to find additional transport mutants only revealed mutations in *fhuA* and *tonB exbB exbD*, which suggests that CGP 4832 crosses the cytoplasmic membrane by diffusion rather than by transport[19]. The use of FhuA as transporter for CGP 4832 was surprising since CGP 4832 does not contain iron and has no structural resemblance to ferrichrome (Fig 2). Therefore, it was particularly attractive to determine the crystal structure of FhuA loaded with CGP4832[19].

Analysis of the X-ray diffraction data revealed that CGP 4832 largely occupies the site in FhuA that is also used by ferrichrome. Interestingly, three amino acid residues, which also bind ferrichrome, recognize those side chains of CGP 4832 that differ from unmodified rifamycin (Fig 2). Two unique residues also contact such CGP 4832 side chains, whereas the 12 residues bind to sites that CGP 4832 shares with rifamycin.

In contrast to ferrichrome and albomycin, CGP 4832 in the crystal does not cause the large structural change in the periplasmically oriented pocket of FhuA. This does not seem to be caused by restriction of FhuA movements in the crystal since binding of CGP 4832 to FhuA in solution does not result in intrinsic FhuA tryptophan fluorescence quenching[19], as is observed when FhuA binds ferrichrome[19,20]. This finding has an impact on the concept of how FhuA interacts with TonB since, as discussed above, the large structural transition is thought to facilitate interaction of FhuA with TonB. Since transport of CGP 4932 depends on TonB, interaction of TonB with FhuA can also occur in the absence of the structural change. Analysis of a FhuA deletion derivative described below may provide a hint of how CGP 4832 is transported without substrate-induced enhancement of FhuA binding to TonB.

## 4.    FhuAΔ5–160, WHICH LACKS THE CORK, UNEXPECTEDLY STILL DISPLAYS TonB-DEPENDENT ACTIVITIES

We have deleted the cork to examine whether the residual β-barrel forms a stable protein, and if so, whether FhuAΔ5–160 is exported across the cytoplasmic membrane and incorporated into the outer membrane, and whether it shows any FhuA activities[21]. FhuAΔ5–160 is found in the outer membrane in amounts lower than that of wild-type FhuA, but is as resistant to trypsin and proteinase K as wild-type FhuA. FhuAΔ5–160 forms an open channel, as revealed by unspecific diffusion of compounds across the outer membrane of cells that synthesize FhuAΔ5–160. Such cells display a higher sensitivity to larger antibiotics, such as erythromycin, rifamycin, bacitracin, and vancomycin, and grow on maltotetraose in the absence of LamB, which in wild-type *E. coli* serves as a facilitated diffusion channel for maltodextrins. Higher concentrations of ferrichrome support growth of a *tonB* mutant that synthesizes FhuAΔ5–160. However, growth of a *tonB* wild-type strain occurs at low ferrichrome concentrations, and ferrichrome is transported with 45% of the wild-type rate despite the lack of those ferrichrome binding sites provided by the cork (Arg-81, Gly-99, Gln-100, Tyr-116). FhuAΔ5–160 confers sensitivity to the phages and colicin M at levels similar to that of wild-type FhuA. The activity of FhuAΔ5–160 still depends on TonB, although the mutant lacks the TonB box (residues 7 to 11) implicated in the interaction of FhuA with TonB[9,10]. TonB mutants of cells that contain FhuAΔ5–160 in their outer membrane no longer transport ferrichrome and are resistant to albomycin, rifamycin CGP 4832, colicin M, and the TonB-dependent phages T1 and φ80, but are sensitive to the TonB-independent phage T5, as are cells that contain wild-type FhuA. Apparently, FhuAΔ5–160 still functions as a specific transporter and responds to TonB, which implies that sites in addition to the TonB box are involved in the TonB-mediated reaction of FhuA to the proton gradient of the cytoplasmic membrane. This finding may also explain why, despite the lack of a structural transition in the periplasmic portion of the cork upon binding of rifamycin CGP 4832, the antibiotic is transported in a TonB-dependent way. The data also indicate that the mechanism of ferrichrome and antibiotic transport still has to be unraveled, taking the precise structural information into consideration. Even less clear is how biopolymers, phage DNA, and colicin M are transported through FhuA[22]. This would afford movement of the entire cork out of the FhuA β-barrel into the periplasm for which more energy is required than can probably be provided by the proton-motive force.

## ACKNOWLEDGMENTS

The authors work was supported by the Deutsche Forschungsgemeinschaft (SFB 323, project B1, Graduiertenkolleg Mikrobiologie (M.B.) and the Fonds der chemischen Industrie. We also thank the x-ray crystal structure analysis group of W. Welte, Biophysics, University of Constance, for excellent cooperation.

## REFERENCES

1. Braun, V., Hantke, K., and Köster, W., 1998, Bacterial iron transport: mechanisms, genetics, and regulation. In *Metal ions in biological systems* (A. Sigel and H. Sigel, eds.) Vol. 35, Marcel Dekker, Inc. New York, pp. 67–145.

2. Wyckoff, E.E., Duncan, D., Torres, A.G., Mills, M., Maase, K., and Payne, S.M., 1998, Structure of the *Shigella dysenteriae* haem transport locus and its phylogenetic distribution in enteric bacteria. *Mol. Microbiol.* **28:** 1139–1152.

3. Boos, W., and Lucht, J.M., 1996, Periplasmic binding protein-dependent ABC transporters. In *Escherichia coli* and *Salmonella. Cellular and molecular biology* (F.C. Neidhardt, ed.) ASM Press, Washington. pp. 1175–1209.

4. Mademidis, A., Killmann, H., Kraas, W., Flechsler, I., Jung, G., and Braun, V., 1997, ATP-dependent ferric hydroxamate transport system in *Escherichia coli*: periplasmic FhuD interacts with a periplasmic and with a transmembrane/cytoplasmic region of the integral membrane protein FhuB, as revealed by competitive peptide mapping. *Mol. Microbiol.* **26:** 1109–1123.

5. Braun, V., and Killmann, H., 1999, Bacterial solutions to the iron supply problem. *Trends in Biochem. Sci.* **24:** 104–109.

6. Ferguson, A.D., Hofmann, E., Coulton, J.W., Diederichs, K, and Welte, W., 1998, Structural basis for siderophore-mediated iron transport: crystal structure of FhuA with bound lipopolysaccharide. *Science* **282:** 2215–2220.

7. Locher, K., Rees, B., Koebnik, R., Mitschler, A., Moulinier, L., Rosenbusch, J.P., and Moras, D., 1998, Transmembrane signaling across the ligand-gated FhuA receptor: crystal structures of free and ferrichrome-bound states reveal allosteric changes. *Cell* **95:** 771–778.

8. Killmann, H., Videnov, G., Jung, G., Schwarz, H., and Braun, V., 1995, Identification of receptor binding sites by competitive peptide mapping: phages T1, T5, and φ80 and colicin M bind to the gating loop of FhuA. *J. Bacteriol.* **177:** 694–698.

9. Braun, V., 1995, Energy-coupled transport and signal transduction through the gram-negative outer membrane via TonB-ExbB-ExbD - dependent receptor proteins. *FEMS Microbiol. Rev.* **16:** 295–307.

10. Schöffler, H., and Braun, V., 1989, Transport across the outer membrane of *Escherichia coli* K12 via the FhuA receptor is regulated by the TonB protein in the cytoplasmic membrane. *Mol. Gen. Genet.* **217:** 378–383.

11. Rohrbach, M.R., Braun, V, and Köster, W., 1995, Ferrichrome transport in *Escherichia coli* K-12: altered substrate specificity of mutated periplasmic FhuD and interaction of FhuD with the integral membrane protein FhuB. *J. Bacteriol.* **177:** 7186–7193.

12. Benz, G., Schröder, T., Kurz, J., Wünsche, C., Karl, W., Steffens, G., Pfitzner, J., and Schmidt, D., 1982, Konstitution der Desferriform der Albomycine $\partial_1$, $\partial_2$, ε. *Angew. Chem.* **Suppl.** 1322–1335.

13. Hartmann, A., Fiedler, H.-P., and Braun, V., 1979, Uptake and conversion of the antibiotic albomycin by *Escherichia coli* K-12. *Eur. J. Biochem.* **99:** 517–524.

14. Braun, V., Günther, K., Hantke, K., and Zimmermann, L., 1983, Intracellular activation of albomycin in *Escherichia coli* and *Salmonella typhimurium*. *J. Bacteriol.* **156:** 308–315.

15. Ferguson, A.D., Braun, V., Fiedler, H.-P., Coulton, J.W., Diederichs, K., and Welte, W., 2000, Crystal structure of the antibiotic albomycin in complex with the outer membrane transporter FhuA. Submitted.

16. Wehrli, W., Zimmermann, W., Klump, W., Tosch, W., Fischer, W., and Zak, O., 1987, CGP 4832, a semisynthetic rifamycin derivative highly active against some gram-negative bacteria. *J. Antibiotics* **40:** 11733–1739.

17. Kadner, R.J., Heller, K., Coulton, J.W., and Braun, V., 1980, Genetic control of hydroxamate-mediated iron uptake in *Escherichia coli*. *J. Bacteriol.* **143:** 256–264.

18. Pugsley, P.A., Zimmermann, W., and Wehrli, W., 1987, Highly efficient uptake of a rifamycin derivative via FhuA-TonB-dependent uptake route in *Escherichia coli*. *J. Gen. Microbiol.* **133:** 3505–3511.

19. Ferguson, A.D., Ködding, J., Diederichs, K., Walker, G., Coulton, J.W., Braun, V., and Welte, W., 2000, Crystal structure of FhuA with a semisynthetic rifamycin derivative. Submitted.

20. Locher, K.P., and Rosenbusch, J.P., 1997, Oligomeric states and siderophore binding of the ligand-gated FhuA protein that forms channels across the *Escherichia coli* outer membranes. *Eur. J. Biochem.* **247:** 770–775.

21. Braun, M., Killmann, H. and Braun, V., 1999, The β-barrel domain of FhuAΔ5–160 is sufficient for TonB-dependent FhuA activities of *Escherichia coli*. *Mol. Microbiol.* **33:** 1037–1049.

22. Braun, V., 1998, Pumping iron through cell membranes. *Science* **282:** 2202–2203.

# THE CYTOTOXIC NECROTIZING FACTOR 1 (CNF1) FROM UROPATHOGENIC *ESCHERICHIA COLI*

Patrice Boquet

*INSERM U452 Faculté de Médecine, 28 avenue de Valombrose, Nice, 06100, France*

## 1.     INTRODUCTION

*Escherichia coli* are an important cause of intestinal infections. These bacteria, become highly pathogenic upon acquision of genes coding for virulence factors. In the case of urinary tract infections (UTIs), *E. coli* strains often express exotoxins, such as hemolysin and cytotoxic necrotizing factor 1 (CNF1) together with colonization factors such as Pap or Afa adhesins [1,2,3,4,5,6]. Genes coding for these virulence factors are linked on the chromosome of uropathogenic *E. coli* J96 strains[5,6] clustered within chromosomal DNA which have been called pathogenicity islands (PAIs)[7,8.] CNF1 is a toxin of 110 kDa[9] which induces, in cultured cells, a reorganization of actin microfilaments[10] by activation of the 21-kDa Rho GTP-binding protein[11,12].

## 2.     FREQUENCY OF CNF1-PRODUCING *E. COLI*

CNF1 is chromosomally encoded in *E. coli* by a single structural gene[13]. The GC percent of CNF1 (and CNF2) (35%) gene is lower than that of the *E. coli* genome[12,13]. CNF1 belongs to a pathogenicity island [5,6]. In the J96 strain two pathogenicity islands have been mapped to the 64-min (PAI IV) and 94- min (PAI V) regions of *E. coli* K12. Only the PAI V contains

*Genes and Proteins Underlying Microbial Urinary Tract Virulence*
Edited by L. Emödy *et al.*, Kluwer Academic/Plenum Publishers, 2000

45

the CNF1 gene[5,6]. In the J96 strain the gene of CNF1 is located between the operons coding for the hemolysin alpha operon, and the fimbriae adhesin protein Prs[6]. They are about 1 Kbp upstream the start codon of CNF1 and the stop codon of the *hly C* gene[13]. The vast majority (76%) of uropathogenic *E. coli hly* and *cnf1 positive* are associated with *pap/prs* together with *S-fimbriae (sfa)* genes[14]. In the same study, 4O % of these *E. coli* had only the *S-fimbriae* adhesin gene[14]. Only 12% of uropathogenic *E. coli* harbouring *hly* and *cnf1* genes contain the *pap/prs* and also 12% does not contain genes coding for adhesins[14]. This demonstrates that the PAI containing the *cnf1* gene is strictly associated with the *hly* operon but might vary in term of adhesins. The CNF1 protein does not contain an identifiable signal sequence and therefore it is excluded that this toxin uses a sec-dependent type 2 secretion mechanism. Furthermore, the *cnf1* gene does not belong to an operon, like the *hly* operon, which codes for the hemolysin structure and also for the secretion apparatus (type 1) of this pore-forming toxin and the post-translational activation of this toxin by acylation[15].

Frequency of *E. coli* producing CNF1 among uropathogenic *E. coli* is now documented. In a survey of 175 uropathogenic *E. coli* strains, at the University Hospital of Nice, 33% of these strains were found to produce CNF1[14] confirming the previous findings[16]. When the causative bacteria were separated on the basis of the urinary infectious process (cystisis, acute pyelonephritis or asymptomatic bacteriuria) exactly the same percentage of CNF1-producing *E. coli* was found in each group[14].

## 3.    CELLULAR EFFECTS OF *E. COLI* CNF1

CNF1 is a single chain protein toxin[13] with a predicted molecular mass of 113 kDa (1014 amino acids). The toxin is produced at very low level in wild-types pathogenic *E. coli* strains such as the J96. CNF1 has been described first as a dermonecrotic toxin upon injection in the rabbit skin and as inducing multinucleation in cultured HeLa cells[17]. The observation that CNF1 was able to induce the formation of actin stress fibers and membrane ruffling[10] led to the suspicion that this toxin was operating via the regulation of the actin cytoskeleton[10]. The induction of membrane actin folding and multinucleation by CNF1 are electively observed in epithelial HEp-2 cells whereas in fibroblastoid cells such as Vero or 3T3 mouse cells are the best cell models for actin stess fibers formation. After membrane actin folding induction, CNF1 allows spreading of epithelial cells such as HEp-2 and this is observed after 10 up to 24 h.

# 4.    MOLECULAR MECHANISM OF ACTION OF CNF1

CNF1 induces cell actin cytoskeleton reorganization by stimulating permanently the Rho protein. The first hint for this activity has been shown as follows: when the cytosol from HEp-2 cells previously incubated with CNF1 was ADP-ribosylated with exoenzyme C3 it was observed that the Rho protein had a molecular weight shifted to a slightly higher value. This result indicated a possible post-translational modification of the GTP-binding protein in CNF1 treated[11,12]. CNF1 was shown then to modify directly *in vitro* Rho without the need of cellular co-factors[18]. Microsequencing of CNF1-modified Rho showed that there was a single modification in the CNF1-treated GTPase compared to the wild type. Rho glutamine 63 was changed into glutamic acid[18]. Therefore, CNF1 exerts a specific deamidase activity. An identical activity for CNF1 on Rho was reported concomitantly using mass spectrometry[19].

The equivalent amino acid of Rho glutamine 63 in p21 Ras is glutamine 61. Rho glutamine 63 is known to be an important residue for the intrinsic and RhoGAP-mediated GTPase of Rho[20]. Both CNF1-treated Rho and mutated Rho on glutamine 63 into glutamic acid (RhoQ63E) exhibit a mobility shift, upon electrophoresis, identical to CNF1-treated[18,19]. CNF1-treated Rho and RhoQ63E nucleotide dissociation rate was increased by 2 orders of magnitude but the RhoGAP activity was totally impaired on both CNF1-treated Rho and RhoQ63E[18,19]. RhoGAP has been shown to activate GTP-hydrolysis of Rho by introducing into the regulatory molecule an elongated domain that contains an arginine residue in the[20]. This structure called an «arginine finger» allows the stabilization of the Rho glutamine 63 during the catalytic GTPase transition state and thus increases the intrinsic GTPase activity of Rho. By modifying Q63 into E63 in Rho, CNF1 impairs the role of the arginine finger of RhoGAP. Thus CNF1 allows Rho to be permanently bound with GTP, enhancing the activity on Rho effectors.

# 5.    STRUCTURE-FUNCTION RELATIONSHIPS OF CNF1

By using gluthathione S-transferase (GST) gene-fusion method to produce recombinant N-terminal 33 kDa (GST-CNF1Nter) and C-terminal 31, 5 kDa (GST-CNF1Cter) regions of the CNF1 the functional organization of this toxin has been studied[21]. These experiments clearly showed that the catalytic deamidase activity of CNF1 is located to the CNF1 C-ter region whereas the cell binding properties of the toxin are on its N-ter domain[21].

Recently, it has been reported that CNF1 possesses *in vitro* transglutaminase, in addition to deamidase, activity[22]. This was shown by the ability of CNF1 to incorporate on RhoA Q 63 alkylamines[22]. However the transglutaminase activity of CNF1 appears to be much lower that the deamidase activity[22]. As reported previously[21] the amino acid sequence 855-888 was found to contain an essential cysteine residue (cysteine 866, belonging to the consensus sequence LSGCTT) for the catalytic deamidase activity[22].

The amino-terminal domain of CNF1 (amino acids 1 to 299) contains the cell binding region of CNF1[21]. This has been shown by the fact that a GST-fusion protein containing this CNF1 polypeptide competes with CNF1 on the cell receptor[21]. More works are now necessary to further localize the CNF1 cell binding site. Finally, the CNF1 domain encompassing amino acids 299 to 720 that contain two hydrophobic domains (H1 and H2) are supposed to allow translocation of CNF1 across the cell membrane as does the translocating domain of diphtheria toxin.

We know actually nothing about the nature of the cell receptor of CNF1. CNF1 upon cell binding enters into the endocytic pathway by non clathrin-coated vesicles (Contamin et al., submitted). Then CNF1 must be transferred to an acidic compartment most likely late endosomes (Contamin et al., submitted). Acidification of CNF1 triggers its translocation through the lipidic membrane in the same manner than diphtheria toxin (Contamin et al., submitted).

## 6.     IS CNF1 A VIRULENCE FACTOR?

Secretion of CNF1 by the producing *E. coli* remains totally speculative. One hypothesis will be that CNF1 is not secreted by the bacteria but simply released when there is a lysis of *E. coli*. At the present time, we must thus be prudent to assimilate CNF1 with a virulence factor for uropathogenic *E. coli*. However incubation of CNF1 with different cell systems has shown that this toxin might behave like a bacterial virulence factor. For instance, CNF1 induces in non-professional phagocytic cells such as epithelial cells an active macropinocytic activity[23], it interferes with the transepithelial migration of polymorphonuclear lymphocytes across[24], it protects epithelial cells against apoptosis[25,26], it modifies epithelium permeability made of certain cells[27], and finally it changes the activity of phagocytosis of human macrophages[28].

Induction of a phagocytic behaviour in epithelial cells by CNF1 evokes a possible role of virulence factor to this toxin[23]. Bacterial invasion is a process by which a microbe can find a shelter against the host defenses and an advantageous milieu for its growth. Furthermore, invasion of epithelial cells can lead to the passage of bacteria from the lumen of mucosa to the bloodstream. A very interesting observation was that induction of phagocytosis by CNF1 could be correlated with the ability of the toxin to protect cells against apoptotic stimuli (such as ultraviolet radiation, UVB)[25]. The significant inverse correlation between the two phenomena, suggests that they could be part of a pathogenic mechanism used by bacteria. In the mechanism used by CNF1 to hinder apoptosis, proteins of the Bcl-2 family as well as the mitochondrial homeostasis, play a pivotal role. We have indeed shown that CNF1 was capable of reducing the mitochondrial membrane depolarization induced by UVB and to modulate the intracellular expression of some Bcl-2 related proteins. In particular, the amount of death antagonist Bcl-2 and Bcl-X, increased following exposure to CNF1 while the amount of the death agonist Bax remained substantially unchanged[26]. Mitochondria and the Bcl-2 family proteins have an essential role in apoptosis[29], and they are linked to each other. By modulating the expression of proteins of Bcl-2 family (probably *via* Rho activation), CNF1 may operate on one of the main regulatory systems which drive a cell towards death or survival.

CNF1 was also shown to reduce the transmigration of polymorphonuclear lymphocytes (PMNs) in intestinal T84 epithelial cell monolayers[24]. CNF1 effaced the intestinal microvilli (viewed by transmission electron micoscopy), induced a strong reorganization of the actin cytoskeleton especially at the baso lateral face of cells, and reduced the transmigration of PMNs induced by the chemoattractant N-formyl-Met-Leu-Phe either in the baso to apical or apico to basal[24]. Thus, CNF1 might decrease PMNs transmigration by remodelling of the cell actin cytoskeleton without gross modification of tight junction permeability. This mechanism would provide an advantage to the colonizing bacteria by reducing the ability of PMNs to cross the paracellular pathway.

CNF1 has been shown recently also to induce dramatic morphological changes and a profound reorganization of the actin cytoskeleton in human monocytic cells which impaired the CR3 phagocytosis but not the FcR-mediated ingestion[28]. By limiting integrin-mediated uptake of microbes (CR3), thus in an independent fashion from an immune specific response, CNF1 may prevent the phagocytosis of *Escherichia coli* producing this toxin.

In conclusion, CNF1 is the first toxin shown to act in the cytosol by deamidation of a glutamine residue belonging to a small GTP-binding protein. The role of CNF1 as a virulence factor for uropathogenic *Escherichia coli* is not established however, this toxin is a useful reagent to study the mode of action of Rho GTPases.

# REFERENCES

1.  Caprioli, A., Falbo, V., Ruggeri, F.M., Baldassari, L., Bisicchia, R., Ippolito, G., Romoli, E., and Donelli, G., 1987, Cytotoxic necrotizing factor production by hemolytic strains of Escherichia coli causing extra-intestinal infections. J. Clin. Microbiol. 25: 146-149.
2.  Caprioli, A., Falbo, V., Ruggeri, F.M., Minelli, F., Orskov, I., and Donelli, G., 1989, Relationships between cytotoxic necrotizing factor production and serotype in hemolytic *Escherichia coli*. *J. Clin. Microbiol.* **27**: 758-761.
3.  Falbo, V., Famiglieti, M. and Caprioli, A.,1992, Gene block encoding production of cytotoxic necrotizing factor 1 and hemolysin in *Escherichia coli* isolates from extra intestinal infections. *Infect. Immun.* **60**: 2182-2187.
4.  Blanco, J., Blanco, M., Alonso, M. P., Blanco, J.E., Gonzalez, E.A.and Garabal, J.I., 1992, Characteristics of haemolytic *Escherichia coli* with particular reference to production of cytotoxic necrotizing factor type 1 (CNF1). *Res. Microbiol.* **143**: 869-878.
5.  Blum, G., Falbo, V., Caprioli, A., and Hacker, J., 1995, Gene clusters encoding the cytotoxic necrotizing factor type 1, Prs-fimbriae and alpha hemolysin from the pathogenicity island II of the uropathogenic *Escherichia coli* strain J96. *FEMS Microbiol. lett.***126**: 189-195.
6.  Swenson, D.L., Bukanov, N.O., Berg, D.E., and Welch, R.A., 1996, Two pathogenicity islands in uropathogenic *Escherichia coli* J96: cosmid cloning and sample sequencing. *Infect. Immun.* **64**: 3736-3743.
7.  Groisman, E.A. and Ochman H., 1996, Pathogenicity islands: bacterial evolution in quantum leaps. *Cell*, **87**: 791-794.
8.  Hacker, J., Blum-Oehler, G., Mühldorfer, H., and Tschäpe, H., 1997, Pathogenicity islands of virulent bacteria: structure, function and impact on microbial evolution. *Mol. Microbiol.* **23**: 1089-1097.
9.  Caprioli, A., Falbo, V., Roda, L.G., Ruggeri, F.M., and Zona, C., 1983, Partial purification and characterization of an *Escherichia coli* toxic factor that induces morphological cell alterations. *Infect. Immun.* **39**: 1300-1306.
10. Fiorentini, C., Arancia, G., Caprioli, A., Falbo, V., Ruggeri, F.M. and Donelli, G., 1988, Cytoskeletal changes induced in Hep-2 cells by the cytotoxic necrotizing factor of *Escherichia coli*. *Toxicon* **26**: 1047-1056.
11. Fiorentini, C., Giry, M., Donelli, G., Falzano, L., Aullo, P., and Boquet, P., 1994, *Escherichia coli* cytotoxic necrotizing factor 1 increases actin assembly via the p21 Rho GTPase. *Zentrabl. Bakteriol Suppl.* **24**: 404-405.
12. Oswald, E. Sugai, M., Labigne, A., Wu, H.C., Fiorentini, C., Boquet, P. and O'Brien, A.D., 1994 Cytotoxic necrotizing factor type 2 produced by virulent *Escherichia coli* modifies the small GTP-binding protein Rho involved in assembly of actin stress fibers. *Proc. Natl. Acad. Sci. USA* **91**: 3814-3818.
13. Falbo, V., Pace, T., Picci, L., Pizzi, E., and Caprioli, A., 1993, Isolation and nucleotide sequence of the gene encoding cytotoxic necrotizing factor 1 of *Escherichia coli*. *Infect. Immun.* **61**: 4909-4914.
14. Landraud, L., Gauthier, M., Fosse, T., and Boquet, P., 1999, Frequency of *Escherichia coli* strains producing the cytotoxic necrotizing factor (CNF1) in nosocomial urinary tract infections. *Lett. Appl. Microbiol.* **29**: in press.
15. Koronakis, V., and Hughes, C.. 1996, Synthesis, maturation and export of the *E. coli* hemolysin. *Med. Microbiol. Immunol.* **185**: 65-71.
16. Blanco, M., Blanco, J.E., Alonso, M. and Blanco, J., 1996, Virulence factors and O groups of *Escherichia coli* isolates from patients with acute pyelonephritis, cystitis and asymptomatic bacteriuria. *Eur. J. Epidemiol.* **12**: 191-198.

17. Caprioli, A., Donelli, G., Falbo, V., Possenti, L., Roda, G., Roscetti, G. and Ruggeri, F.M.. 1984, A cell division active protein from *Escherichia coli*. *Biochem. Biophys. Res. Commun.* **118**: 587-593.

18. Flatau, G., Lemichez, E., Gauthier, M., Chardin, P., Paris, S., Fiorentini, C. and Boquet, P., 1997, Toxin-induced activation of the G-protein p21 Rho by deamidation of glutamine. *Nature* **387**: 729-733.

19. Schmidt, G., Sehr, P, Wilm, M., Selzer, J., Mann, M. and Aktories, K., 1997, Rho gln 63 is deamidated by *Escherichia coli* cytotoxic necrotizing factor 1. *Nature* **387**: 725-729.

20. Rittinger, K., Walker, P.A., Eccleston, J.F., Smerdon, S.J. and Gamblin, S.J., 1997, Structure at 1,65 A of RhoA and its GTPase-activating protein in complex with a transition state analogue. *Nature* **389**: 753-762.

21. Lemichez, E., Flatau, G., Bruzzone, M., Boquet, P. and Gauthier, M., 1997, Molecular localization of the *Escherichia coli* cytotoxic necrotizing factor 1 cell binding and catalytic domains. *Mol. Microbiol.* **24**: 1061-1070.

22. Schmidt G., Selzer, J., Lerm, M. and Aktories, K., 1998, The Rho-deamidating cytotoxic necrotizing factor 1 from *Escherichia coli* possesses transglutaminase activity. *J. Biol. Chem.* **273**: 13669-13674.

23. Falzano, L., Fiorentini, C., Donelli, G., Michel, E., Kocks, C., Cossart, P., Cabanié, L., Oswald, E., and Boquet, P., 1993, Induction of phagocytic behaviour in human epithelial cells by *Escherichia coli* cytotoxic necrotizing factor 1. *Mol. Microbiol.* **9**: 1247-1254.

24. Hofman, P., Flatau, G., Selva, E., Gauthier, M., Le Negrate, G., Fiorentini, C., Rossi, B. and Boquet, P., 1998, *Escherichia coli* cytotoxic necrotizing factor 1 effaces microvilli and decreases transmigration of polymorphonuclear leukocytes in intestinal T84 epithelial cell monolayers. Infect. *Immun.* **66**: 2494-2500.

25. Fiorentini, C., Fabbri, A., Matarrese, P., Falzano, L., Boquet, P., and Malorni, W., 1997, Hinderance of apoptosis and phagocytic behaviour: induced by *Escherica coli* necrotizing factor (CNF1): two related activities in epithelial cells. *Biochem. Biophys. Res. Comm.* **241**: 341-346.

26. Fiorentini, C., Matarrese, P., Straface, E., Falzano, L., Fabbri, A., Donelli, G., Cossarizza, A., Boquet, P., and Malorni, W., 1998, Toxin-induced activation of Rho GTP-binding protein increases Bcl-2 expression and influences mitochondrial homeostasis. *Exp. Cell. Res.* **242**: 341-350.

27. Gerhard R, Schmidt G, Hofmann F and Aktories K., 1998, Activation of Rho GTPases by *Escherichia coli* cytotoxic necrotizing factor 1 increases intestinal permeability in caco-2 cells. *Infect. Immun.* **66**: 5125-5131.

28. Capo, C., Sangueldoce, M.V., Meconi, S., Flatau, G., Boquet, P. and Mége, J.L., 1998, Effect of cytotoxic necrotizing factor 1 on actin cytoskeleton in human monocytes: role in the regulation of integrin-dependent phagocytosis. *J. Immunol.*. **161**: 4301-4308.

29. Green, D.R., 1998, Apoptotic pathways: the road to ruin. Cell **94**: 695-698.

# GENETIC CHARACTERIZATION OF THE UROPATHOGENIC *E. COLI* STRAIN 536 - A SUBTRACTIVE HYBRIDIZATION ANALYSIS

Britta Janke, Jörg Hacker and Gabriele Blum-Oehler
*Institut für Molekulare Infektionsbiologie der Universität Würzburg, Röntgenring 11, D-97070 Würzburg*

## 1.      THE UROPATHOGENIC *E. COLI* STRAIN 536

Usually *Escherichia coli* is a normal inhabitant of the gut flora. Variants of *E. coli* are able to cause extraintestinal infections e.g. urinary tract infections or newborn meningitis. For the colonization and the infectious processes pathogenic bacteria need several virulence factors.

The uropathogenic *E. coli* strain 536 (O6:K15:H31) was isolated from a patient suffering from acute pyelonephritis and is characterized by the production of certain virulence factors such as α-hemolysin (*hly*), fimbrial adhesins e.g. type 1, P-related and S fimbriae (*fim, prf, sfa*), the siderophores enterobactin (*ent*) and yersiniabactin (*ybt*)[1]. In the early 1980s uropathogenic *E. coli* strains have been shown to contain distinct blocks of DNA carrying closely linked virulence genes so-called pathogenicity islands (PAIs). PAIs are generally characterized as follows: these structures are present in the genome of pathogenic isolates but absent from non pathogenic variants. Their G+C content differs from the G+C content of the rest of the bacterial genome. Often they are inserted in or near by tRNA sequences. The acquisition of PAIs may have occurred by horizontal gene transfer[2]. The *E. coli* strain 536 carries four pathogenicity islands of sizes from ~25 to 190 kb. The PAI I and II of the *E. coli* strain 536 (PAI I$_{536}$ and PAI II$_{536}$) can spontaneously and independently be deleted from the chromosome possibly by the involvement of the flanking direct repeats in homologous recombination. The deletion of PAI III$_{536}$ and PAI IV$_{536}$ has not been detected yet.

*Genes and Proteins Underlying Microbial Urinary Tract Virulence*
Edited by L. Emödy  *et al.*, Kluwer Academic/Plenum Publishers, 2000

## 2. SUBTRACTIVE HYBRIDIZATION AS AN APPROACH TO ANALYSE THE *E. COLI* STRAIN 536

In order to distinguish between pathogenic and non pathogenic bacteria the properties of the pathogenic bacteria have to be further analysed. In the genome of the *E. coli* K-12 strain MG1655 none of the classical virulence associated genes were identified. Therefore this strain was important for the analysis of pathogenic *E. coli* variants.

For the identification of sequences which are present in one strain (so-called tester-strain) and absent in another strain (driver-strain) a suppressive subtractive hybridization technique based on a publication of Diatchenko et al.[3] was used. A schematic overview of the subtractive hybridization is given in Fig 1.

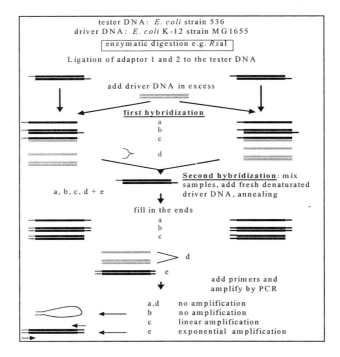

*Figure 1.* Schematic overview of the subtractive hybridization method modified by Akopyants et al.[4]. Black lines represent the digested tester DNA and grey lines represent the digested driver DNA. The two different adaptor sequences are given in dotted and hatched thin lines.

In our case the genome of the *E. coli* strain 536 (tester) was compared to the *E. coli* K-12 strain MG1655 (driver) with respect to sequence differences. The genomic DNA from the bacterial strains of interest were digested with a suitable four base cutting restriction enzyme. The tester DNA was subdivided in two portions and ligated with two different adaptors. Then two hybridization steps were performed followed by two PCR reactions. A pattern of different PCR bands was obtained and further analysed.

# 3.  IDENTIFICATION OF NEW DNA-SEQUENCES SPECIFIC FOR *E. COLI* STRAIN 536

The resulting DNA fragments after the nested PCR were analysed in Southern blot experiments with chromosomal DNA of the *E. coli* K-12 strain MG1655 in order to test their specificity for the strain 536. Additionally we used PAI $I_{536}$ and PAI $II_{536}$ negative strains to identify the position of these fragments on particular PAIs.

Using the subtractive hybridization approach we obtained 22 *E. coli* 536 specific DNA fragments (see Table 1). Five of these fragments showed a homology to already known virulence determinants like α-hemolysin (*hly*) and the P-related fimbriae (*prf*). For two fragments sequence similarities to genes which are important for the LPS-biosynthesis were identified. Additionally we have found a DNA fragment which shows a homology to a capsule protein, a siderophore receptor and a protein which is probably important for the fimbrial biogenesis.

Eight of the obtained DNA fragments have no homology to known DNA or protein sequences. These fragments may be part of PAI $III_{536}$ or PAI $IV_{536}$ or of new pathogenicity islands.

*Table 1.* Subtractive hybridization fragments derived from the *E. coli* strain 536 and their properties

| Presence on the K-12 genome | Presence on PAI $I_{536}$ or PAI $II_{536}$ | Sequence homology | No. of fragments |
|---|---|---|---|
| - | PAI $I_{536}$ and PAI $II_{536}$ | α-hemolysin | 3 |
| - | PAI $II_{536}$ | P-fimbriae | 2 |
| - | - | LPS biosynthesis | 2 |
| - | - | capsule protein | 1 |
| - | - | siderophore receptor | 1 |
| - | PAI $I_{536}$ | fimbrial biogenesis | 1 |
| - | ? | others | 12 |

## 4. CONCLUSIONS

The species *E. coli* comprises non pathogenic variants and other strains which are able to cause infectious diseases. In order to identify DNA fragments which are present in the pathogenic *E. coli* strain 536 but absent from the non-pathogenic *E. coli* strain MG1655 we have performed a subtractive hybridization analysis.

We obtained diverse DNA fragments specific for the *E. coli* strain 536. Sequence data of several cloned subtractive hybridization fragments showed a homology to known virulence genes. Other *E. coli* strain 536 specific DNA fragments showed no homology to already known DNA or protein sequences and may represent new virulence genes on PAIs.

In conclusion subtractive hybridization is a successful method for the identification of strain specific DNA sequences. It is a useful approach to complement other genomic approaches such as proteome analysis or differential RNA display analysis.

## REFERENCES

1.  Hacker, J., Blum-Oehler, G., Janke, B., Nagy, G., and Goebel, W., Pathogenicity islands of extraintestinal Escherichia coli. In: *Pathogenicity islands and other mobile elements* (J. Kaper and J. Hacker, eds.). ASM Press 1999. pp. 59- 76.
2. Hacker, J., Blum-Oehler, G., Mühldorfer, I., and Tschäpe, H., 1997, Pathogenicity islands of virulent bacteria: structure, function and impact on microbial evolution. *Mol. Microbiol.* **23:**1089-1097.
3.  Diatchenko, L., Lau, Y.F., Campell, A.P., Chenik, A., Moqadam, F., Huang, B., Lukyanov, S., Lukyanov, K., Gurskaya, N., Sverdlov, E.D., and Siebert, P.D., 1996, Suppression subtractive hybridization: a method for generating differentially regulated or tissue-specific cDNA probes and libraries. *Proc. Natl. Acad. Sci. U SA* **93:** 6025-6030.
4.  Akopyants, N.S., Fradkov, A., Diatchenko, L., Hill, J.E., Siebert, P.D., Lukyanov, S.A., Sverdlov, E.D., and Berg, D.E., 1998, PCR-based subtractive hybridization and differences in gene content among strains of Helicobacter pylori. *Proc. Natl. Acad. Sci. USA* **95:** 13108-1313.

# ANALYSIS OF THE HEMOLYSIN DETERMINANTS OF THE UROPATHOGENIC *ESCHERICHIA COLI* STRAIN 536

[1]Gábor Nagy, [1]Ulrich Dobrindt, [1]Gabriele Blum-Oehler, [2]Levente Emődy, [3]Werner Goebel and [1]Jörg Hacker

[1]*Institut für Molekulare Infektionsbiologie der Universität Würzburg, Germany.* [2]*Department of Medical Microbiology and Immunology, University Medical School of Pécs, Hungary* [3]*Lehrstuhl für Mikrobiologie der Universität Würzburg, Germany*

## 1.  THE UROPATHOGENIC *E. COLI* STRAIN 536

*Escherichia coli* is by far the most common causative agent of urinary tract infections. The ability of uropathogenic strains to produce certain virulence factors distinguishes them from commensal and intestinal pathogenic strains. Pathogenicity factors, such as fimbriae, ferric uptake systems, toxins, O-, K- and flagellar antigens enable these strains to colonize the urinary tract, to avoid host defense mechanisms and in severe cases to reach the blood-stream by destroying tissue barriers. Virulence factors of uropathogenic *E. coli* are often parts of so-called pathogenicity islands (PAIs), that are large, unstable chromosomal DNA-regions carrying at least one, but often several virulence determinants.

The uropathogenic *E. coli* strain 536 (O6:K15:H31) was isolated from a patient suffering from pyelonephritis. It carries four PAIs on its chromosome possessing the genetical determinants for P-related- (PAI $II_{536}$) and S- (Pai $III_{536}$) fimbriae, yersiniabactin (Pai $IV_{536}$) as well as two distinct copies of the α-hemolysin (*hly*) gene cluster (*hlyI* and *hlyII* are located on PAI $I_{536}$ and PAI $II_{536}$, respectively)[1].

*Genes and Proteins Underlying Microbial Urinary Tract Virulence*
Edited by L. Emődy *et al.*, Kluwer Academic/Plenum Publishers, 2000

## 2.    TRANSCRIPTIONAL ORGANIZATION OF THE HEMOLYSIN OPERON

α-hemolysin is the best characterized representative of the so-called RTX toxin family, which is disseminated among members of the *Enterobacteriaceae*. Determinants encoding the synthesis and secretion of the toxin can be located on plasmids, or in human pathogenic strains, on the chromosome. The genes encoding the synthesis (*hlyA*) and activation (*hlyC*) of the toxin are cotranscribed with the genes responsible for its secretion (*hlyB* and *hlyD*). The expression of these genes, however, can be uncoupled due to a rho-independent terminator sequence located between *hlyA* and *hlyB*. The expression polarity of the operon is suppressed by *trans-* (*rfaH*) and *cis*-acting (such as *hlyR* in the upstream region of the plasmid encoded hemolysin) sequences through inhibition of termination [2,3,4]. In this way the transcripts are allowed to elongate into the genes encoding the secretion proteins.

Up to this point two α-hemolysin operons of *Escherichia coli* have been completely sequenced: one from the well characterized human uropathogenic strain J96, and that of the plasmid pHly152 carried by animal pathogenic strains. Interestingly, while the DNA sequence of the four *hly* genes is highly conserved, the 5' flanking sequences differ considerably among various *hly* determinants of *E. coli*[5].

## 3.    EXPRESSION OF THE TWO HEMOLYSIN DETERMINANTS OF STRAIN 536

Using mutant strains lacking either PAI $I_{536}$ or PAI $II_{536}$, we were able to determine the hemolytic activity originating from *hlyI* and *hlyII*, separately (Fig. 1) While the loss of PAI $I_{536}$ caused a 40-fold reduction of both secreted- and intracellular hemolytic activity, the loss of PAI $II_{536}$ resulted only in a moderate decrease compared to the wildtype. The mutant lacking both PAI $I_{536}$ and PAI $II_{536}$ had a non-hemolytic phenotype. Inactivation of the *rfaH* gene resulted in a 10-fold decrease of hemolytic activity, indicating that this locus plays a major role in the regulation of the hemolysin operon(s).

In order to determine if the different hemolytic activity is due to different expression of the operons we performed Northern blot analysis from total cellular RNA. The results are shown in Fig. 2. While the long *hlyCABD* transcripts were not detectable, the probe hybridized with a fragment of about 4 kb. This size corresponds the short *hlyCA* transcript. While the quantity of the *hly* transcripts of the PAI $I_{536}^-$ mutant (536-114) was significantly decreased, that of the PAI $II_{536}^-$ (536-225) strain seemed to be not altered compared to the wild type strain.

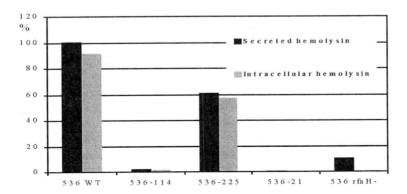

*Figure 1.* Secreted- and intracellular hemolytic activity of 536 wild type (PAI I$_{536}$$^+$, PAI II$_{536}$$^+$) and its derivatives 536-114 (PAI I$_{536}$$^-$, PAI II$_{536}$$^+$), 536-225 (PAI I$_{536}$$^+$, PAI II$_{536}$$^-$) and 536-21 (PAI I$_{536}$$^-$, PAI II$_{536}$$^-$).

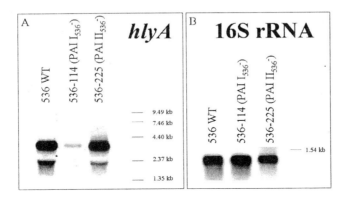

*Figure 2.* A: Northern blot-analysis of the *hly* transcript from the strain 536 (PAI I$_{536}$$^+$, PAI II$_{536}$$^+$) and its derivatives 536-114 (PAI I$_{536}$$^-$, PAI II$_{536}$$^+$) and 536-225 (PAI I$_{536}$$^+$, PAI II$_{536}$$^-$) B: Detection of the 16S rRNA as an internal standard.

## 4.    SEQUENCING OF THE HEMOLYSIN DETERMINANTS OF STRAIN 536

We performed the sequencing of both *hly* operons of strain 536 using cosmid clones of a genomic library as templates. DNA sequences were determined by using the so-called primer walking method. Assembling of the sequences was performed by the ABI Prism AutoAssembler 2.1 program. The homology search with the hemolysin nucleotide sequence of the uropathogenic *E. coli* strain J96 and the naturally occurring hemolytic plasmid pHly152 revealed a very high degree of homology (95-98%) over the entire operon among these gene clusters and those of 536[6]. The 5' flanking regions, however, differed considerably between the two determinants of strain 536. While the upstream region of *hlyI* was 96% homologous to that of strain J96, the same region of *hly II* showed only very week similarity to *hlyR*, a proposed enhancer sequence for the plasmid encoded hemolysin. The recently described 8 bp-long operon polarity suppressor (*ops*) motif  could be identified in the upstream regions[4]. Interestingly, in case of *hlyII$_{536}$* it is overlapped by the *hlyR* sequence (such as that of the plasmid encoded hemolysin). The distance between the *ops* and the start codon of *hlyC* is also different concerning the two *hly* determinants of strain 536 (334 bp in *hlyI*; 654 bp in *hlyII*).

## 5.    *IN VIVO* VIRULENCE TESTS

The *in vivo* virulence of the wild type strain compared to the mutant that lost both PAIs carrying the hemolysin determinants (536-21) was investigated in mouse models. Loss of  both PAIs resulted in a completely avirulent phenotype as shown in intravenous, respiratory and nephrovirulence assays (Table 1).

*Table 1. In vivo* virulence of strain 536 and its mutant 536-21 (PAI I$_{536}$⁻, PAI II$_{536}$⁻)

| Strain | Intravenous lethality* | Respiratory virulence** | Nephrotoxicity*** |
|--------|------------------------|-------------------------|-------------------|
| 536 WT | 50/50 | 80 | nephrovirulent |
| 536-21 | 0/50 | 0 | avirulent |

\*      death within 3 days after intravenous infection with 2.5 x 10$^8$ bacteria

\*\*     % death within 24 hours after intranasal instillation of 5.0 x 10$^7$ bacteria

\*\*\*    increase of bacterial counts in the kidney, and decrease in the other organs 8 hours after intravenous infection with 2.5 x 10$^8$ bacteria

## 6. CONCLUSION

The *in vitro* hemolytic activity directed by the two *hly* operons of strain 536 differ significantly, which is probably the effect of the different transcriptional rate.

While the coding regions of the two *hly* determinants are 96% homologous, no similarity can be found in the 5' flanking regions (except the 8 bp *ops* motif). The dissimilar upstream elements may explain the different expression of the operons.

Loss of the pathogenicity islands carrying the hemolysin determinants results in an avirulent phenotype.

## REFERENCES

1. Hacker, J., Blum-Oehler, G., Mühldorfer, I., and Tschäpe, H., 1997, Pathogenicity islands of virulent bacteria: structure, function and impact on microbial evolution. *Mol. Microbiol.* **23:** 1089-97.
2. Vogel, M., Hess, J., Then, I., Juarez, A., and Goebel, W., 1988, Characterization of a sequence (hlyR) which enhances synthesis and secretion of hemolysin in *Escherichia coli. Mol. Gen. Genet.* **212:** 76-84
3. Koronakis, V., Cross, M., and Hughes, C., 1989, Transcription antitermination in an *Escherichia coli* hemolysin operon is directed progressively by cis-acting DNA sequences upstream of the promoter region. *Mol. Microbiol.* **3:** 1397-1404.
4. Bailey, M.J., Hughes, C., Koronakis, V., 1997, Rf*a*H and the ops element, components of a novel system controlling bacterial transcription elongation. *Mol. Microbiol.,* **26:** 845-851.
5. Hess, J., Wels, W., Vogel, M., Goebel, W., 1986, Nucleotide sequence of a plasmid-encoded hemolysin determinant and its comparison with corresponding chromosomal hemolysin sequence. *FEMS Microbiology Letters* **34:** 1-11
6. Hacker, J., Blum-Oehler, G., Janke, B., Nagy, G., and Goebel, W., 1999, Pathogenicity islands of extraintestinal *Escherichia coli.* In Pathogenicity Islands and Other Mobile Virulence Elements (J.B. Kaper and J. Hacker, eds.), American Society for Microbiology., Washington D.C., pp. 59-76.

# FUNCTIONAL VARIABILITY OF TYPE 1 FIMBRIAE OF *ESCHERICHIA COLI*

[1]Riitta Pouttu, [1]Terhi Puustinen, [1]Maini Kukkonen, [1]Ritva Virkola, [1]Minni Laurila, [2]Jörg Hacker, [3]Per Klemm and [1]Timo K. Korhonen
[1]*Division of General Microbiology, Department of Biosciences, University of Helsinki, Finland:*
[2]*Institut für Molekulare Infektionsbiologie, Würzburg, Germany:* [3]*Department of Microbiology, Technical University of Denmark, Lyngby, Denmark*

## 1. INTRODUCTION

Type 1 fimbriae are filamentous protein structures that are commonly found on the surfaces of bacteria belonging to the *Enterobacteriaceae* family. Type 1 fimbriae are characterized by their binding to mannose containing oligosaccharides that are common constituents in eucaryotic glycoproteins. The chromosomal *fim*-gene-cluster composed of nine genes encodes for the expression of type 1 fimbrial proteins. The type 1 fimbrial filament is composed predominantly of the major protein FimA, three minor proteins FimF, FimG and FimH are also present[1]. The mannose sensitive binding of type 1 fimbriae to targets is mediated by the FimH-adhesin[2, 3]. It is remarkable that the FimH-lectin binds to mannoproteins as well as proteins lacking carbohydrate, such as the N-terminus of human fibronectin[3]. This binding is inhibited by mannose, which upon binding, probably changes the FimH conformation.

The adherence of invasive bacterial pathogens to mammalian extracellular matrix- and basement membrane-components, like the poorly glycosylated collagens, is thought to enhance bacterial colonization and invasion into subepithelial tissues[4] and contribute to the initiation of systemic infection[5, 6]. Bacterial expression of receptors for plasminogen, a precursor of the serine protease plasmin, potentiates the generation of bacterium bound plasmin

*Genes and Proteins Underlying Microbial Urinary Tract Virulence*
Edited by L. Emődy *et al.*, Kluwer Academic/Plenum Publishers, 2000

activity by plasminogen activators. Plasmin activity on adhesive bacteria can be directed against host structures that function as tissue barriers, thus enabling the penetration of bacteria into tissues or circulation[7, 8].

## 2.   COLLAGEN ADHERENCE

The adherence of *E. coli* -strains IHE3034, IHE3034-2, IHE3034 (pRPO-1)[9] and HB101(pPKL4)[10] to collagens and BSA immoblized on glass was characterized[9, 11] as previously described[12] (Fig 1).

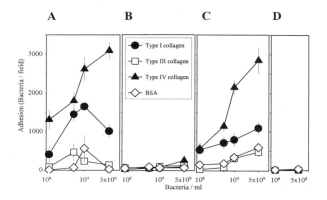

*Figure 1.* Adhesion to type I, type III, type IV collagen and to BSA by *E. coli* IHE3034 (A), IHE3034-2 (B), IHE3034-2(pRPO-1) (C)l, and HB101(pPKL4) (D). (Modified from reference 9).

The strain IHE3034 adhered efficiently to type IV collagen, more weakly to type I collagen, but not to type III collagen or BSA. The *fimA::cat* mutant strain IHE3034-2 failed to adhere, while the IHE3034-*fim*-complemented strain IHE3034-2(pRPO-1) exhibited adherence pattern similar to that of the wild type strain IHE3034[9]. We found that the type 1 fimbriae of *E. coli* PC31, expressed by HB101(pPKL4) did not bind to collagens[11] (Fig 1). This indicated that the two fimbriae differ functionally.

The sequences of mature FimH-proteins *of E. coli* -strains IHE3034[9] and PC31[13] were compared. The amino acid sequence of FimH of IHE3034 differed from that of PC31 at five positions[9] (Fig 2).

To analyze the role of the differing amino acid residues between FimH of IHE3034 and PC31 for the collagen adherence, each one of the five differing residues in the IHE3034 FimH was individually substituted by PCR mutagenesis to the corresponding one in the PC31 FimH[9] and expressed in the *E. coli fimH*-null-strain MS4[14].The wild type FimH-proteins from strains

IHE3034 and PC31 were expressed similarly[9,14] and the adherence of the *fimH*-complemented strains to type I and to type IV collagens and to BSA was tested[9] (Fig 3).

**PC31 FimH**

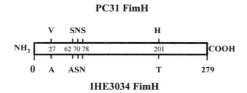

**IHE3034 FimH**

*Figure 2.* Location of the amino acid sequence differences in the mature FimH-proteins of *E. coli* PC31 and IHE3034. (Modified from reference 9).

MS4(pRPO-2) expressing the IHE3034 FimH adhered efficiently to type IV and to type I collagen, but not to BSA. The mutations A27V, S70N, N78S and T201H had little or no effect on the adherence to collagens, whereas the mutation A62S in the IHE3034-FimH reduced the collagen adhesiveness to the level seen with MS4(pMAS4) expressing the PC31-FimH. The importance for the collagen binding of the amino acid residue Alanine-62 in the FimH-adhesin was further demonstrated by enhanced collagen adherence of MS4(pRPO-3) expressing the PC31-FimH with the mutation S62A (Fig 3).

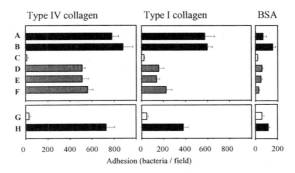

*Figure 3.* Adhesion of the fimH-null-strain E. coli MS4 expressing FimH-derivatives originating from IHE3034-FimH (bars A - F) or from PC31-FimH (bars G and H). The constructs are: MS4(pRPO-2) expressing IHE3034 FimH (A), MS4(pRPO-21) with the substitution A27V(B), MS4(pRPO-22) with the substitution A62S (C), MS4(pRPO-23) with the substitution S70N (D), MS4(pRPO-24) with the substitution N78S (E), MS4(pRPO-25) with the substitution T201H (F), MS4(pMAS4) expressing PC31 FimH (G), and MS4(pRPO-3) with the substitution S62A (H). (Modified from reference 9).

## 3.      PLASMINOGEN RECEPTOR FUNCTION

Binding of plasminogen and enhancement of plasminogen activation were studied as previously described[15,16] using purified type 1 fimbriae of *E. coli* - strains IHE3034 and PC31 as well as laminin as a positive and BSA as a negative control (Fig 4).

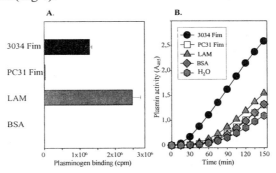

*Figure 4.* Binding of plasminogen (A) and enhancement of tPA-catalyzed plasminogen activation (B) by purified type 1 fimbriae of E. coli -strains IHE3034 and PC31 and by laminin and BSA.

Type 1 fimbriae of *E. coli* IHE3034 immobilized plasminogen and enhanced its tPA-catalyzed activation into plasmin; i.e. they functioned as plasminogen receptors. This was not observed with the type 1 fimbriae of *E. coli* PC31. Sequence comparison of Fim-proteins of IHE3034 and PC31 showed differences in amino acid residues potentially important for plasminogen binding (data not shown), and we are currently locating the residues important for plasminogen immobilization on the fimbriae.

## 4.      CONCLUSIONS

Type 1 fimbriae and the FimH-adhesins of *E. coli* differ in adhesive functions: those of a meningitis isolate IHE3034 mediate adhesion to collagens whereas those of an avirulent K-12 strain PC31 do not. Amino acid residue Alanine-62 in the FimH is critical for the collagen binding ability: substitution of $Ala^{62}$ of IHE3034 FimH into serine abolishes collagen adhrence whereas substitution of $Ser^{62}$ of PC31 FimH into alanine restores the binding.

Fimbriae also are targets for binding of functionally important host proteins. Type 1 fimbriae of *E. coli* differ in plasminogen receptor function:

those of the strain IHE3034 mediate plasminogen receptor function while those of the strain PC31 do not. The Fim-protein(s) and the critical amino acids involved in plasminogen receptor function remain to be identified.

# REFERENCES

1. Soto, G.E., and Hultgren, S.J., 1999, Bacterial adhesins: common themes and variations in architecture and assembly. *J. Bacteriol.* **181**: 1059-1071.
2. Krogfelt, K.A., Bergmans, H., and Klemm, P., 1990, Direct evidence that the FimH protein is the mannose-specific adhesin of *Escherichia coli* type 1 fimbriae. *Infect. Immun.* **58**: 1995-1998.
3. Sokurenko, E.V., Courtney, H.S., Ohman, D.E., Klemm, P., and Hasty, D., 1994, FimH family of type 1 fimbrial adhesins: functional heterogeneity due to minor sequence variations among *fimH* genes. *J. Bacteriol.* **176**: 748-755.
4. Westerlund, B., and Korhonen, T.K., 1993, Bacterial proteins binding to the mammalian extracellular matrix. *Mol. Microbiol.* **9**: 687-694.
5. Tamm, A., Tarkkanen, A.-M., Korhonen, T.K., Kuusela, P., Toivanen, P., and Skurnik, M., 1993, Hydrophobic domains affect the collagen-binding specificity and surface polymerization as well as the virluence potential of the YadA protein of *Yersinia enterocolitica. Mol. Microbiol.* **10**: 995-1011.
6. Roggenkamp., A., Neuberger; H.-R., Flugel, A., Schmoll, T., and Heeseman, J., 1995, Substitution of two histidine residues in YadA protein of *Yersinia enterocolitica* abrogates collagen binding, cell adherence and mouse virulence. *Mol. Microbiol.* **16**: 1207-1219.
7. Korhonen, T.K., Virkola, R., Lähteenmäki, K., Björkman, Y., Kukkonen, M., Raunio, T., Tarkkanen, A.-M., and Westerlund, B., 1992, Penetration of fimbriate enteric bacteria through basement membranes: a hypothesis. *FEMS Microbiol. Lett.* **100**: 307-312.
8. Lähteenmäki, K., Virkola, R., Pouttu, R., Kuusela, P., Kukkonen, M., and Korhonen, T.K., 1995, Bacterial plasminogen receptors: *in vitro* evidence for a role in degradation of the mammalian extracellular matrix. *Infect. Immun.* **63**: 3659-3664.
9. Pouttu, R., Puustinen, T., Virkola, R., Hacker, J., Klemm, P., and Korhonen, T.K., 1999, Amino-acid residue Ala-62 in the FimH fimbrial adhesin is critical for the adhesiveness of meningitis-associated *Escherichia coli* to collagens. *Mol. Microbiol.* **31**: 1747-1757.
10. Klemm, P., Jörgensen, B.J., van Die, I., de Ree, H., and Bergmans, H., 1985, The *fim* genes responsible for synthesis of type 1 fimbriae in *Escherichia coli*, cloning and genetic organization. *Mol. Gen. Genet.* **199**: 410-414.
11. Kukkonen, M., Raunio, T., Virkola, R., Lähteenmäki, K., Mäkelä, P.H., Klemm, P., Clegg, S., and Korhonen, T.K., 1993, Basement membrane carbohydrate as a target for bacterial adhesion: binding of type 1 fimbria of *Salmonella enterica* and *Escherichia coli* to laminin. *Mol. Microbiol.* **7**: 229-237.

12. Toba, T., Virkola, R., Westerlund, B., Björkman, Y., Sillanpää, J., Vartio, T., Kalkkinen, N., and Korhonen, T.K.,1995, A collagen-binding S-layer protein in Lactobacillus crispatus. *Appl. Environ. Microbiol.* **61**: 2467-2471.

13. Klemm, P., and Christiansen, G., 1987, Three *fim* genes required for the regulation of length and mediation of adhesion of *Escherichia coli* type 1 fimbriae. *Mol. Gen. Genet.* **208**: 439-445.

14. Schembri, M.A., Pallesen, L., Connel, H., Hasty, D.L., and Klemm, P., 1996, Linker insertion analysis of the FimH adhesin of type 1 fimbriae in an *Escherichia coli fimH-*null background. *FEMS Microbiol. Lett.* **137**: 257-263.

15. Parkkinen, J., and Korhonen, T.K., 1989, Binding of plasminogen to *Escherichia coli* adhesion proteins. *FEBS Lett.* **250**: 437-440.

16. Parkkinen, J., Hacker, J., and Korhonen, T.K., 1991, Enhancement of tissue plasminogen activator catalyzed plasminogen activation by *Escherichia coli* S fimbriae associated with neonatal septicaemia and meningitis. *Thromb. Haemost.* **65**: 483-486.

# HPI OF HIGH-VIRULENT *YERSINIA* IS FOUND IN *E. COLI* STRAINS CAUSING URINARY TRACT INFECTION
*Structural, Functional Aspects, and Distribution*

Sören Schubert, Johanna L. Sorsa, Sonja Cuenca, Daniela Fischer, Christoph
A. Jacobi, and Jürgen Heesemann
*Max von Pettenkofer-Institut für Hygiene und Medizinische Mikrobiologie der LMU,
Pettenkoferstr. 9a, 80336 München, Germany*

## 1.     INTRODUCTION

Recently, the concept of pathogenicity islands (PAIs) as large mobile genomic elements has led to new insights in the evolution of microbial pathogenicity[1]. PAIs have been found in a wide variety of bacterial species including *Salmonella enterica, Yersinia spp., Escherichia coli, Helicobacter pylori* and *Vibrio cholerae*. The PAI of yersiniae has been termed a high-pathogenicity island (HPI), because it is associated with the mouse lethal phenotype of *Y. pestis, Y. pseudotuberculosis* and *Y. enterocolitica* biogroup 1B. As with many PAIs of other species, the *Yersinia* HPI is inserted adjacent to a *tRNA* gene, namely the *asn tRNA,* and flanked by 17- to 20-bp direct repeats (DR) representing a duplication of the 3´-end of *asn t-RNA*.

The 5´-extremity of the HPI associated with the *asn tRNA* gene consists of a P4-like integrase gene (*int*) and is followed by a cluster of 11 genes involved in regulation (*ybtA*), biosynthesis (*irp1-5,9*) and transport (*irp6,7, fyuA*) of the siderophore yersiniabactin. This part encompasses about 30-kb and can be defined as the functional "core" of the HPI. Downstream of this functional core, a 5- to 13-kb AT-rich region could be characterized in *Y. pseudotuberculosis* and *Y. enterocolitica*, respectively[2].

*Genes and Proteins Underlying Microbial Urinary Tract Virulence*
Edited by L. Emödy *et al.*, Kluwer Academic/Plenum Publishers, 2000

We have demonstrated previously that the HPI of *Y. pestis* is frequently found in *E. coli* strains isolated from blood cultures of septic patients as well as in enteroaggregative *E. coli* (EAggEC), a novel enteric pathotype of *E. coli*[3]. Whether the presence of the HPI in *E. coli* contributes to virulence or to ecological fitness of the bacteria has not yet been demonstrated. The aims of this study were (i) to characterize the integration site, structure, and boundaries of the HPI in *E. coli* to gain more insight into the evolutionary aspects of HPI distribution and (ii) to examine the functional expression of *irp* and *fyuA* genes, as well as production of the yersiniabactin siderophore system in uropathogenic *E. coli*.

## 2.       STRUCTURAL FEATURES OF THE *YERSINIA*-HPI IN UROPAHTOGENIC *E. COLI*

By using Southern hybridization (probes E6, E8.8, E3.5) and PCR approaches the structure of the HPI in *E. coli* has been defined (Fig 1). Thus, the *E. coli* HPI consists of the conserved core part of the HPI, encoding for genes involved in synthesis (*irp1-5,9*) and uptake (*irp6,7, fyuA*) of the siderophore yersiniabactin, as well as for an integrase gene (*int*). Nucleotide sequence comparison of *E. coli* and *Yersinia* revealed >98.8% identity for *fyuA* and *irp2* of *Y. pestis*[3] .

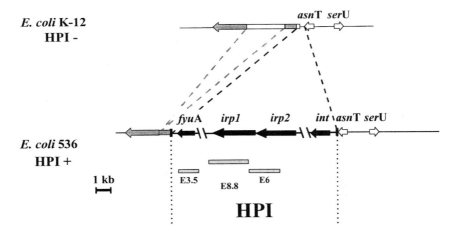

*Figure 1.* Insertion locus of the HPI within the *asn-tRNA* locus of the *E. coli* chromosome. Dark filled arrows indicate genes located on the HPI (*intB, irp2, irp1, fyuA*). Dotted boxes indicate the position of the probes E6, E8.8 and E3.5. Deletions within the *E. coli* chromosome neighbouring the *fyuA* boundary of the HPI are depicted by dotted lines[4].

A PCR-approach (LA-PCR-Cloning, TakaRa Inc.) was performed in order to determine the exact insertion locus within the *E. coli* chromosome. We demonstrated that in 30 *E. coli* isolates investigated, the HPI is associated with the *asnT tRNA* (5'-prime extremity) and truncated in the AT-rich region (3'-prime extremity) since the 17-bp direct repeat (DR) of the *asn tRNA* that flanks the HPI in *Yersina* is missing in *E. coli* (Fig 1. and 2). Moreover, in comparison to HPI-negative *E. coli* K-12 strain, an uniform deletion must have taken place in the *E. coli* chromosome adjacent to the 3'-prime border of the HPI[4].

## 3.     FUNCTIONAL ASPECTS OF THE *E. COLI* HPI

In *E. coli* (EAggEC, EPEC, UPEC and *E. coli* isolated from septicemia) the polypeptides encoded by *fyuA*, *irp1* (HMWP1) and *irp2* (HMWP2) genes of the HPI could be detected by SDS-PAGE and immunoblotting whereas mutants generated by insertional mutagenesis of *irp1* or *irp2* lack expression of HMWP1/2[3].

To demonstrate the production of yersiniabactin by uropathogenic *E. coli* 536, a bioassay using the *gfp* reporter gene was used. For this, a *Y. enterocolitica irp1* mutant deficient in yersiniabactin production was transformed with plasmid pCJG3.3N carrying *fyuA* (encoding the yersiniabactin outer membrane receptor FyuA) fused to *gfp* reporter gene[5]. Expression of *fyuA-gfp* is regulated by ferricyersiniabactin through the AraC-like activator YbtA. Yersiniabactin in bacterial supernatants (NBD medium) was applicated to the reporter strain and lead to increased expression of the *fyuA-gfp* fusion as measured by flow cytometry (manuscript in preparation). Figure 2 shows the results of seven independent experiments using supernants of *E. coli* strain 536 and the isogenic *irp1* mutant strain 536*irp1* both grown in iron starved medium. The culture supernatant of HPI positive *E. coli* strain 536 revealed a significantly enhanced fluorescence signal compared to *E. coli* K-12 (P<0.001) indicating the production of yersiniabactin (manuscript in preparation).

## 4.     DISTRIBUTION OF THE HPI IN *E. COLI*

PCR and colony hybridisation were applied to determine the distribution of *Yersinia* HPI among *E. coli* strains and other gram negative rods isolated from urine samples and blood cultures. 74,6% of 238 clinical isolates of *E. coli* were found to be HPI positive. All 34 uropathogenic *E. coli* strains (UPEC, serotype O6) carried the HPI (manuscript in preparation).

The HPI could be detected in 25% of environmental *E. coli* isolates and in about 55% of *E. coli* stool isolates obtained of healthy individuals.

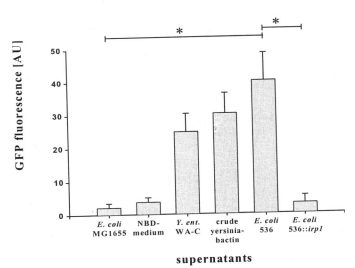

*Figure 2.* Yersiniabactin detection by GFP-reporter assay.

## 5. CONCLUSION

The *E. coli* HPI consists of a well vonserved core part, encoding for the yersiniabactin siderophore system (*irp/fyuA* genes) and for the P4-like integrase (*int* gene). We could demonstrate that genes as *fyuA* or *irp1* and *irp2* encoded by the HPI are expressed in *E. coli*. Moreover, HPI positive *E. coli* strains were shown to produce the siderophore yersinibactin, indicating the functional integrity of the HPI core in *E. coli*. Further studies are required to define the impact of the *E. coli* HPI on virulence and/or fitness.

## ACKNOWLEDGMENTS

The work from our laboratory was supported by a grant from the Deutsch Forschungsgemeinschaft to J.H. (HE 1297/8-1).

# REFERENCES

1. Hacker, J., Blum Oehler, G., Muhldorfer, I., Tschape, H., 1997, Pathogenicity islands of virulent bacteria: structure, function and impact on microbial evolution. *Mol. Microbiol.* **23:** 1089-1097.
2. Rakin, A., Noelting, C., Schubert, S., Heesemann, J., 1999, Common and specific characteristics of the high-pathogenicity island of *Yersinia enterocolitica*. *Infect. Immun.* **67:** 5265-5274.
3. Schubert, S., Rakin, A., Karch, H., Carniel, E., Heesemann, J., 1998, Prevalence of the "high-pathogenicity island" of *Yersinia* species among *Escherichia coli* strains that are pathogenic to humans. *Infect. Immun.* **66:** 480-485,
4. Schubert, S., Rakin, A., Fischer, D., Sorsa, J., Heesemann, J., 1999, Characterization of the integration site of *Yersinia* high-pathogenicity island in *Escherichia coli*. *FEMS Microbiol. Lett.* **179:** 409-414.
5. Pelludat, C., Rakin, A., Jacobi, C.A., Schubert, S., Heesemann, J., 1998, The yersiniabactin biosynthetic gene cluster of *Yersinia enterocolitica*: organization and siderophore-dependent regulation. *J. Bacteriol.* **180:** 538-546.

# AGGREGATION SUBSTANCE OF *ENTEROCOCCUS FAECALIS*: A MULTIFUNCTIONAL ADHESIN

[1]Albrecht Muscholl-Silberhorn, [2]Eva Rozdzinski and [1]Reinhard Wirth
*[1]Universität Regensburg, Institut für Mikrobiologie NWFIII, Universitätsstr. 31, D-93053 Regensbur; [2]Universitätsklinik Ulm, Abteilung für Medizinische Mikrobiologie und Hygiene, Robert-Koch-Str. 8, D-89081 Ulm*

## 1.    INTRODUCTION

The Gram-positive species *Enterococcus faecalis* commonly inhabits the mammalian intestine, where it belongs to the predominant flora immediately after birth and remains present in considerable amounts during all life. However, it can also grow in other habitats such as plant surfaces or diary products and survive even heavy stress conditions during a prolonged period of time. The latter fact contributes to the increasing incidence of *E. faecalis* in nosocomial infections of, e.g., the urinary tract, endocardium, or blood. The high intrinsic resistance to high temperatures (62 °C), desiccation, high osmolarity (9 % NaCl), low pH (3.2), ultraviolet irradiation, oxigen radicals (20 mM $H_2O_2$, 0.05 % NaOCl), ethanol (17 %), etc.[1], promotes the rapid spread of clinical strains within hospitals. A second feature of *E. faecalis* important in this context is the frequency of mobile genetic elements such as conjugative plasmids or transposons, which readily transfer between *E. faecalis* strains and even to other species. Therefore, *E. faecalis* is considered as a central 'gene pool' for the interspecific transfer of antibiotic resistances among bacteria of the digestive tract[2]. Some strains of *E. faecalis*, similarly to *Staphylococcus aureus*, are meanwhile resistant to most of the therapeutically relevant antibiotics including vancomycin.

*Genes and Proteins Underlying Microbial Urinary Tract Virulence*
Edited by L. Emődy *et al.*, Kluwer Academic/Plenum Publishers, 2000

In contrast to these primary prerequisites for its success as a pathogen there is only a limited knowledge on the molecular strategies used by *E. faecalis* during infection. Several possible virulence factors have been described (Table 1.); for a hemolysin/bacteriocin determinant a correlation with virulence could be established[3]. For most other factors the role in pathogenicity is deduced primarily from their statistically higher occurrence among clinical strains when compared to non-clinical isolates.

## 2.    SEX PHEROMONE PLASMID-ENCODED AGGREGATION SUBSTANCE

### 2.1    The Role of Aggregation Substance in Conjugative Plasmid Transfer

In one case, the sex pheromone plasmid-encoded aggregation substance, several experiments have been carried out underlining its function for the attachment to host tissues (see below). However, though generally detected in clinical strains, the great interest in aggregation substance originally was not due to its interaction with host cells, but to the fact that it plays an additional important role in the conjugative transfer of the sex pheromone plasmid on which it is encoded[4].

*Table 1.* Presumptive virulence factors of *E. faecalis* and their probable or actual functions

| Virulence factor | Function for pathogenicity |
|---|---|
| Lipoteichoic acid | induction of cytokine secretion? |
| Hyaluronidase | damage of connective tissues? |
| Gelatinase ($Zn^{2+}$-endopeptidase) | proteolytic cleavage of, e.g., collagen and haemolysin |
| Oligopeptides (sex pheromones) | chemo-attractants for neutrophils |
| cytolysin (hemolysin/bacteriocin) | lysis of various cell types |
| EfaA surface protein | antigen coupled to endocarditis |
| Esp surface antigen | increased frequency in clinical isolates |
| aggregation substance | - attachment to matrix proteins<br>- attachment to and invasion of epithelial cells and macrophages via $\beta_2$-integrins<br>- suppression of respiratory burst |

The characteristic feature of this conjugation system is the involvement of a highly specific oligopeptide, the so-called sex pheromone, secreted by plasmid-free cells and inducing plasmid-bearing cells in extremely low amounts (down to $10^{-11}$ M). The first visible effect is the expression of the just mentioned aggregation substance on the cell-surface, which adheres to the constitutive „binding substance" present on both donor and recipient cells. This binding substance consists of lipoteichoic acid (the characteristic Lancefield group D antigen) and a proteinaceous component not yet precisely defined[5]. The resulting physically very tight cell/cell contact, visible as large clumps in nutrient broth, is responsible for the efficient intraspecific plasmid transfer with a frequency of up to $10^{-1}$ per recipient cell. However, transferability seems to be confined to *E. faecalis*, excluding the possibility that sex pheromone plasmids might be the major tool for the interspecific or intergeneric dissemination of antibiotic resistances; this function should rather be attributed to the conjugative broad host-range plasmids, such as pAMβ1, also frequently found in *E. faecalis*.

Aggregation substance is a 137 kDa protein of unique structure, i.e., there are few similarities to other known adhesins in addition to the signal peptide and cell wall anchor corresponding to typical Gram-positive surface proteins. We tried to get information on the protein domains of aggregation substance, Asa1, involved in the clumping reaction[6]. Two major approaches were chosen:

1. A variety of in-frame deletions covering great part of the protein were introduced into *asa1* and the derivatives expressed in *E. faecalis* by a plasmid complementation system using a sex pheromone plasmid defective in aggregation substance. It could be shown that the C-terminal half (and at least a small N-terminal section) of Asa1 seems to be dispensable for cell aggregation.

2. Various Asa1 fragments were combined with a N-terminal „his-tag" by use of a special cloning vector (pQE30 series from Qiagen). The fragments were expressed in *E. coli*, purified and bound to $Ni^{2+}$-NTA-coated microwells. Afterwards, binding capacity of *E. faecalis* to the immobilized peptides was monitored. Only a fragment covering the complete N-terminal two thirds of aggregation substance showed a significant effect, whereas the next shorter peptide lacking about 300 further amino acids did not at all.

A combination of the results from 1. and 2. implies that a small central section of about 90 amino acids is responsible for the clumping reaction. Of course, this does not rule out the possibility that other parts of the protein might also play a minor role in aggregation.

## 2.2    The Role of Aggregation Substance in Host/bacterium Interaction

First hints to a function of aggregation substance as an adhesin for the attachment to host tissues came from experiments with pig renal tubular cells which showed that an *E. faecalis* strain constitutively expressing aggregation substance binds sevenfold better to this cell type than a plasmid-free (as well as a non-induced plasmid-bearing) control strain[7]. Since the adhesin contains two RGD (arg/gly/asp) motifs shown for other proteins to mediate interaction with integrins, this function was also predicted for aggregation substance. Indeed, binding capacity could be reduced by the addition of RGDS peptide to the co-incubated cells.

Recent experiments[8,9,10] carried out with other cell types confirmed the specific interaction between the RGD motifs with $ß_2$ type integrins. By quantifying the binding of *E. faecalis* expressing aggregation substance and competing this interaction with RGD peptides or anti-$ß_2$-integrin antibodies, respectively, we could show that both the adhesion to human macrophages is mediated by $ß_2$ integrins. Aggregation substance was also found to promote phagocytosis of *E. faecalis* and its intracellular survival. Interestingly, aggregation substance also reduced the respiratory burst triggered by macrophages, indicating that the adhesin serves as a defence mechanism against the chemical immunoresponse.

Aggregation substance not only interacts with integrins but also is able to adhere to different matrix proteins, first of all fibronectin. By immobilizing each fragment of the modular fibronectin dimer to latex beads and checking the aggregation substance-mediated attachment of *E. faecalis* the 45 kDa fragment of the smaller subunit turned out to be the major target of interaction. The result was confirmed by competing the adhesion to immobilized fibronectin with soluble fragments thereof; again, the 45 kDa fragment reduced binding most efficiently.

To analyse which part of aggregation substance - in addition to the obviously involved RGD motifs - is responsible for the attachment to these eukaryotic proteins, the Asa1 derivatives used for the investigation of the clumping-mediating domain (see above) were used in the various binding assays. Surprisingly, the C-terminal third of the protein (containing one of the RGD motifs) seems to be largely dispensable for all known adhesive functions of aggregation substance. Correspondingly, a fragment covering great part of the N-terminus had the best competitive effects on binding.

With respect to the *in vivo* relevance of aggregation substance during infection, only its involvement in the development of endocarditis has been investigated by several groups; results vary considerably with the animal model used. While two independent studies with rabbits[11,12] revealed a striking correlation between mortality and the presence of aggregation substance, this was not the case for a rat model[13]. The studies, however, are not perfectly comparable since different *E. faecalis* strains and sex pheromone plasmids were used differing, e.g., in their hemolytic activity which rather than aggregation substance might play the dominant role in the development of endocarditis.

## 2.3 Asa373, a Novel Representative of Aggregation Substance

All experiments described above were carried out with Asa1, which is a representative of 'classical' aggregation substance constituting a family of closely related adhesins. For one particular aggregation substance, Asa373, encoded on sex pheromone plasmid pAM373, no similarities to this 'classical' aggregation substance could be detected by Southern or Western blots using Asa1-specific DNA-probes/antibodies[14]. Another special feature of this adhesin is the fact that it is induced by a pheromone produced not only by *E. faecalis* itself but also by coagulase-positive *S. aureus* (explanations for this phenomenon are still highly speculative)[15,16].

Determination of the Asa373 sequence seemed advantageous for several reasons: Due to the low similarity to the other aggregation substances any conserved amino acid residues within Asa373 may be restricted to functional domains essential for this type of adhesin with respect to both the clumping reaction and the attachment to host cells. Furthermore, database searches might reveal additional motifs linking Asa373 to adhesins of other bacterial species; thus, the isolated position of aggregation substance might be broken and insights in the evolution of this adhesin class become possible. Finally, the sequence might allow conclusions on a possible function of Asa373 for *S. aureus* (see above).

A fragment of pAM373 covering the *asa373* gene was amplified by use of degenerate primers deduced from i) a regulatory region found on all sex pheromone plasmids and ii) the cell wall anchor motif conserved for most Gram-positive surface proteins including aggregation substance[17]. Sequence analysis of the PCR product revealed a high conformity with sex pheromone plasmid pPD1; however, similarities between an 1.8 kb open reading frame encoding a presumptive cell surface protein and the pPD1-encoded (i.e. 'classical') aggregation substance were largely confined to the signal peptide and cell wall anchor (Fig 1). The identity of this open reading frame with *asa373* was proven by knock-out mutation of the gene - the resulting strain failed to aggregate - and expressing the protein by use of a newly designed expression vector which conferred a clumping phenotype to *E. faecalis* strains lacking any further pAM373 sequences.

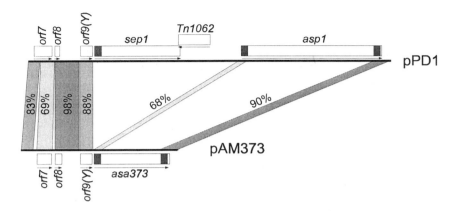

*Figure 1.* Sequence similarities between pAM373 and pPD1 in a region containing the genes for aggregation substance, *asp1* and *asa373*, respectively. (Reproduced from reference 17, with kind permission from the publisher.)

A comparison of Asa373 with database sequences revealed some moderately conserved amino acid motifs related to both 'classical' aggregation substance and other bacterial adhesins. Especially striking is the similarity of an extended motif to the so-called AgI/II type polypeptides of oral Streptococci (Fig 2)[18]. In analogy to aggregation substance-dependent cell clumping these adhesins mediate cell aggregation in the presence of soluble salivary agglutinin. Other properties of these adhesins are their ability to attach to collagen, to confer invasion into human root dentinal tubules, and the fact that some epitopes cross-react with anti-IgG antibodies. The relevance of these properties for Asa373 remains to be analysed.

| | | |
|---|---|---|
| asa1 | (*E. faecalis*) | DQLQKEQ//KAELKAKNEKIAK |
| asa373 | (*E. faecalis*) | SIQAVDSENAEIKKRNADALAKYQKAKAELDAKNAKIKA |
| sspB | (*S. gordonii* M5) | KLAAYQTELARVQKANADAKATYEKAVEDNKAKNAAIKA |
| sspB | (*S. gordonii* DL1) | KLAAYQAELARVQKANADAKAAYEKAVEENTAKNTAIQA |
| sr/pac/spaP | (*S. mutans*) | KLTAYQTELARVQKANADAKAAYEAAVAANNAANAALTA |
| pag | (*S. sobrinus*) | AKEAYDKELARVQAANAAAKKEYEEALAANTTKNEQIKA |
| spaA | (*S. sobrinus*) | KKAAYEQELARVQAANAAAKQAYEQALAANSAKNAQITA |

| | | |
|---|---|---|
| asa373 | (*E. faecalis*) | SANSTTEKVSEQATTGEQTKPVEEQPTVDTPEKEETKKAAEEPKPEEKTPEV |
| omlA | (*A. pleuropneumoniae*) | SSGSSSKPNSELTPKVDMSAPKAEQPKKEEVPQADNSKAEEPK--EMAPQV |

| | | |
|---|---|---|
| asa373 | (*E. faecalis*) | PVEEQPTVDTPEKEETKKAEEPKPEEKTPE...PSKEEADK-DFKEQENKVK |
| strH | (*S. pneumoniae*) | P-EAPKTVETETPATDKVASLPKTEEKPQE...PKKEEAKEVDSKES-NTDK |

*Figure 2.* Alignment of Asa373 with similar motifs of various surface proteins. (Reproduced from reference 17, with kind permission from the publisher.)

Another amino acid motif is interesting in that the corresponding sequence on 'classical' aggregation substance maps within the 90 amino acid section shown above to be essential for the clumping reaction. The idea that these conserved amino acids might represent the predicted universal clumping-mediating motif presupposes that the corresponding binding substance on the *E. faecalis* surface is the same for both Asa373 and 'classical' aggregation substance. This, however, could be largely excluded since expression of Asa373 - in contrast to Asa1 - in a binding substance-deficient strain[19] did not abolish clumping ability.

## 3. CONCLUDING REMARKS

The many data available on the multiple functions of aggregation substance (a survey is given in Table 2) indicate that this adhesin indeed plays an important role in host infection. On the other hand, though more frequently found in clinical strains than in isolates from healthy persons or the environment, it cannot be looked upon as an indispensable prerequisite for pathogenicity, since 40 - 80 % of arbitrarily selected clinical strains lack any sex pheromone plasmid and therefore aggregation substance. The same holds true for the other presumptive virulence factors of Table 1.

Therefore, it is not possible at the present time to clearly distinguish between potentially infectious and totally avirulent *E. faecalis* strains - if such a differentiation should be possible at all. Similarly, the importance of sex pheromone plasmids for *E. faecalis* in addition to encoding aggregation substance remains unclear. Some of the very large plasmids (37 - 91 kb) code for cytolysin or antibiotic resistances, but in many cases no detectable function can be found. Therefore, many aspects of this interesting plasmid class remain to be elucidated.

*Table 2.* Survey on the multiple functions of aggregation substances (AS)

| AS | Function | Target cells / structures | Active part of AS | Binding partner |
|---|---|---|---|---|
| Asa1 | aggregation and conjugative plasmid transfer | all *E. faecalis* cells | 90 amino acid central section | 'binding substance' (= lipoteichoic acid + protein(s)) |
| | attachment to host tissues | extracellular matrix | N-terminus | 45 kDa domain of fibronectin; thrombospondin, etc. |
| | attachment and invasion | endothelial cells (renal tubuli, umbilical cord, endocardium etc.) | RGD motifs | β2-integrins |

| AS | Function | Target cells / structures | Active part of AS | Binding partner |
|---|---|---|---|---|
| Asa373 | attachment and invasion; inhibition of respiratory burst conjugative transfer of pAM373 attachment to host tissues? | macrophages<br><br>all (?) *E. faecalis* cells; other bacterial species? ? | RGD motifs; ?<br><br>?<br><br>motifs similar to other bacterial adhesins? | β2-integrins; ?<br><br>'binding substance' different from that of 'classical' AS ? |

# REFERENCES

1. Hartke, A., Giard, J.-C., Laplace, J.-M., and Auffray, Yanick, 1998, Survival of *Enterococcus faecalis* in an oligotrophic microcosm: Changes in morphology, development of general stress resistance, and analysis of protein synthesis. *Appl. Env. Microbiol.* **64**: 4238-4245.
2. Clewell, D.B., 1981, Plasmids, drug resistance, and gene transfer in the genus *Streptococcus*. *Microbiol. Rev.* **45**: 409-436.
3. Jett, B.D., Huycke, M.M., Gilmore, M.S, 1994, Virulence of Enterococci. *Clin. Microbiol. Rev.* **7**: 426-478.
4. Wirth, R., 1994, The sex pheromone system of *Enterococcus faecalis*: more than "just" a plasmid collection mechanism? *Eur. J. Biochem.* **222**: 235-246.
5. Bensing, B., and Dunny, G., 1993, Cloning and molecular analysis of genes affecting expression of binding substance, the recipient-encoded receptor(s) mediating mating aggregate formation in *Enterococcus faecalis*. *J. Bacteriol.* **175**: 7421-7429.
6. Muscholl-Silberhorn, A.B., 1998, Analysis of the clumping-mediating domain(s) of sex pheromone plasmid pAD1-encoded aggregation substance. *Eur. J. Biochem.* **258**: 515-520.
7. Kreft, B., Marre, R., Schramm, U., and Wirth, R., 1992, Aggregation substance of *Enterococcus faecalis* mediates adhesion to cultured renal tubular cells. *Infect. Immun.* **60**: 25-30.
8. Rozdzinski, E., Muscholl, A., Wirth, R., and Marre, R., 1996, Fibronectin binding of *Enterococcus faecalis* is mediated by aggregation substance. 36th Interscience Conference on Antimicrobial Agents and Chemotherapie, New Orleans, Lousiana. (manuscript in preparation)
9. Süßmuth, S., Muscholl, A., Wirth, R., Marre, R., and Rozdzinski, E., 1997, Aggregation substance (AS) of *Enterococcus faecalis* mediates adherence to and entry into macrophages by interacting with β2-integrins. DGHM-meeting, Jena. (manuscript in preparation)
10. Rozdzinski, E., Susa, M., Muscholl, A., Wirth, R., and Marre, R., 1997, *Enterococcus faecalis* adherence to and internalization by endothelial cells is promoted by aggregation substance (AS). DGHM-meeting, Jena. (manuscript in preparation)
11. Chow, J.W., Thal, L.A., Perri, M.B., Vazquez, J.A., Donabedian, S.M., Clewell, D.B., and Zervos, M.J., 1993, Plasmid-associated hemolysin and aggregation substance

production contribute to virulence in experimental enterococcal endocarditis. *Antimicrob. Agents. Chemother.* **37**: 2474-2477.

12. Schlievert, P.M., Gahr, P.J., Assimacopoulos, A.P., Dinges, M.M., Stoehr, J.A., Harmala, J.W., Hirt, H., and Dunny, G.M., 1998, Aggregation and binding substances enhance pathogenicity in rabbit models of *Enterococcus faecalis* endocarditis. *Infect. Immun.* **66**: 218-223.

13. Berti, M., Candiani, G., Kaufhold, A., Muscholl, A., and Wirth, R., 1998, Does aggregation substance of *Enterococcus faecalis* contribute to development of endocarditis? *Infection* **26**: 48-53.

14. Hirt, H., Wirth, R., and Muscholl, A., 1996, Comparative analysis of eighteen sex pheromone plasmids: detection of a new insertion element on pPD1 and implications for the evolution of this plasmid family. *Mol. Gen. Genet.* **252**: 640-647.

15. Clewell, D.B., An, F.Y., White, B.A., and Gawron-Burke, C., 1985, *Streptococcus faecalis* sex pheromone (cAM373) also produced by *Staphylococcus aureus* and identification of a conjugative transposon (*Tn918*). *J. Bacteriol.* **162**: 1212-1220.

16. Muscholl-Silberhorn, A.B., Samberger, E., and Wirth, R., 1997, Why does *Staphylococcus aureus* secrete an *Enterococcus faecalis*-specific pheromone? *FEMS Microbiol. Lett.* **157**: 261-266.

17. Muscholl-Silberhorn, A.B., 1999, Cloning and expression of Asa373, a novel adhesin unrelated to the other sex pheromone plasmid-encoded aggregation substances of *Enterococcus faecalis. Mol. Microbiol.* **34**: 620-630.

18. Jenkinson, H.F., and Demuth, D.R., 1997, Structure, function and immunogenicity of streptococcal antigen I/II polypeptides. *Mol. Microbiol.* **23**: 183-190.

19. Trotter K.M., and Dunny, G.M., 1990, Mutants of *Enterococcus faecalis* deficient as recipients in mating with donors carrying pheromone-inducible plasmids. *Plasmid* **24**: 57-67.

# A ROLE FOR THE $\sigma^S$ SUBUNIT OF RNA POLYMERASE IN THE REGULATION OF BACTERIAL VIRULENCE

Regine Hengge-Aronis
*Department. of Biology – Microbiology, Freie Universität Berlin, Königin-Luise-Str. 12-16, 14195 Berlin, Germany*

## 1.     INTRODUCTION

The sigma factor is the subunit that confers sequence-specific DNA binding properties to RNA polymerase (RNAP). Within the RNAP holoenzyme, sigma binds to promoters and is crucial for open complex formation, i.e. the initiation of transcription. Besides the vegetative sigma factor, which recognizes the "standard" promoter, many bacteria also possess alternative sigmas that confer altered promoter specificity upon RNAP[1]. Alternative sigmas are synthesized or activated in response to certain environmental conditions. By partially and/or temporarily replacing the vegetative sigma, they are thus crucial for many stress responses[2]. In general, bacterial species with a very variable lifestyle tend to have larger numbers of sigma factors. The enteric bacterium *Escherichia coli* has seven sigmas, one of which is $\sigma^S$ (RpoS), which is essential for survival of many different stress conditions[3-5].

## 2.     THE GENERAL STRESS SIGMA FACTOR $\sigma^S$

While discovered in *E.coli*, $\sigma^S$ has also been found in other enteric bacteria, in the various pseudomonads, and other bacteria within the gamma

*Genes and Proteins Underlying Microbial Urinary Tract Virulence*
Edited by L. Emödy *et al.*, Kluwer Academic/Plenum Publishers, 2000

branch of the proteobacteria. These include a number of important pathogens, such as pathogenic *E.coli, Salmonella, Shigella, Yersinia, Legionella, Pseudomonas aeruginosa* and others. So far, $\sigma^S$ has not been described in $\alpha$-proteobacteria or other phylogenetically more distant species.

Since 1991, $\sigma^S$ has been known as the master regulator of the *E.coli* starvation or stationary phase response[6]. Since then, research on $\sigma^S$ has been extraordinarily fruitful in many respects. First, in recent years it has become clear that the importance of $\sigma^S$ goes far beyond survival of starvation, and that $\sigma^S$ in fact is the top regulator of a general stress regulatory network that allows cells to cope with many different stress conditions. Moreover, work with $\sigma^S$ has demonstrated that our current concept of promoter recognition is too simple. In addition, the regulation of $\sigma^S$ itself is intriguingly complex, especially with respect to post-transcriptional control. And finally, recent investigations have begun to reveal a role for $\sigma^S$ also in bacterial virulence.

## 2.1    The Physiological Function of $\sigma^S$: A General Stress Sigma Factor

Growing cells that are not subject to any particular stress, contain only very little $\sigma^S$ and most $\sigma^S$-dependent stress-protective genes are not expressed. However, in response to a variety of quite diverse stress conditions, the intracellular levels of $\sigma^S$ increase between 5 and 20fold. Besides starvation (for carbon, nitrogen or phosphorus sources or amino acids) also shifts to high osmolarity, high or low temperature or acidic pH result in $\sigma^S$ accumulation[7-11]. As a consequence, numerous $\sigma^S$-dependent genes are activated (more than 50 of these genes have been identified so far). The phenotypic output of this response are strongly increased multiple stress resistance including crossprotection, morphological and structural alterations, the accumulation of storage and protective substances and metabolic alterations - in other words, rather dramatic physiological and morphological changes, that allow the cells to survive conditions that would be instantaneously lethal for rapidly growing cells[3,4,12].

## 2.2    Promoter Recognition by $\sigma^S$

The general concept of promoter recognition is that each sigma factor has its own concensus promoter sequence, and that therefore, exchange of one sigma for another reprograms RNAP to recognize a different kind of promoter sequence. $\sigma^S$, however, turned out to have the same promoter sequence recognition specificity in vitro as the "housekeeping" $\sigma^{70}$. In vivo, however, $\sigma^S$ and $\sigma^{70}$ control distinct genes. This "$\sigma^S/\sigma^{70}$" promoter recognition paradox" has clearly shown that the one-sigma/one-concensus concept is too simple. In fact, RNAP does not "see" naked linear promoter DNA, but complex nucleoprotein structures, in which DNA can be bent, over- or underwound, wrapped around and partially occluded by proteins. Often such proteins are so-called histone-like proteins (H-NS, Lrp, etc.)[13,14]. What seems to matter for recognition by RNAP containing either $\sigma^S$ or $\sigma^{70}$, are the small differences between these holoenzymes in dealing with these non-ideal and promoter-specific in-vivo arrangements of DNA[15].

## 2.3    $\sigma^S$ Regulation

How can so many different stress conditions (starvation, high osmolarity, non-optimal temperatures and acidic pH) affect a single parameter, i.e. the cellular $\sigma^S$ content? The basic answer to this signal integration problem is that different stresses affect different levels in the control of $\sigma^S$, with post-transcriptional control mechanisms being of special importance. Translation of pre-existing *rpoS* mRNA is stimulated by high osmolarity, during late exponential phase (above a certain cell density), or by shift to low temperature. On the other hand, in rapidly growing cells $\sigma^S$ is also very unstable protein, with this turnover being inhibited by starvation, high osmolarity, or shifts to high temperature or acidic pH (summarized in ref.4).

Significant progress has been made recently in the elucidation of the underlying regulatory mechanisms. *rpoS* mRNA seems to fold into a secondary structure, in which the ribosomal binding site and the initiation codon are base-paired, and therefore not accessible for ribosomes[16] (and D. Traulsen and R. Hengge-Aronis, unpublished). In addition, the RNA-binding protein Hfq is essential for *rpoS* translation[17], whereas H-NS protein has an inhibitory influence on translation[18,19]. The small regulatory DsrA RNA is essential for low temperature stimulation of *rpoS* translation, and acts by an anti-antisense mechanism[20,21].

Degradation of $\sigma^S$ requires ClpXP protease[22]. In addition, the response regulator RssB is absolutely essential for $\sigma^S$ proteolysis[23,24]. RssB was recently shown to act as a direct recognition factor for $\sigma^S$, which binds to the "turnover element" within $\sigma^S$, a small patch of amino acids that overlaps region 2.4/2.5, i.e. a region within $\sigma^S$ that is crucial for promoter recognition. RssB affinity for $\sigma^S$ is modulated by phosphorylation, suggesting that environmental stress affects RssB phosphorylation and thereby controls primary recognition of $\sigma^S$ by the proteolytic system[25]. Under certain conditions, RssB can also inhibit $\sigma^S$ activity as a transcription factor, which lead to the proposal that RssB may be a former stress-regulated anti-sigma factor that has been recruited to serve as a recognition factor for the proteolytic machinery[26].

## 3.    A ROLE FOR $\sigma^S$ IN BACTERIAL VIRULENCE?

A number of recent studies have now provided initial evidence that $\sigma^S$ may also play a role in bacterial pathogenicity. This subject is still in its experimental infancy, but when put into a common perspective, the already existing investigations seem to suggest that further work in this field may be extremely rewarding.

### 3.1    Overlap Between the Control of Stress-Responsive Genes and Virulence Genes

Virulence genes are often controlled in complex ways by environmental conditions (temperature, osmolarity, growth phase, pH). This is especially so for "early" virulence genes that play a role during the early stages of infection, or genes that have to be activated in specific organelles during intracellular growth. By contrast, "late" virulence genes, that have to be active after contract with specific host cells has been established, can be expected to be controlled by specific host cell-produced signals. During infection of a mammalian host, bacteria may have to cope with acid (in the stomach), a switch to alkaline pH (in the small intestine), high osmolarity (in the gastrointestinal tract, as well as other body fluids such as urine), nutrient limitation (due to intensive competition with commensals), high bacterial cell densities, etc. Intriguingly, these are exactly the conditions that when applied in vitro result in $\sigma^S$ induction (see above).

### 3.2    Is $\sigma^S$ Expressed *in vivo*, i.e. in Bacteria Associated with a Mammalian Host?

Even though virulence genes are often controlled by the same environmental signals that induce $\sigma^S$, it has not been studied systematically, whether $\sigma^S$ is present at high cellular levels during infection. There is, however, a recent report demonstrating that high *rpoS* mRNA levels are present in *Pseudomonas aeruginosa* from chronically infected cystic fibrosis patients[27]. Because of extensive post-transcriptional control of $\sigma^S$, a putative high $\sigma^S$ protein level in these cells would have to be shown directly, but the mRNA data indicate that these cells are at least in a state that allows to increase their $\sigma^S$ level extremely rapidly.

## 3.3 Does $\sigma^S$ Play a Role in Survival of "Host-Provided" Stress?

For in-vitro grown enteric bacteria and various pseudomonads, it has been shown that $\sigma^S$ is crucial for resistance against and therefore survival of starvation, high osmolarity, acidic pH, and oxidative stress[6,9,28]. There is no reason to assume that $\sigma^S$ is less important for survival of these conditions when encountered inside a host, especially since these conditions are basically identical to the stresses that the host provides or even specifically produces, such as macrophage oxidative bursts. In *Salmonella*, the inducible oxidative stress stress responses mediated by the OxyR and SoxRS systems do not seem to protect against macrophage killing[29]. This indicates that systems that are already induced before macrophage contact, such as the general stress-induced $\sigma^S$ regulon, which is essential for *Salmonella* virulence (see below), may be more important. Relevant $\sigma^S$-dependent gene products may be Dps, a DNA-binding protein that protects against hydrogen peroxide[30], exonuclease III (encoded by *xthA*)[31], and flavohemoglobin[32], which detoxifies nitric oxide[33]. It has long been known that nutrient depletion produces higher resistance against phagocytosis and serum killing[34] as well as reduced antibiotic susceptibility[35]. Moreover, it was also shown that in log phase cells, increased resistance could be produced by temperature downshift[36]. Both nutrient depletion and temperature downshift are $\sigma^S$-inducing conditions, but unfortunately, an involvement of $\sigma^S$ in such host-related phenotypes has not yet been tested directly.

## 3.4 Is $\sigma^S$ Essential for Virulence?

$\sigma^S$ is clearly essential for virulence of *S.typhimurium* in a mouse model. *rpoS* mutants[37] or $\sigma^S$ overproducing strains[38] are avirulent. The avirulent *S.typhimurium* laboratory strain LT2 also carries a mutation in *rpoS*[39], and so does the vaccine strain Ty2 of *S.typhi*[40]. By contrast, an *rpoS* mutant of *Yersinia enterocolitica* does not seem to be impaired in virulence in a mouse model[41]. However, a mutation in *nlpD*, which is probably polar on *rpoS* due to the operon structure of the two genes[42], affects survival of *Y.enterocolitica* in mice[43].

Another interesting case is that of *Legionella pneumophila*. Here, $\sigma^S$ is not essential for stationary phase-associated stress resistance of cells grown in vitro, and $\sigma^S$ is also not required for replication within and killing of human macrophages. However, $\sigma^S$ is essential for survival and growth in the environmental host, i.e. amoeba such as *Acanthamoeba castellanii*[44]. *L.pneumophila* cells isolated either from macrophages or from amoeba exhibit smaller morphology (a typical $\sigma^S$-dependent phenotype) and increased resistance against antibiotics and host defense mechanisms[45]. This may suggest that $\sigma^S$, while being dispensible for survival within isolated macrophages, could play a role in survival in the host organism.

Biofilm formation (associated with reduced antibiotic susceptibility) is often part of the host-associated phase in the life cycles of pathogenic bacteria[46]. There is evidence that *rpoS* mutants of *E.coli* are also impaired in biofilm formation[47].

## 3.5 Virulence Genes Under $\sigma^S$ Control

While reduced virulence of *rpoS* mutants may in part be due to general stress sensitivity and therefore inability to cope with host-associated stress, recent evidence demonstrates that $\sigma^S$ also controls specific virulence genes. A well-documented case is of the virulence plasmid-encoded *spv* genes in *S.typhimurium*, which are essential for colonization of spleen and liver. *spv* expression depends on a local regulator, SpvR, as well as on $\sigma^S$ for expression[48-50]. In enterohemorrhagic *E.coli* (EHEC), the *esp* operon, which encodes a type III secretion system crucial for adhesion to epithelial cells, is under $\sigma^S$ control[51]. $\sigma^S$ also influences the expression of fimbriae. These include curli in *E.coli* (also termed thin aggregative fimbriae in *Salmonella*), which require $\sigma^S$ for expression[52,53], as well as type 1 fimbriae, which are under negative control of $\sigma^S$ which results in switching off their expression in stationary phase[54]. In *P.aeruginosa*, a number of virulence-associated factors are influenced by $\sigma^S$. *rpoS* mutants exhibit reduced production of exotoxin and alginate, whereas pyocyanin and pyoverdin were found in increased amounts[28].

## 4. PERSPECTIVES

Questions concerning the role of $\sigma^S$ during infection by pathogenic bacteria have not yet been addressed systematically. However, recent evidence clearly indicates that $\sigma^S$ plays a role in virulence of certain pathogenic bacteria and some specific virulence genes under $\sigma^S$ control have now been identified. The data obtained so far suggest that more systematic analyses of the role of $\sigma^S$ in bacterial pathogenicity are clearly warranted. In particular, expression of $\sigma^S$ in host-associated bacteria, its role in survival of host-provided stress conditions, and its regulatory role in the expression of specific virulence genes should be studied in detail. The finding that *rpoS* mutant strains are good candidates for vaccine development[40], indicate that such studies may have practical applications, which may also include the use of sigma factors in general or of $\sigma^S$ in particular as novel targets for antibiotic development.

## REFERENCES

1. Gross, C. A., Chan, C. L. & Lonetto, M. A. A structure/function analysis of *Escherichia coli* RNA polymerase. *Phil. Trans. R. Soc. Lond. B* **351**, 475-482 (1996).
2. Storz, G. & Hengge-Aronis, R. (eds.) *Bacterial Stress Responses* (ASM Press, Wahsington, D.C., 2000) (in press).
3. Hengge-Aronis, R. in *Escherichia coli and Salmonella typhimurium: Cellular and Molecular Biology* (ed. Neidhardt, F. C.) 1497-1512 (American Society for Microbiology, Washington D.C., 1996).
4. Hengge-Aronis, R. in *Bacterial Stress Responses* (eds. Storz, G. & Hengge-Aronis, R.) (in press) (ASM Press, Washington, D.C., 2000) (in press).
5. Loewen, P. C. & Hengge-Aronis, R. The role of the sigma factor $\sigma^S$ (KatF) in bacterial global regulation. *Annu. Rev. Microbiol.* **48**, 53-80 (1994).
6. Lange, R. & Hengge-Aronis, R. Identification of a central regulator of stationary-phase gene expression in *Escherichia coli*. *Mol. Microbiol.* **5**, 49-59 (1991).
7. Gentry, D. R., Hernandez, V. J., Nguyen, L. H., Jensen, D. B. & Cashel, M. Synthesis of the stationary-phase sigma factor $\sigma^S$ is positively regulated by ppGpp. *J. Bacteriol.* **175**, 7982-7989 (1993).
8. Lange, R. & Hengge-Aronis, R. The cellular concentration of the $\sigma^S$ subunit of RNA-polymerase in *Escherichia coli* is controlled at the levels of transcription, translation and protein stability. *Genes Dev.* **8**, 1600-1612 (1994).
9. Lee, I. S., Lin, J., Hall, H. K., Bearson, B. & Foster, J. W. The stationary-phase sigma factor $\sigma^S$ (RpoS) is required for a sustained acid tolerance response in virulent *Salmonella typhimurium*. *Mol. Microbiol.* **17**, 155-167 (1995).
10. Muffler, A., Traulsen, D. D., Lange, R. & Hengge-Aronis, R. Posttranscriptional osmotic regulation of the $\sigma^S$ subunit of RNA polymerase in *Escherichia coli*. *J. Bacteriol.* **178**, 1607-1613 (1996).
11. Muffler, A., Barth, M., Marschall, C. & Hengge-Aronis, R. Heat shock regulation of $\sigma^S$ turnover: a role for DnaK and relationship between stress responses mediated by $\sigma^S$ and $\sigma^{32}$ in *Escherichia coli*. *J. Bacteriol.* **179**, 445-452 (1997).
12. Hengge-Aronis, R. in *Prokaryotic gene expression* (ed. Baumberg, S.) 169-193 (Oxford University Press, Oxford, 1999).
13. Colland, F., Barth, M., Hengge-Aronis, R. & Kolb, A. Sigma factor selectivity of *Escherichia coli* RNA polymerase at the *osmY* promoter: role for CRP, IHF and Lrp transcription factors (1999) (submitted).
14. Marschall, C. *et al.* Molecular analysis of the regulation of *csiD*, a carbon starvation-inducible gene in *Escherichia coli* that is exclusively dependent on $\sigma^S$ and requires activation by cAMP-CRP. *J. Mol. Biol.* **276**, 339-353 (1998).
15. Hengge-Aronis, R. Interplay of global regulators in the general stress response of *Escherichia coli*. *Curr. Op. Microbiol.* **2**, 148-152 (1999).
16. Brown, L. & Elliott, T. Mutations that increase expression of the *rpoS* gene and decrease its dependence on *hfq* function in *Salmonella typhimurium*. *J. Bacteriol.* **179**, 656-662 (1997).
17. Muffler, A., Fischer, D. & Hengge-Aronis, R. The RNA-binding protein HF-I, known as a host factor for phage Qβ RNA replication, is essential for the translational regulation of *rpoS* in *Escherichia coli*. *Genes Dev.* **10**, 1143-1151 (1996).

18. Barth, M., Marschall, C., Muffler, A., Fischer, D. & Hengge-Aronis, R. A role for the histone-like protein H-NS in growth phase-dependent and osmotic regulation of $\sigma^S$ and many $\sigma^S$-dependent genes in *Escherichia coli*. *J. Bacteriol.* **177**, 3455-3464 (1995).

19. Yamashino, T., Ueguchi, C. & Mizuno, T. Quantitative control of the stationary phase-specific sigma factor, $\sigma^S$, in *Escherichia coli*: involvement of the nucleoid protein H-NS. *EMBO J.* **14**, 594-602 (1995).

20. Majdalani, N., Cunning, C., Sledjeski, D., Elliott, T. & Gottesman, S. DsrA RNA regulates translation of RpoS message by an anti-antisense mechanims, independent of its action as an antisilencer of transcription. *Proc. Natl. Acad. Sci. USA* **95**, 12462-12467 (1998).

21. Lease, R. A., Cusick, M. E. & Belfort, M. Riboregulation in *Escherichia coli*: DsrA RNA acts by RNA:RNA interaction at multiple loci. *Proc. Natl. Acad. Sci. USA* **95**, 12456-12461 (1998).

22. Schweder, T., Lee, K.-H., Lomovskaya, O. & Matin, A. Regulation of *Escherichia coli* starvation sigma factor ($\sigma^S$) by ClpXP protease. *J. Bacteriol.* **178**, 470-476 (1996).

23. Muffler, A., Fischer, D., Altuvia, S., Storz, G. & Hengge-Aronis, R. The response regulator RssB controls stability of the $\sigma^S$ subunit of RNA polymerase in *Escherichia coli*. *EMBO J.* **15**, 1333-1339 (1996).

24. Pratt, L. A. & Silhavy, T. J. The response regulator, SprE, controls the stability of RpoS. *Proc. Natl. Acad. Sci. USA* **93**, 2488-2492 (1996).

25. Becker, G., Klauck, E. & Hengge-Aronis, R. Regulation of RpoS proteolysis in *Escherichia coli*: The response regulator RssB is a recognition factor that interacts with the turnover element in RpoS. *Proc. Natl. Acad. Sci. USA* **96**, 6439-6444 (1999).

26. Becker, G., Klauck, E. & Hengge-Aronis, R. The response regulator RssB, a recognition factor for $\sigma^S$ proteolysis in *Escherichia coli*, can act like an anti-$\sigma^S$ factor. *Mol. Microbiol.*, (being revised for publication) (1999).

27. Foley, I., Marsch, P., Wellington, E. M. H., Smith, A. W. & Brown, M. R. W. General stress response master regulator *rpoS* is expressed in human infection: a possible role in chronicity. *J. Antimicrob. Chemother.* **43**, 164-165 (1999).

28. Suh, S.-J. *et al.* Effect of *rpoS* mutation on the stress response and expression of virulence factors in *Pseudomonas aeruginosa*. *J. Bacteriol.* **181**, 3890-3897 (1999).

29. Fang, F. C., Vazquez-Torres, A. & Xu, Y. The transcriptional regulator SoxS is required for resistance of *Salmonella typhimurium* to paraquat but not for virulence in mice. *Infect. Immun.* **65**, 5371-5375 (1997).

30. Martinez, A. & Kolter, R. Protection of DNA during oxidative stress by the nonspecific DNA-binding protein Dps. *J. Bacteriol.* **179**, 5188-5194 (1997).

31. Sak, B. D., Eisenstark, A. & Touati, D. Exonuclease III and the catalase hydroperoxidase II in *Escherichia coli* are both regulated by the *katF* product. *Proc. Natl. Acad. Sci. USA* **86**, 3271-3275 (1989).

32. Membrillo-Hernandez, J., Cook, G. M. & Poole, R. K. Roles of RpoS ($\sigma^S$), IHF and ppGpp in the expression of the *hmp* gene encoding the flavohemoglobin (Hmp) of *Escherichia coli* K-12. *Mol. Gen. Genet.* **254**, 599-603 (1997).

33. Gardner, P. R., Gardner, A. M., Martin, L. A. & Salzman, A. L. Nitric oxide dioxygenase: an enzymic function for flavohemoglobin. *Proc. Natl. Acad. Sci. USA* **95**, 10378-10383 (1998).

34. Finch, J. E. & Brown, M. R. W. Effect of growth environment on *Pseudomonas aeruginosa* killing by rabbit polymorphonuclear leukocytes and cationic proteins. *Infect. Immun.* **20**, 340-346 (1978).

35. Brown, M. R. W. Nutrient depletion and antibiotic susceptibility. *J. Antimicrob. Chemother.* **3**, 198-201 (1977).

36. Anwar, H. & Brown, M. R. W. Effect of nutrient depletion on sensitivity of *Pseudomonas cepacia* to phagocytosis and serum bactericidal activity at different temperatures. *J. Gen. Microbiol.* **129**, 2021-2027 (1983).
37. Fang, R. C. *et al.* The alternative σ factor KatF (RpoS) regulates *Salmonella* virulence. *Proc. Natl. Acad. Sci. USA* **89**, 11978-11982 (1992).
38. Bearson, S. M. D., Benjamin Jr., W. H., Swords, W. E. & Foster, J. W. Acid shock induction of RpoS is mediated by the mouse virulence gene *mviA* of *Salmonella typhimurium. J. Bacteriol.* **178**, 2572-2579 (1996).
39. Wilmes-Riesenberg, M. R., Foster, J. W. & Curtiss III, R. An altered *rpoS* allele contributes to the avirulence of *Salmonella typhimurium* LT2. *Infect. Immun.* **65**, 203-210 (1997).
40. Coynault, C., Robbe-Saule, V. & Norel, F. Virulence and vaccine potential of *Salmonella typhimurium* mutants deficient in the expression of the RpoS ($\sigma^S$) regulon. *Mol. Microbiol.* **22**, 149-160 (1996).
41. Badger, J. L. & Miller, V. L. Role of RpoS in survival of *Yersinia enterocolitica* to a variety of environmental stresses. *J. Bacteriol.* **177**, 5370-5373 (1995).
42. Lange, R. & Hengge-Aronis, R. The *nlpD* gene is located in an operon with *rpoS* on the *Escherichia coli* chromosome and encodes a novel lipoprotein with a potential function in cell wall formation. *Mol. Microbiol.* **13**, 733-743 (1994).
43. Darwin, A. J. & Miller, V. L. Identification of *Yersinia enterocolitica* genes affecting survival in an animal host using signature-tagged transposon mutagenesis. *Mol. Microbiol.* **32**, 51-62 (1999).
44. Hales, L. M. & Shuman, H. A. *Legionella pneumophila rpoS* is required for growth within *Acanthamoeba castellanii. J. Bacteriol.* **181**, 4879-4889 (1999).
45. Barker, J., Scaife, H. & Brown, M. Intraphagocytic growth induces an antibiotic-resistant phenotype of *Legionella pneumophila. Antimicrob. Agents Chemother.* **39**, 2684-2688 (1995).
46. Costerton, J. W., Lewandowski, Z., Caldwell, D. E., Korber, D. R. & Lappin-Scott, H. M. Microbial biofilms. *Annu. Rev. Microbiol.* **49**, 711-745 (1995).
47. Adams, J. L. & MacLean, R. J. C. Impact of *rpoS* deletion on *Escherichia coli* biofilms. *Appl. Environ. Microbiol.* **65**, 4285-4287 (1999).
48. Heiskanen, P., Taira, S. & Rhen, M. Role of *rpoS* in the regulation of *Salmonella* plasmid virulence (*spv*) genes. *FEMS Microbiol. Lett.* **123**, 125-130 (1994).
49. Norel, F., Robbe-Saule, V., Popoff, M. Y. & Coynault, C. The putative sigma factor KatF (RpoS) is required for the transcription of the *Salmonella typhimurium* virulence gene *spvB* in *Escherichia coli. FEMS Microbiol. Lett.* **99**, 271-276 (1992).
50. RobbeSaule, V., Schaeffer, F., Kowarz, L. & Norel, F. Relationships between H-NS, $\sigma^S$, SpvR and growth phase in the control of spvR, the regulatory gene of the *Salmonella* plasmid virulence operon. *Mol. Gen. Genet.* **256**, 333-347 (1997).
51. Beltrametti, F., Kresse, A. U. & Guzmán, C. A. Transcriptional regulation of the *esp* genes of enterohemorrhagic *Escherichia coli. J. Bacteriol.* **181**, 3409-3418 (1999).
52. Römling, U., Bian, Z., Hammar, M., Sierralta, W. D. & Normark, S. Curli fibers are highly conserved between *Salmonella typhimurium* and *Escherichia coli* with respect to operon structure and regulation. *J. Bacteriol.* **180**, 722-731 (1998).
53. Olsén, A., Arnqvist, A., Hammar, M., Sukupolvi, S. & Normark, S. The RpoS sigma factor relieves H-NS-mediated transcriptional repression of *csgA*, the subunit gene of fibronectin binding curli in *Escherichia coli. Mol. Microbiol.* **7**, 523-536 (1993).
54. Dove, S. L., Smith, S. G. & Dorman, C. J. Control of *Escherichia coli* type 1 fimbrial gene expression in stationary phase: a negative role for RpoS. *Mol. Gen. Genet.* **254**, 13-20 (1997).

# TRANSCRIPTIONAL ORGANISATION AND REGULATION OF *E. coli* GROUP 2 CAPSULE EXPRESSION

Ian S. Roberts

*School of Biological Sciences, Stopford Building, Oxford Road, University of Manchester, M13 9PT*

## 1.    INTRODUCTION

The production of an extra cellular polysaccharide capsule is a common feature of many bacteria. The capsule, which often constitutes the outermost layer of the cell, mediates the interaction between the bacterium and its immediate surroundings and plays a crucial role in the survival of bacteria in hostile environments. One such environment is the human host where interactions between the capsule and the host's immune system may be vital in deciding the outcome of an infection[1, 2]. In the absence of specific antibody a capsule offers protection against the non-specific arm of the host's immune system by conferring increased resistance to complement-mediated killing and complement-mediated opsonophagocytosis[2, 3, 4]. A small set of capsular polysaccharides which resemble polysaccharide moieties present in host tissue are poorly immunogenic[5,6]. The *E. coli* K1 and *Neisseria meningitidis* group B capsules, both of which contain N-acetyl-neuraminic acid and the heparin-like *E. coli* K5 capsule, all elicit a poor antibody response in infected individuals and confer some measure of resistance to the host's adaptive humural response[7]. Aside from direct interactions with the host's immune system, capsules may promote the formation of biofilms and the colonisation of a variety of ecological niches, including indwelling catheters, prostheses and the formation of alginate-rich biofilms in the lungs of cystic fibrosis patients[8]. In such instances the polysaccharide may present a permeability barrier to antibiotics and hinder the effective eradication of the bacteria[9].

*Genes and Proteins Underlying Microbial Urinary Tract Virulence*
Edited by L. Emődy *et al.*, Kluwer Academic/Plenum Publishers, 2000

95

*Escherichia coli* produces more than 80 chemically and serologically distinct capsules, called K antigens[10]. These capsules have been separated into four groups (1-4) on the basis of chemical composition, molecular weight, intergenic relationships and regulation of expression[11, 12, 13]. The majority of extra-intestinal isolates of *E. coli* associated with invasive disease express group 2 capsules, with particular capsules being associated with certain diseases[14]. Typical of many virulence factors, expression of group 2 capsules in *E. coli* is regulated by temperature with group 2 capsules only being expressed at temperatures above 20°C[12,13]. Environmental regulation of virulence gene expression is well documented in a broad range of pathogenic bacteria[15] and it is likely that this offers a mechanism by which pathogenic bacteria may adapt to particular niches encountered within the host. The regulation of virulence gene expression by temperature provides a means by which bacteria may selectively express virulence determinants upon entry into the host.

## 2.    GENETIC ORGANISATION OF GROUP 2 CAPSULE GENE CLUSTERS

Group 2 capsule gene clusters have a common organisation consisting of three regions[11, 12, 13]. A central, capsule-specific region, region 2, encoding the enzymes for polysaccharide biosynthesis[12, 13] flanked by regions 1 and 3, which are common to all of the group 2 capsule gene clusters. Regions 1 and 3 encode the eight Kps proteins which constitute the common export pathway for the transport of group 2 polysaccharides out of the cell[12, 13, 16, 17] Region 1 consists six genes *kpsFEDUCS* organised in a single transcriptional unit with a sigma (σ)[70] promoter which is located 225 bp 5' of *kpsF*[18] (Fig. 1). Two Integration Host Factor (IHF) binding site consensus sequences are present 110 bp 5' and 130 bp 3' of the transcription start site[17]. Transcription from the promoter 5' of *kpsF* generates an 8.0-kb polycistronic transcript, that is then processed to generate a separate, 1.3 kb *kpsS* transcript (Fig. 1) which may enable the differential expression of the KpsS protein[17]. The role of RNaseE or RNaseIII in the processing of the region 1 mRNA awaits elucidation.

Region 3 contains two genes *kpsM* and *kpsT* which are organised as a single transcriptional unit with a σ[70] promoter 741 bp 5' of the start of *kpsM*[19] (Fig. 1). An *ops* sequence, which is conserved in RfaH regulated genes is located 30 bp 5' to the initiation codon of *kpsM* and mutations in *rfaH* or deletion of the *ops* sequence result in a lack of capsule expression[18](see below).

The size of serotype-specific region 2 can be correlated with the complexity of the encoded polymer[12]. In the case of the K5 capsule gene cluster, region 2 contains four genes *kfiA-D* all of which are transcribed in the same direction as region 3 (Fig. 1). Weak promoters were identified 5' to the *kfiA*, *kfiB* and *kfiC* genes[20] which, in the absence of read through transcription from the region 3 promoter, do not generate sufficient transcription to yield detectable levels of Kfi proteins and expression of a K5 capsule[18].

## 3. THE BIOCHEMISTRY OF GROUP II CAPSULE EXPRESSION

The functions of the proteins encoded by regions 1 and 3 are beginning to emerge. The KpsM and T proteins are members of the superfamily of ATP-binding cassette (ABC)-type transporters and comprise a cytoplasmic membrane polysaccharide transport system[12, 13, 21]. It is likely that the KpsMT transporter consists of two molecules of KpsM, possibly forming some form of cytoplasmic membrane spanning pore, associated with two molecules of KpsT, which hydrolyse ATP to energise the transport process[20]. The KpsE and D proteins play key roles in the transport of group II polysaccharides across the periplasmic space linking the KpsMT transporter in the cytoplasmic membrane with the cell surface[13]. The KpsC and S proteins are believed to be involved in the attachment of phosphatidyl-Kdo to the reducing end of the polysaccharide, and this substitution may be the stage at which the nascent polysaccharide molecule becomes committed to the export pathway and docks with the KpsMT transporter[12]. In addition, the KpsC and S proteins play key roles in the assembly of the capsule biosynthetic complex on the inner-face of the cytoplasmic membrane[22]. The KpsU protein is a CMP-Kdo synthetase which provides the CMP-Kdo for substitution of the polysaccharide chain with phosphatidyl-Kdo[23]. The function of the KpsF protein is as yet unknown[13].

The functions for three of the four Kfi proteins have been determined. The KfiA protein is a GlcNAc transferase which acts to initiate K5 polysaccharide biosynthesis, KfiC is the glycosyl transferase which then adds alternate GlcA and GlcNAc residues to synthesise the K5 polymer[24] and KfiD is a UDP-Glc dehydrogenase which catalyses the formation of UDP-GlcA[24, 25] an essential substrate for K5 biosynthesis. No role has yet been established for the KfiB protein. The Kfi proteins function together with the Kps proteins to form a biosynthetic/transport complex which is assembled on the inner-face of the cytoplasmic membrane[21].

## 4. REGULATION OF GROUP II CAPSULE GENE EXPRESSION

Previously using the K5 capsule gene cluster as a paradigm we had shown that at $20^0C$ there is no transcription from either the region 1 or 3 promoter indicating that temperature regulation of regions 1 and 3 is at the level of transcription[17, 25]. No changes in the organisation of the capsule gene cluster could be detected in cells grown at $20^0C$ as compared to $37^0C$, indicating that temperature regulation does not involve genetic rearrangements. The effects of known global regulatory genes on the expression of the K5 capsule at 37°C and 20°C was studied. Mutations in *topA, lrp, rcsA, rcsB, hha, hupA, hupB, rimJ, ropS, rpoN, rpoH* and *crp* had no detectable effect on K5 capsule expression at either temperature as measured by K5 phage sensitivity, K5 membrane transferase activity, Western blot analysis and reporter gene expression[25, 26]. Mutations in the *himA* or *himD* genes which encode the two subunits of IHF, whilst not abolishing capsule production at 37°C, led to a five fold reduction in the expression of KpsE at 37°C[17]. IHF is a member of the family of bacterial architectural proteins including HU, FIS and H-NS that act as global regulators of gene expression[27]. Generally IHF acts in concert with other transcriptional factors and it is believed that it acts to bend the DNA within the promoter region and that the correct DNA deformation is important in permitting the appropriate DNA/protein interactions necessary for transcriptional activation[27]. Recently we have demonstrated by band shift analysis that IHF binds to the region 1 promoter and that deletion of the IHF binding sites reduces transcription of region 1 two fold at 37°C but had no effect on transcription at 20°C. Therefore in the case of the region 1 promoter IHF is probably playing a architectural role in facilitating the formation of the correct nucleoprotein complex at the region 1 promoter for the activation of transcription at 37°C by as yet unidentified regulatory proteins.

Mutations in the *rfaH* gene abolished group II capsule expression at 37°C[18]. In other systems, perhaps best studied in the *E. coli hlyCABD* operon, it has been shown that RfaH can act as a transcription elongation factor to allow transcription to proceed over long distances[29]. In the case of the K5 capsule gene cluster we were able to show that RfaH was essential for transcription originating from the region 3 promoter to proceed into region 2 (Fig. 1)[18]. In the absence of RfaH, transcription terminates 3' to *kpsT*, resulting in insufficient expression of the region 2 encoded *kfi* genes and a lack of K5 capsule. The *ops* sequence 5' to *kpsM* is typical for genes regulated by RfaH and deletion of the *ops* sequence results in a loss readthrough transcription into region 2 and lack of capsule expression[18]. The role of the *ops* sequence in RfaH regulation is unclear but it may act in the nascent RNA to recruit RfaH to the RNA polymerase complex to allow transcription elongation to proceed[28].

Therefore the transcriptional organisation of the K5 capsule gene cluster can be regarded as two large convergent transcripts (Fig. 1). One of which originates from the region 1 promoter and covers region 1, the other of which originates from the region 3 promoter and, in the presence of RfaH, spans regions 2 and 3 (Fig. 1). In this case the temperature regulation of the K5 capsule gene expression will be principally mediated by the temperature regulation of the region 1 and 3 promoters.

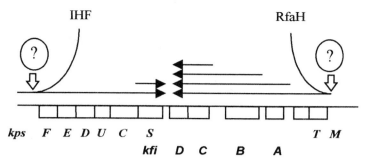

*Figure 1*. The transcriptional organisation of the K5 capsule gene cluster. The boxes beneath the line define the genes whilst the arrows denote the transcripts. The site of action of RfaH and IHF are shown. The circles depic unknown transcriptional activators necessary for transcription at 37°C.

## 5. CONCLUSION

Therefore as a consequence of our studies to date a picture is beginning to emerge of a complex integrated regulatory system involving a number of interacting regulatory proteins and over-arching regulatory control circuits (Fig. 1). The key questions that we need to address are how is transcription from the region 1 and 3 promoters co-ordinated? What is the role of global regulators such as H-NS in repressing transcription at 20°C? How is capsule expression regulated *in vivo* and is capsule expression co-ordinated with the expression of other cell surface structures involved in disease? Answering these questions represents a fascinating biological problem.

## ACKNOWLEDGEMENTS

Work in the laboratory of ISR is supported by the BBSRC of the UK, the Wellcome Trust and the Lister Institute of Preventive Medicine.

## REFERENCES

1.  Whitfield, C. , and Valvano, M., 1993, Biosynthesis and expression of cell surface polysaccharides in gram-negative bacteria. *Adv. Micro Phyiol.* **35:** 135-246.
2.  Moxon, E.R., and Kroll, J.S. , 1990, The role of bacterial polysaccharide capsules as virulence factors. *Curr. Top. Microbiol. Immunol.* **150:** 65-86.
3.  Cross, A.S., (1990, The biologic significance of bacterial encapsulation. *Curr. Top. Microbiol. Immunol.* **150:** 87-95.
4.  Michalek, M., Mold, C., and Bremer, E., 1988, Inhibition of the alternative pathway of human complement by structural analogues of sialic acid. *J. Immunol.* **140:** 1588-1599.

5. Finne, J. , 1982, Occurrence of unique polysialosyl carbohydrate units in glycoproteins of developing brain. *J. Biol. Chem* **257:** 11966-11970.

6. Lindahl, U., Lidholt, K., Spillmann, D., and Kjellen, L. , 1994, More to "heparin" that anticoagulation. *Thrombin Res.* **75:** 1-32.

7. Lifely, M.R., Moreno, C., Lindon, J.C., 1987, An integrated molecular and immunological approach towards a meningococcal group B vaccine. *Vaccine* **5:** 11-26.

8. Costerton, J.W., Chjeng, K-J, Geesey, G.G., Ladd, T.I., Nickel, J.C., Dasgupta, M., and Marrie T., 1987, Bacterial biofilms in nature and disease. *Ann. Rev. Microbiol.* **41:** 435-64.

9. Lam, J., Cham, R., Lam, K., and Costeron, J.W., 1980, Production of mucoid microcolonies by *Pseudomonas aeruginosa* within infected lungs in cystic fibrosis. *Infect. Immunol.* **28:** 546-556.

10. Jann, K., and Jann, B., 1992, Capsules of *Escherichia coli* expression and biological significance. *Can J. Microbiol.* **38:** 705-10.

11. Roberts, I.S., 1995, Bacterial polysaccharides in sickness and in health. *Microbiology* **141:** 2023-2031.

12. Roberts I.S., 1996, The biochemistry and genetics of capsular polysaccharide production in bacteria. *Ann. Rev. Microbiol.* **50:** 285-315.

13. Whitfield, C., and Roberts, I.S., 1999, Structure, assembly and regulation of expression of capsules in *Escherichia coli*. *Mol. Microbiol.* **31:** 1307-1320.

14. Gransden, W.R., Eykyn, S.J., Phillips, I., and Rowe, B., 1990, Bactermia due to *Escherichia coli*: a study of 861 episodes. *J. Infect. Dis.* **12:** 1008-1018.

15. Mekalanos, J., 1992, Environmental signals controlling expression of virulence determinants in bacteria. *J. Bacteriol.* **174:** 1-7.

16. Pazzani, C., Rosenow, C., Boulnois, G.J., Jann, K., and Roberts, I.S., 1993, Molecular analysis of region 1 of the *Escherichia coli* K1. *J. Biol. Chem.* **269:** 20149-20158.

17. Simpson, D., Hammarton, T., and Roberts, I.S., 1993, Transcriptional organisation and regulation of expression of region 1 of the *Escherichia coli* K5 capsule gene cluster. *J. Bacteriol.* **178:** 6466-6474.

18. Stevens, M.P., Clarke, B.R., and Roberts, I.S., 1997, Regulation of the *Escherichia coli* K5 capsule gene cluster by transcription anitermination. *Mol. Microbiol.* **24:** 1001-1012.

19. Petit, C., Rigg, G.P., Pazzani, C., Smith, A., Sieberth, V., Stevens, M., Boulnois, G.J., Jann, K., and Roberts, I.S., 1995, Region 2 of the *Escherichia coli* K5 polysaccharide. *Mol. Microbiol.* **17:** 611-620.

20. Bliss, J.M., and Silver, R.P., 1996, Coating the surface: a model for expression of capsular polysialic acid in *Escherichia coli* K1. *Mol. Microbiol.* **21:** 221-231.

21. Rigg, G.P., Barrett, B., and Roberts, I.S., 1998, The localisation of KpsC, S and T and KfiA, C and D proteins involved in the biosynthesis of the *Escherichia coli* K5 capsular polysaccharide: evidence for a membrane-bound complex. *Microbiology* **144:** 2905-2914.

22. Rosenow, C., Roberts, I.S., and Jann, K., 1995, Isolation from recombinant *Escherichia coli* and characterisation of CMP-Kdo synthetase, involved in the expression of the capsular K5 polysaccharide (K-CKS). FEMS Microbiol. Lett **125:** 159-164.

23. Griffiths, G., Cook, N.J., Gottfridson, E., Lind, T., Lidholt, K., and Roberts, I.S., 1998, Characterisation of the glycosyltransferase enzyme from the *Escherichia coli* K5 capsule gene cluster and identification and characterisation of the glucuronyl active site. *J. Biol. Chem.* **273:** 11752-11757.

24. Sieberth, V., Rigg, G., Roberts, I.S., and Jann, K., 1995, Expression and characterisation of UDPGlc dehydrogenase (KfiD), which is encoded in the type-specific region 2 of the *Escherichia coli* K5 capsule genes. J. Bacteriol. **177:** 4562-4565.

25. Stevens, M., 1995, PhD Thesis *Regulation of Escherichia coli K5 capsule production.* University of Leicester.
26. Stevens, M., Hanfling, P., Jann, B., Jann, K., and Roberts, I.S., 1994, Regulation of *Escherichia coli* K5 capsular polysaccharide expression: evidence for involvement of RfaH in the expression of group II capsules. *FEMS Microbiol. Letts.* **124**: 93-98.
27. Goosen, N., and van de Putte, P., 1995, The regulation of transcription initiation by integration host factor. *Mol. Microbiol.* **16**: 1-7.
28. Bailey, M.J., Hughes, C., and Koronakis, V., 1997, RfaH and the *ops* element, components of a novel system controlling bacterial transcription elongation. *Mol. Microbiol.* **26**: 845-851.

# MOLECULAR BASIS OF CATHETER ASSOCIATED INFECTIONS BY STAPHYLOCOCCI

[1]Friedrich Götz, [2]Christine Heilmann and [1]Sarah E. Cramton
[1]*Mikrobielle Genetik, Waldhäuser Str. 70/8, 72076 Tübingen, Germany; [2]Institut für Medizinische Mikrobiologie, Domagk Str. 10, 48149 Münster, Germany*

## 1.     INTRODUCTION

The first reports that slime-producing *Staphylococcus epidermidis* strains are involved in catheter-associated sepsis and infections came from the groups of Peters[1], Christensen[2], and Costerton[3]. Mostly *S. epidermidis*, but sometimes also mixed cultures, have been isolated from colonized catheters recovered from patients. In 1981, intravenous catheters infected with staphylococci by perfusion were investigated by scanning electron microscopy (SEM) to demonstrate the mode of adhesion[4]. Bacterial cells, primarily those of staphylococci, followed by *Acinetobacter calcoaceticus* and *Pseudomonas aeruginosa*, were shown to be attached to the inner surface of the catheter. The thickest bacterial layers were found in catheters infected by coagulase-negative staphylococci (CNS). The bacteria appeared to be closely packed and cemented together by a slimy matrix[1].

These early observations and pioneering work indicated that the skin bacterium *S. epidermidis*, once considered to be harmless, is an opportunistic pathogen that can cause chronic staphylococcal infection and that certain strains produce slime, an extracellular polysaccharide, that contributes to the formation of a confluent "biofilm". The virulent character of slime is

*Genes and Proteins Underlying Microbial Urinary Tract Virulence*
Edited by L. Emödy *et al.*, Kluwer Academic/Plenum Publishers, 2000

supported by data from many groups. Biofilms have been demonstrated on nearly all kinds of catheters, including right heart flow-directed catheters, urinary catheters, arterial catheters, and central venous catheters, as well as other medical devices, such as endocardial pacemaker leads. In addition to *S. epidermidis, Staphylococcus aureus* and *Candida parapsilosis* are also able to form a biofilm, which indicates that bacteria and yeasts colonize intravascular catheters by an adherent biofilm mode of growth[5]. Both *S. aureus* and *Enterococcus faecalis* have been isolated from biofilm; occasionally, fungal cells or *Proteus mirabilis* have been identified[6].

## 2. ADHERENCE OF STAPHYLOCOCCI TO VARIOUS SYNTHETIC POLYMERS USED AS PROSTHETIC DEVICES

As soon as it became obvious that durable catheters and implants are frequently a source of sepsis and infections, mainly due to slime-producing and biofilm-forming CNS, the question arose whether there are materials with a lower incidence of biofilm formation. It was soon realized that adherence (attachment) of microorganisms is the first step in biofilm formation, and various methods have been worked out to determine adherence and biofilm formation on a given polymer surface. Pulverer et al.[7] investigated the adhesion of a slime-positive CNS strain, KH11, to 12 different polymers. None of the tested polymers with different organic additives were able to prevent bacterial adhesion and some of the polymers, such as cellulose acetate, polycarbonate, and polyesterurethane, even provoked massive biofilm and slime formation. Metal devices did not perform better than plastic materials. *S. aureus* has been recovered from the surface of pacemaker leads recovered from patients with an *S. aureus* bacteremia. The metal tip, the inner surface, and the internal wires were covered with a heavy biofilm. Only the outer silastic surface did not have a biofilm, but did have well-spaced bacterial cells[3]. It was thought that the bactericidal properties of cyanoacrylate (n-butyl-2-cyanoacrylate) might prevent biofilm formation. However, in an *in vitro* study using a modified Robbins device, it was found that *S. epidermidis* rapidly colonized the polymer surface, producing an extensive amorphous biofilm, which indicates that the bactericidal properties of the polymer to this species were weak or absent[8]. Even Teflon (e.g., on catheters) does not prevent adherence and biofilm formation[9]. *S. aureus* forms a biofilm that can be seen by ruthenium red staining, on silk threads *in vitro,* and in a mouse skin model[10]. The biofilm appeared *in vitro* only in the presence of silk threads, and was enhanced by the presence of mouse plasma.

## 3.     MOLECULAR BASIS OF ADHERENCE TO A HYDROPHOBIC SURFACES

It was assumed that CNS form biofilms on prosthetic devices in two steps: 1) the attachment of bacterial cells to the polymer surface, which occurs very quickly, and 2) the accumulation of multilayered cell clusters within a slimy matrix. In order to identify the genes responsible for these phenotypes, biofilm-negative transposon-insertion mutants of *S. epidermidis* O-47 were isolated and analyzed. In this approach, two classes of mutants were isolated: class A mutants are defective in the attachment to a polystyrene surface and class B mutants are defective in slime production and are unable to accumulate in multilayered cell clusters[11]. For the first time, the two steps in biofilm formation could be genetically verified. The characteristics of the two mutant classes are briefly described.

Class A mutants are unable to form a biofilm on a polystyrene surface, but form a biofilm on a glass surface. The number of cells that adhere to the hydrophobic polystyrene surface is 50-fold lower than that of the isogenic wild-type strain. This phenotype occurs concomitantly with other characteristics, such as a decreased hydrophobicity, the formation of large cell clusters, and the absence of a number of surface proteins in the range of 120 to 38 kDa. Mapping of the transposon insertion site indicated that transposition is accompanied by an 8-kb deletion. The nucleotide sequence of the corresponding wild-type region revealed a gene that encodes a protein of 1335 amino acids with a predicted molecular mass of 148 kDa[12]. The amino acid sequence exhibits a high similarity (61% identity) to the *atl* gene product of *S. aureus*[13], which is the major autolysin; therefore, the open reading frame was designated *atlE*. By analogy to the *S. aureus* autolysin, AtlE is composed of two bacteriolytically active domains — a 60-kDa amidase and a 52-kDa glucosaminidase domain, which are generated by proteolytic processing. The 60-kDa amidase catalyzes the last step in cell division — the separation of the two daughter cells. It is therefore not surprising that the AtlE mutant cells form cell clusters in which the daughter cells are still covalently bound to each other. Additionally, AtlE exhibits vitronectin-binding activity, indicating that AtlE plays a role in adherence to uncoated polystyrene surfaces. Since the mutant is still able to adhere to a hydrophilic glass surface and to form a biofilm, it is evident that adherence to glass and polystyrene is mediated by different surface compounds.

## 4.    CHEMICAL COMPOSITION OF POLYSACCHARIDE INTERCELLULAR ADHESIN (PIA)

The most reliable work with respect to the chemical structure and composition of slime was carried out by Mack et al.[14]. They purified a specific polysaccharide antigen of the biofilm-producing strains *S. epidermidis* 1457 and RP62A and were able to distinguish two polysaccharide fractions. Polysaccharide I (>80%) is a linear homoglycan of at least 130 residues consisting of β-1,6-linked *N*-acetylglucosamines, 15–20% of which are de-acetylated and therefore positively charged. Polysaccharide II (<20%) is structurally related to polysaccharide I, but has a lower content of non-*N*-acetylated D-glucosaminyl residues and contains phosphate and ester-linked succinate, rendering it anionic. The acetylated amino group of the D-glucosaminyl residues is important for reactivity with the specific antiserum. The structure of this polysaccharide is unique and, according to its function in cellular aggregation, it is referred to as polysaccharide intercellular adhesin (PIA)[14].

## 5.    MOLECULAR BASIS OF SLIME PRODUCTION AND CELL AGGREGATION

In an early review by Peters[15], it is mentioned that during the course of polymer colonization, staphylococcal cells produce large amounts of extracellular slime in which the cells are imbedded and finally completely covered. Electron microscopy studies have revealed that slime is an extensive, diffuse polyanionic matrix that surrounds the cells[1,2].

Our analyzed class B mutants are not defective in adherence to polystyrene, but lack several traits, such as the ability to form a biofilm on polystyrene and glass surfaces, cell aggregation, and PIA production. The cell-surface-associated protein pattern and hydrophobicity are unchanged[11]. The PIA-negative mutants could also be differentiated on congo red agar. The wild-type and class A mutants form black colonies (positive reaction), while the colonies of class B mutants are red (negative reaction)[16]. The class B transposon-insertion mutants could be complemented to slime (PIA) production by the corresponding wild-type DNA cloned on plasmid pCN27. The nucleotide sequence of the insert revealed an operon, named *ica* for intercellular adhesion[17]. The operon is composed of the *icaR* (regulatory) gene and *icaADBC* (biosynthesis) genes.

With PIA-specific antibodies and by immunofluorescence studies, it was shown that PIA is located mainly on the cell surface. Transfer of pCN27 into the heterologous cloning host *S. carnosus* leads to the formation of large cell aggregates, the formation of a biofilm on a glass surface, and PIA production. The presence of the *ica* operon in *S. carnosus* leads to the production of PIA, and the isolated slime material reacts with PIA-specific antibodies. The function of the IcaABCD proteins is currently under investigation. IcaA contains four potential transmembrane helices, indicative of a membrane location. The deduced IcaA amino acid sequence shows similarity to that of polysaccharide-polymerizing enzymes, especially to an *N*-acetylglucosaminyl transferase of *Rhizobium meliloti*, which is involved in lipo-chitin biosynthesis (22.5% overall identity and 37.4% overall similarity). To study the function of the individual genes, we have established an *in vitro* assay using UDP-*N*-acetylglucosamine as a substrate for PIA biosynthesis, and analyzed the products by thin-layer chromatography and mass spectrometry. IcaA alone exhibits a low N-acetylglucosaminyl transferase activity and is the catalytic enzyme. Coexpression of *icaA* with *icaD* leads to a significant increase in activity. The function of the other genes is currently under investigation.

## 6.    PIA-RELATED SLIME MATERIAL

It appears that SAA[18] and PS/A[19], formerly described as a *N*-acetylglucosamine- and galactose/glucosamine-predominating polymer, respectively, very likely are PIA. The group of G. Pier found that *S. carnosus* (pCN27), which produces PIA, reacts not only with PIA-specific[17], but also with PS/A-specific antibodies[20], which indicates that PIA and PS/A share common immunological activity and also intercellular adhesion and biofilm formation. The only chemical difference between PIA isolated from *S. epidermidis* and from the *S. carnosus* (pCN27) clones is the lack of deacetylated acetylglucosamine residues (glucosamines) in the *S. carnosus* clones[20]. Most of the glucosamines are succinylated or acetylated. However, in *in vitro* synthesis studies with extracts of *S. carnosus* expressing various *ica* genes, all the oligomers produced were composed of *N*-acetylglucosamine residues[21]. The components of PIA (and PS/A) from *S. carnosus* (pCN27) have not yet been fully characterized. Recently, a PIA-related substance was isolated from *S. aureus* MN8; the substance is referred to as poly-*N*-succinyl β-1,6-glucosamine (PNSG), and strains producing PNSG exhibit properties similar to those of PIA- or PS/A-positive staphylococcal strains[22]. The *N*-acetylglucosamine residues of this preparation of PNSG are completely succinylated. This compound apparently also has the main characteristic of PIA, namely the β-1-6 linkage, although a convincing chemical proof for this linkage is still lacking.

## 7.          PREVALENCE OF *ICA* OPERON IN *S. AUREUS*

A variety of *S. aureus* strains have been screened for the presence of the *ica* determinant; the corresponding genes were present in all strains tested, but only some strains were able to form biofilms *in vitro*. The *S. aureus*-specific *ica* locus was cloned and its sequence compared with that of the *S. epidermidis ica* genes. The corresponding proteins reveal a 59–78% amino acid identity. Deletion of the *ica* locus in *S. aureus* results in the loss of the ability to form biofilms, to produce PIA, and to mediate *N*-acetylglucosaminyl transferase activity *in vitro*. Cross-species hybridization experiments revealed the presence of *icaA* in several other staphylococcal species, which suggests that cell–cell adhesion and the potential to form biofilms is conserved within this genus[23], albeit with various expression levels.

## 8.          DISCUSSION

Over time it became more and more clear that in most of the cases the chemical basis of slime, in connection with biofilm formation, is PIA or a PIA derivative. The basic structure of PIA is a β-1,6-linked *N*-acetylglucosamine polymer that can be to a variable degree deacetylated and *N*-succinylated, depending on the staphylococcal strain or species from which it is isolated. In most cases, it is PIA, sometimes together with released teichoic acids, which is responsible for biofilm formation by staphylococci. Many cells produce large amounts of this extracellular slime in which the cells are imbedded and finally completely covered. The genetic analysis confirm that biofilm formation involves two steps: 1) the adherence of the bacterial cells to the polymer surface, and 2) the accumulation in multilayered cell clusters in a slimy matrix (Fig 1). Slime-producing CNS are more prevalent among clinical isolates than on the skin of healthy persons. In numerous animal models, slime-positive *S. epidermidis* strains were more virulent, and it took longer to clear these strains from host tissues than to cure slime-negative variants. In patients suffering from a chronic polymer-associated infection, the removal of the colonized device is frequently the only therapeutic means of combating the infection. Therefore, numerous studies have aimed at studying the effect of antibiotics in prevention and curing of biofilm-related infection. In general, slime-producing staphylococci are more resistant than non-slime producing variants to the majority of antibiotics. In the future, there is a great need for the development of a proficient therapeutic regimen. Vaccination with PIA or PNSG might solve some problems. What is really needed, however, are new anti-infective drugs that inhibit adherence and slime formation and that eradicate already-formed biofilms on implants. The search for materials that are inert to adherence of blood proteins and bacteria should also be continued.

## Biofilm

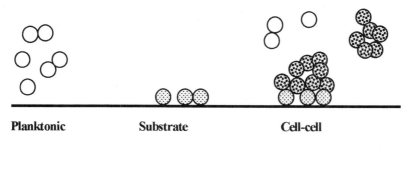

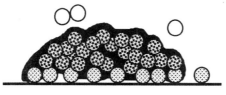

**Biofilm**

*Figure 1.* Two-step model of staphylococcal biofilm formation. The first step in biofilm formation is the adherence of planktonic bacterial cells (open circles) to the substrate surface (grey circles). The second step is the adhesion of cells to each other (stippled circles) and the embedding of the cells in a thick slime matrix (black), forming a biofilm. One component of a biofilm has been identified as PIA. Within this biofilm, cells appear to have reduced physiological activity, an anoxic environment and exhibit a decreased sensitivity to many antibiotics compared to their planktonic counterparts.

## ACKNOWLEDGEMENTS

The authors' work was supported by the German Bundesministerium für Bildung Wissenschaft, Forschung und Technologie (DLR: 01KI9751/1) and an NRSA postdoctoral fellowship (AI09626) from the National Institute of Allergy and Infectious Diseases to S.E.C.

# REFERENCES

1 .Peters, G., Locci, R., and Pulverer, G., 1981, Microbial colonization of prosthetic devices. II. Scanning electron microscopy of naturally infected intravenous catheters. *Zentralbl. Bakteriol. Mikrobiol. Hyg. [B].* **173**: 293-299.

2. Christensen, G.D., Simpson, W.A., Bisno, A.L.,and Beachey, E.H., 1982, Adherence of slime-producing strains of *Staphylococcus epidermidis* to smooth surfaces. *Infect. Immun.* **37**: 318-326.

3. Marrie, T.J., Nelligan, J.,and Costerton, J.W., 1982, A scanning and transmission electron microscopic study of an infected endocardial pacemaker lead. Circulation. **66**: 1339-1341.

4. Locci, R., Peters, G.,and Pulverer G., 1981, Microbial colonization of prosthetic devices. III. Adhesion of staphylococci to lumina of intravenous catheters perfused with bacterial suspensions. *Zentralbl Bakteriol Mikrobiol Hyg [B].* **173**: 300-307.

5. Marrie, T.J., and Costerton. J.W., 1984, Scanning and transmission electron microscopy of in situ bacterial colonization of intravenous and intraarterial catheters. *J. Clin. Microbiol.* **19**: 687-693.

6. Reed, W.P., Moody, M.R., Newman, K.A., Light, P.D., and Costerton. J.W., 1986, Bacterial colonization of Hemasite access devices. *Surgery.* **99**: 308-317.

7. Ludwicka, A., Locci, R., Jansen, B., Peters, G., and Pulverer, G., 1983, Microbial colonization of prosthetic devices. V. attachment of coagulase-negative staphylococci and "slime"-production on chemically pure synthetic polymers. *Zentralbl. Bakteriol. Mikrobiol. Hyg. [B].* **177**: 527-532.

8. Olson, M.E., Ruseska, I., and Costerton, J.W., 1988, Colonization of N-butyl-2-cyanoacrylate tissue adhesive by *Staphylococcus epidermidis. J Biomed. Mater. Res.* **22**: 485-495.

9. Shibl, A.M., Ramadan, M.A., and Tawfik, A.F., 1994. Differential inhibition by clindamycin on slime formation, adherence to teflon catheters and hemolysin production by *Staphylococcus epidermidis. .J Chemother.* **6**: 107-10.

10. Akiyama, H., Torigoe, R., and Arata, J., 1993, Interaction of *Staphylococcus aureus* cells and silk threads *in vitro* and in mouse skin. *J. Dermatol. Sci.* **6**: 247-257.

11. Heilmann, C., Gerke, C., Perdreau-Remington, F., and Götz, F., 1996, Characterization of Tn917 insertion mutants of *Staphylococcus epidermidis* affected in biofilm formation. Infect. Immun. **64**: 277-282.

12. Heilmann, C., Hussain, M., Peters, G., and Götz, F., 1997, Evidence for autolysin-mediated primary attachment of *Staphylococcus epidermidis* to a polystyrene surface. Mol Microbiol. **24**: 1013-1024.

13. Oshida, T., Sugai, M., Komatsuzawa, H., Hong, Y.M., Suginaka, H., and Tomasz, A.,. 1995, A *Staphylococcus aureus* autolysin that has an N-acetylmuramoyl-L- alanine amidase domain and an endo-beta-N-acetylglucosaminidase domain: cloning, sequence analysis, and characterization. *Proc. Natl. Acad. Sci. USA* **92**: 285-289.

14. Mack, D., Fischer, W., Krokotsch, A., Leopold, K., Hartmann, R.,. Egge, H., and Laufs, R., 1996, The intercellular adhesin involved in biofilm accumulation of *Staphylococcus epidermidis* is a linear beta-1,6-linked glucosaminoglycan: purification and structural analysis. *J. Bacteriol.* **178**: 175-183.

15. Peters, G., 1984,[Pathogenesis of staphylococcal infections of implanted plastics and intravascular catheters. *Infection* **12**: 235-239.

16.Heilmann, C., and Götz, F., 1998, Further characterization of *Staphylococcus epidermidis* transposon mutants deficient in primary attachment or intercellular adhesion. *Zentralbl. Bakteriol.* **287**: 69-83.

17. Heilmann, C., Schweitzer, O., Gerke, C., Vanittanakom, N., Mack, D., and Götz F., 1996, Molecular basis of intercellular adhesion in the biofilm-forming *Staphylococcus epidermidis. Mol. Microbiol.* **20:** 1083-1091.

18. Baldassarri, L., Donnelli, G., Gelosia, A., Voglino, M.C., Simpson, A.W., and Christensen, G.D., 1996, Purification and characterization of the staphylococcal slime-associated antigen and its occurrence among *Staphylococcus epidermis* clinical isolates. *Infect. Immun.* **64:** 3410-3415.

19. Tojo, M., Yamashita, N., Goldmann, D.A., and Pier, G.B., 1988, Isolation and characterization of a capsular polysaccharide adhesin from *Staphylococcus epidermidis.* [published erratum appears in *J. Infect. Dis.* 1988, **158:**268]. *J. Infect. Dis.* **157:** 713-722.

20. McKenney, D., Hubner, J., Muller, E., Wang, Y., Goldmann, D.A., and PierG.B.., 1998, The ica locus of *staphylococcus epidermidis* encodes production of the capsular Polysaccharide/Adhesin [In Process Citation]. *Infect. Immun.* **66:** 4711-4720.

21. Gerke, C., Kraft, A., Sussmuth, R., Schweitzer, O., and Götz, F., 1998, Characterization of the N-acetylglucosaminyltransferase activity involved in the biosynthesis of the *Staphylococcus epidermidis* polysaccharide intercellular adhesin. *J. Biol. Chem.* **273:** 18586-18593.

22. McKenney, D., Pouliot, K.L., Wang, Y., Murthy, V., Ulrich, M., Döring, G., Lee, J.C., Goldmann, D.A., and Pier, G.B., 1999, Broadly protective vaccine for *Staphylococcus aureus* based on an in vivo-expressed antigen. *Science* **284:** 1523-1527.

23. Cramton, S. E., Gerke, C., Schnell, N.F., Nichols, W.W., and Götz, F., 1999, The intercellular adhesion (*ica*) locus is present in *Staphylococcus aureus* and is required for biofilm formation. *Infect. Immun.* **67:** 5427-5433.

# CONTROL MECHANISMS IN THE PAP-PILI SYSTEM

Bernt Eric Uhlin, Carlos Balsalobre, Kristina Forsman-Semb, Mikael Göransson, Jana Jass, Jörgen Johansson, Saule Naureckiene, Berit Sondén, Jurate Urbonaviciene, and Yan Xia
*Department of Microbiology, Umeå University, S-90187 Umeå, Sweden*

## 1. INTRODUCTION

The genomes of pathogenic variants of a given bacterial species may carry extra genetic information normally not present in non-pathogenic strains. From molecular genetic analyses of bacterial pathogens it is evident that virulence-associated genetic determinants are subject to intricate regulatory mechanisms that may contribute to the ability of bacteria to adapt to altered host environments. The genes for virulence factors occur on plasmids, as part of phage genomes, and in various locations in bacterial chromosomes. For example, in enterobacteria (*e.g.* the genera Escherichia, Salmonella, Shigella, Yersinia) it has been established that a number of genes and operons encoding virulence factors (adhesins, toxins and invasion factors) often are encoded from adjacent gene clusters. The chromosomal regions constituting such genetic determinants found in pathogenic isolates have been referred to as pathogenicity islands (Pais)[1]. Among strains of *Escherichia coli* such Pais were first defined in uropathogenic and enteropathogenic isolates. The polycistronic gene clusters encoding fimbrial adhesins in uropathogenic *E. coli* (UPEC) are commonly found located in Pais.

*Genes and Proteins Underlying Microbial Urinary Tract Virulence*
Edited by L. Emödy *et al.*, Kluwer Academic/Plenum Publishers, 2000

## 2.      EXPRESSION OF FIMBRIAL ADHESINS BY *ESCHERICHIA COLI*

Expression of adhesins by UPEC involves regulation at several different levels and we and others have characterized transcriptional and post-transcriptional features of such operons. Among the aspects that have been studied in the Pap-pili system are:

Transcriptional control
Environmental regulation
Phase variation
Differential gene expression
Post-transcriptional regulation
Co-ordination – crosstalk

The biogenesis of fimbriae depends on regulated and differential expression of individual genes in operons comprising about ten genes.

Transcriptional activation of fimbrial adhesin operons involve several regulatory proteins and the promoter regions are subject to protein-DNA and protein-protein interactions that presumably lead to formation of rather extensive nucleoprotein complexes. There are both operon specific proteins and more globally occurring regulatory proteins. Proteins with also an architectural role in relation to the local DNA conformation may contribute to the intrinsic susceptibility of the regulatory region to respond to different stimuli or environmental cues.

## 3.      THE ROLE OF NUCLEOID-ASSOCIATED BACTERIAL PROTEINS IN VIRULENCE GENE EXPRESSION

A few nucleoid-associated proteins have been found to be important for the regulatory features of many gene systems. Our initial finding with the *pap* fimbrial adhesin genes was that absence of the protein H-NS led to abolished thermoregulation of the transcription[2,3]. Subsequent studies have shown that this protein has a role in the regulatory systems of many different genes and operons[4,5,6,7,8,9]. In several fimbrial adhesin operons the regulatory system include the global regulators Crp and Lrp[8,10]. Together with H-NS and the more recently discovered protein StpA these proteins are involved in a regulatory network that may ensure both coordinated and differential expression of the globally acting proteins[11].

Differences in cellular levels of e.g. the H-NS proteins may influence how tight and responsive the regulatory mechanisms are for certain virulence factors and there is suggestive evidence that such differences are relevant in the case of some pathogenic isolates[5].

## 4. THE ROLE OF ARCHITECTURAL PROTEINS AND DNA CURVATURE IN CONTROL/SILENCING OF ADHESIN GENES

Our results from studies of the *pap* gene system have shown that the promoter region is subject to both pronounced intrinsic, and to protein-induced, DNA bending (Sondén et al., unpublished data). There are binding sites in the intercistronic region between genes *papI* and *papB* for several DNA binding proteins: Crp, PapB, Lrp-PapI. These are transcriptional factors that are needed for positive adhesin expression. Furthermore, some of these proteins (Crp, Lrp) are known to cause bending of DNA while others (PapB oligomers) might stabilize intrinsic curvature. The PapB protein seems to have a somewhat unusual mode of DNA binding in that it appeared to bind to the minor groove and formed oligomeric complexes recognizing AT-rich DNA[12]. There are similar proteins associated with many of the other adhesin gene clusters in enterobacteria and we refer to them as belonging to the PapB protein family. Sofar, only PapB itself has been characterized to any greater extent. We have performed a mutational analysis and identified regions in the protein involved in DNA binding and in oligomer-formation[13] (see also Xia et al., this volume).

Using gelelectrophoretic analysis and electron microscopy we characterized the curvature of this DNA region (Sondén et al., unpublished data). Our in vitro studies showed that the entire intercistronic region is likely forming a loop-structure. Mutations that alter the curvature properties but did not abolish the binding sites for activator proteins gave strong negative effects on expression *in vivo* (Sondén et al, unpublished data). If then the H-NS was lacking due to mutation the expression could be restored to different degrees. It is evident that this type of regulatory DNA region is involved in a rather complex nucleoprotein structure and presumably this makes it responsive to different signals or stimuli.

We have also attempted to define where in the *pap* adhesin regulatory region there is interaction by H-NS. Both DNA binding studies and *in vitro* transcription experiments support the suggestion that there is direct interaction (Sondén et al., unpublished data). It seems that H-NS can bind over rather extended regions encompassing the two divergent promoters. The use of atomic force microscopy in attempts to visualise intermediate type complexes has given us a hint as to how the protein might act at different concentrations (Jass and Uhlin, unpublished data). This has encouraged us that it may be feasible to establish and characterize nucleoprotein complexes *in vitro*.

## 5.    MODULATION OF GENE EXPRESSION BY DNA METHYLATION

As first demonstrated by Low and coworkers[8], the regulatory DNA regions of lectin genes in *E. coli* are often subject to differential methylation by the Dam methylase at certain GATC sequences. This observation correlates with the on-off phase variation that can be monitored with *lac*-fusion constructs in *E. coli* K-12. However, the mechanism behind the effect of such methylation on adhesin gene expression has remained unclear. In our studies of DNA curvature properties we found that methylation at some positions may influence the DNA bending and we hypotesize that modulation of gene expression here might operate at that level (Sondén et al., unpublished data).

## 6.    POST-TRANSCRIPTIONAL MRNA PROCESSING AND DIFFERENTIAL GENE EXPRESSION

The polycistronic gene clusters encoding fimbrial adhesins in uropathogenic *E. coli* are subject to post-transcriptional processing and differential degradation of the mRNA[3,9,11]. We demonstrated that processing and differential decay of the polycistronic mRNA are important for the normal biogenesis of fimbriae and ensures differential expression of individual genes in the operons[14]. The mRNA processing occuring in the promoter-proximal part is mediated by the RNase E endoribonuclease and we identified structural features of the target RNA by *in vitro* analysis and studies of mutated mRNA molecules[15]. We have also studied the other regions of the operon and established that transcription proceeds all through the ten cistrons. There is evidence for additional endonucleolytic cleavages and it seems likely that the RNase E enzyme is involved (Balsalobre and Uhlin, unpublished data; see also Balsalobre et al., this volume). An intriguing aspect in this regard is the recent findings by Mackie[16] that RNase E has inherent vectorial properties and is a 5'-end-dependent endoribonuclease. The question is whether this is the case also when long polycistronic mRNA are substrates and if the cleavage events occurring far apart from each other there are affecting each other. Perhaps the degradosome complex is different in such cases or located in an "alternative compartment".

# 7.    REGULATORY CROSSTALK

As mentioned above, the protein PapB has been subjected to mutagenesis by alanine-scanning and the results have made it possible to define regions important for DNA binding and tetramerization, respectively. The results from this "prototype" protein provided information that is applicable on the other members of the PapB family. Furthermore, we have recently established that there is a role for PapB in regulatory cross-talk between separate adhesin gene clusters. Commonly the *pap* gene cluster occur in strains carrying also the adhesin genes for mannose-specific binding (type 1 fimbriae, *fim* genes) and we have obtained evidence that PapB can affect the expression also of such fimbriae (Xia, Gally, Forsman-Semb and Uhlin, unpublished data). Many naturally occurring *E. coli*, in contrast to the K-12 "laboratory strain", have more than one type of adhesin gene system. This opens the intriguing possibility that when expressed the pyelonephritis (*pap*) associated fimbrial genes may turn off the other adhesin genes and we now have the possibility to directly assess the nature and functional aspects of such regulatory cross-talk.

# REFERENCES

1.    Hacker, J., Blum-Oehler, G., Mühldorfer, I., and Tschäpe, H., 1997, Pathogenicity islands of virulent bacteria: structure, function and impact on microbial evolution. *Mol.. Microbiol.* **23**: 1089-1097.
2.    Göransson, M., Sondén ,B., Nilson, P., Dagberg, B., Forsman,K., Emanuelsson, K., and Uhlin, B.E., 1990, Transcriptional silencing and thermoregulation of gene expression in *Escherichia coli. Nature* **344**: 682-685.
3.    Uhlin, B.E., 1994, Regulation of *E. coli* fimbrial expression. In *Fimbriae: Adhesion, Biogenesis, Genetics and Vaccines* (P. Klemm, eds) CRC Press, Inc., Boca Raton, FL, pp. 171-177.
4.    Atlung, T., and Ingmer, H., 1997, H-NS: a modulator of environmentally regulated geneexpression. *Mol. Microbiol.* **24**: 7-17.
5.    Dagberg, B., and Uhlin, B.E., 1992, Regulation of virulence-associated plasmid genesinenteroinvasive *Escherichia coli. J.Bacteriol.* **174**: 7606-7612.

6.  Johansson, J., Dagberg, B., Richet, E., and Uhlin, B.E., 1998, H-NS and StpA proteins stimulate expression of the maltose-regulon in *Escherichia coli. J. Bacteriol.***180:** 6117-6125.

7.  Jordi, B.A.J.M., Dagberg, B., De Haan, L.A.M., Hamers, A.M., Van der Zeijst, B.A.M., Gaastra, W., and Uhlin, B.E., 1992, The positive regulator CfaD overcomes the repression mediated by histone-like protein H-NS (H1) in the CFA/I fimbrial operon of *Escherichia coli. EMBO J.* **11:** 2627-2632.

8.  Low, D., Braaten, B., and Van der Woude, M., 1996, Fimbriae. In: *Escherichia coli and Salmonella cellular and molecular biology* (eds. F.C. Neidhardt, III.R. Curtiss, J.L. Ingraham, E.C.C. Lin, K.B. Low, B. Magasanik, M. Schaechter and H.E. Umbarger, eds. ) ASM Press, Washington D.C., pp. 146-157.

9.  Morschhäuser J., Uhlin, B.E., and Hacker, J., 1993, Transcriptional analysis and regulation of the *sfa* determi:nt coding for S fimbriae of pathogenic Escherichia coli strains. *Mol.Gen.Genet.* **238:** 97-105.

10.  Sondén, B., 1996, Architectural proteins and DNA curvature in the transcriptional control of fimbrial adhesin genes in *E. coli. Umeå University Medical Dissertations*, New Series No. 488.

11.  Sondén, B., and Uhlin, B.E., 1996, Coordinated and differential expression of histone-like proteins in *E. coli*: Regulation and function of the H-NS analog StpA. *EMBO J.* **15:** 4970-4980.

12.  Xia, Y., Forsnman, K., Jass, J., and Uhlin, B.E., 1998, Oligomeric interaction of the PapB transcriptional regulator with the upstream activating region of pili adhesin gene promoters in *Escherichia coli. Mol. Microbiol.* **30:** 513-523.

13.  Xia, Y., and Uhlin, B.E., 1999, Mutational analysis of the PapB transcriptional regulator in *Escherichia coli.* **274:** 19723-19730.

14.  Nilsson, P., Naureckiene, S., Uhlin, B.E., 1996, Mutations affecting mRNA processing and fimbrial biogenesis in the *Escherichia coli pap* operon. *J. Bacteriol.* **178:** 683-690.

15.  Naureckiene, S., and Uhlin, B.E., 1996, In vitro analysis of mRNA processing by RNase E in the *pap* operon of *Escherichia coli. Mol. Microbiol.* **21:** 55-68.

16.  Mackie, G.A., 1998, Ribonuclease E is a 5'-end-dependent endonuclease. *Nature* **395:** 720-723.

# TRANSCRIPTIONAL ANALYSIS OF THE *SFA* AND *PAP* DETERMINANTS OF UROPATHOGENIC *ESCHERICHIA COLI* STRAINS

[1]Carlos Balsalobre, [2]Joachim Morschhäuser, [2]Jörg Hacker and [1]Bernt Eric Uhlin

[1]*Department of Microbiology, Umeå University, S-90187 Umeå, Sweden;* [2]*Zentrum für Infektionsforschung, Institut für Molekulare Infektionsbiologie, University of Würzburg, Röntgenring 11, D-97070 Würzburg, Germany.*

## 1.  INTRODUCTION

Among the several virulence factors present in *Escherichia coli* uropathogenic strains, the expression of adhesins is necessary for the colonization of the host tissues and the subsequent urinary tract infection. The *pap* and *sfa* determinants code for the P-fimbriae and the S-fimbriae, respectively. These two adhesins are widely spread among the uropathogens. The *pap* and *sfa* determinants consist of eleven and nine genes, respectively, and they share some characteristics in organization and regulation (Fig 1). In the biogenesis of these fimbriae all the proteins coded in these operons take part in a specific stoichiometry.

## 2.  RESULTS

In the present work we studied how the differential expression of the fimbriae-operon genes is carried out. Earlier transcriptional analysis of the proximal genes located close to the promoters in the regulatory region

*Genes and Proteins Underlying Microbial Urinary Tract Virulence*
Edited by L. Emödy *et al.*, Kluwer Academic/Plenum Publishers, 2000

119

showed clear similarities between the two determinants[1,2,3,4]. In both operons, endoribonucleolytic cleavage events of the primary mRNA molecules generated stable transcripts wich contained the sequences for the major subunits of the fimbriae (SfaA and PapA, respectively)[3,4,5,6,7]. We extended the analysis to include the entire determinants.

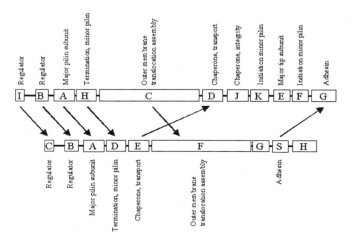

Similarities: - Both operons have been described to be present in PAIs.
- Similar transcriptional regulation pathway by the two regulators coded in the two proximal genes.
- Similar post-transcriptional processes of the transcript coding for the major subunit of the fimbriae, *papA* and *sfaA*, respectively.

Differences: - Different number of genes (11 and 9, respectively).
- The distribution of the genes coding for proteins with homologous function (marked with arrows) is different downstream of the fourth gene.

*Figure 1.* Comparison between *pap* and *sfa* operons.

The transcriptional analysis of the proximal genes of the *sfa* operon indicated that besides the major *sfaA* transcript, one transcript containing the sequences of the four proximal genes located up-stream of the largest *sfaF* gene was generated. Similarly, in previous studies done with the *pap* operon, the presence of one transcript spanning up to the analogous largest gene *papC* was shown. Moreover, our recent results indicated that similar RNA processes occurred in the two determinants with respect to the transcripts corresponding to the central region which included the genes coding for the outer membrane translocation assembly proteins (*papC* and *sfaF,* respectively) (see Fig 2 and Uhlin *et al.*, this volume). However, the transcripts corresponding to the promoter distal genes suggested that post-transcriptional processing occurrs differently in the two determinants.

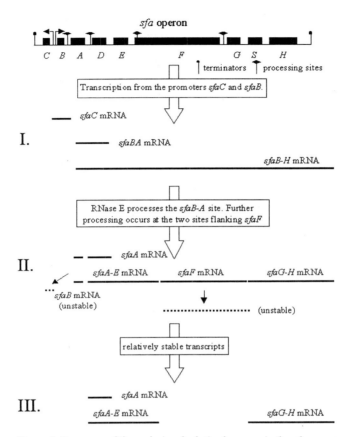

*Figure 2.* Summary of the endorinucleolytic cleavages in the *sfa* operon.

In the case of the *sfa* operon the three distal genes located downstream from *sfaF* were represented by a single transcript. In the *pap* operon the mRNA corresponding to the six genes located downstream from *papC* appeared to be further processed at least at two sites. These RNA processing sites were localized to sequences flanking the *papE* gene, which codes for the major subunit of the tip of the fimbriae. The process of the formation of the P-fimbriae involved a higher expression from the *papE* gene than from the other promoter distal genes. We proposed that post-transcriptional processing and relative stability of the *papE* transcript were important for the biogenesis of the functional fimbrial adhesins.

## 3.    CONCLUSIONS

a) The transcriptional and post-transcriptional events occurring in the proximal part of the *pap* and *sfa* determinants were quite similar. In both cases there was the generation, by mRNA processing, of a major transcript coding for the major fimbrial subunit. Furthermore, the gene coding for the major subunit together with the genes located down-stream out to the longest gene, coding for the outer membrane translocation protein, were represented also by *sfa(B)A-F* and *papA-H* transcripts.

b) In both operons processing of the mRNA at sites flanking the sequences coding for the outer membrane translocation protein (PapC and SfaF) occurred. The resulting transcripts, which should represent such genes, were presumably quickly degraded.

c) The three distal genes of the *sfa* operon were represented by a transcript generated by a cleavage process. The distal part of the *pap* operon contains more genes than the *sfa* operon, and it suffered two more cleavages that generated one distal transcript containing the gene *papE* coding for the major subunit of the fimbria tip.

d) We suggest that several endoribonucleolytic cleavages occur in the mRNA from fimbrial adhesin operons. Such post-transcriptional mRNA processing events result in differential gene expression of importance to adhesin biogenesis.

## REFERENCES

1. Båga, M., Göransson, M., Normark, S. and Uhlin, B.E. 1985. Transcriptional activation of a Pap pilus virulence operon from uropathogenic *Escherichia coli*. *EMBO J.* **4:** 3887-3893.
2. Båga, M., Norgren, M. and Normark, S. 1987. Biogenesis of *E. coli* Pap pili: PapH, a minor pili subunit involved in cell anchoring and length modulation. *Cell* **49:** 241-251.
3. Båga, M., Göransson, M., Normark, S. and Uhlin, B.E. 1988. Processed mRNA with differential stability in the regulation of *E.coli* pilin gene expression. *Cell* **52:** 197-206.
4. Morschhäuser, J., Uhlin, B.E. and Hacker, J. 1993. Transcriptional analysis and regulation of the *sfa* determinant coding for S fimbriae of pathogenic *Escherichia coli* strains. *Mol. Gen. Genet.* **238:** 97-105.
5. Naureckiene, S. and Uhlin B.E. 1996. *In vitro* analysis of mRNA processing by RNase E in the *pap* operon of *Escherichia coli*. *Mol. Microbiol.* **21:** 55-68.
6. Nilsson, P. and Uhlin, B.E. 1991. Differential decay of a polycistronic *Escherichia coli* transcript is initiated by RNase E-dependent endonucleolytic processing. *Mol. Microbiol.* **5:** 1791-1799.
7. Nilsson, P., Naureckiene, S. and Uhlin, B.E. 1996. Mutations affecting mRNA processing and fimbrial biogenesis in the *Escherichia coli pap* operon. *J. Bacteriol.* **178:** 683-690.

# STRUCTURAL AND FUNCTIONAL STUDIES OF THE FIMBRIAL ADHESIN GENE REGULATOR PAPB FROM UROPATHOGENIC *ESCHERICHIA COLI*

[1]Yan Xia , [2]Kristina Forsman-Semb, [1]Jana Jass and [1]Bernt Eric Uhlin
[1]*Department of Microbiology, Umeå University, S-90187 Umeå, Sweden.* [2]*AstraZeneca, Molecular Biology, S-43183 Mölndal, Sweden*

## 1.     INTRODUCTION

Expression of Pap pili in the uropathogenic *E. coli* strain J96 depends on transcription of the major *pap* operon, starting at the *papB* promoter, and the divergent *papI* operon[1]. The *papB* gene product stimulates *pap* operon expression and acts as transcriptional regulator of the *papB* promoter. When the amount of PapB is increased above a certain level, transcription from the *papB* promoter is repressed[2]. Therefore, PapB has an autoregulatory function. There are PapB-like proteins encoded by many fimbrial gene systems. SfaB is a positive regulator which influences the production of the S fimbriae. The products of the *fanA* and *fanB* genes both show resemblance to PapB and are suggested to act as transcriptional antiterminators involved in control of K99 fimbriae production. Biosynthesis of the *E. coli* CS31A surface antigen is negatively controlled by the PapB homolog, ClpB, together with LRP. In the *pef* operon, located on the 90-kb virulence plasmid in *Salmonella typhimurium*, the gene *pefB* is postulated to encode a PapB-like protein. Evidently this family of regulatory proteins occurs in several important pathogens. However, the molecular targets and mode of action of the PapB-like proteins are so far largely unknown. Here we report

*Genes and Proteins Underlying Microbial Urinary Tract Virulence*
Edited by L. Emödy *et al.*, Kluwer Academic/Plenum Publishers, 2000

our studies on the PapB-DNA interaction, and mutational analysis of the PapB protein.

## 2.      THE DNA BINDING MODE OF THE PAPB PROTEIN

We investigated the mode of PapB interaction with site 1 *in vitro*, and the role of this interaction *in vivo* in transcriptional activation of the major *pap* operon[3]. Due to the insertion/deletion of a 9-bp sequence the PapB binding DNA regions are of variable size among the different *pap* operons. This suggested that PapB interacted with several repeated target sequences within these regions. The repeated nucleotide sequence motif $TTT/AAA(N)_6TTT/AAA(N)_6TTT/AAA(N)_6TTT/AAA$ was found in site 1, and the results from mutagenesis of the DNA sequence suggest that PapB binding depends on such repeats. We concluded that PapB recognized a DNA structure including $(T/A)_3$ repeats with 9-bp periodicity rather than a specific DNA sequence. This hypothesis was supported by the observation that an 18-bp insertion into site 1 extended the PapB-footprints by the same number of nucleotides (i.e., strain KS71). The DNase I footprinting analysis of PapB binding to the *foc* regulatory region also showed a 9-bp periodicity in terms of $(T/A)_3$ sequences.

The competition observed for DNA binding between PapB and distamycin, a minor groove DNA binding drug, together with the fact that no effect on PapB binding was obtained with the same amount of the major groove-binder methyl green, suggested that PapB bound to DNA through minor groove interaction.

Considering the size of PapB (104 amino acids) and the length of the DNase I-protected regions (50-70 bp), it seems likely that multiple PapB molecules are required to protect these regions. The DNA binding saturation experiment suggested that 8-10 PapB molecules are required to occupy each J96 site 1, which is consistent with the result of visualization of DNA-PapB complex by Atomic Force Microscopy (AFM). We propose that PapB binds to the neighbouring repeats (with a 9-bp periodicity) in a novel oligomeric fashion.

## 3.   MUTATIONAL ANALYSIS OF THE PAPB PROTEIN

The aa sequence of the PapB protein doesn't contain any obvious recognition motifs that are common in other DNA binding proteins. The computer prediction of the secondary structure of PapB suggested a hydrophilic region (aa 61-70), which, in a comparison with PapB-like proteins from other fimbrial gene systems, seemed to contain several conserved residues and could be important for DNA binding. The gel mobility shift assays with different truncated PapB mutants showed that the predicted hydrophilic region (aa 61-70) is important for DNA binding[4]. The alanine-scanning mutagenesis indicated that the conserved $Arg_{61}$ and $Cys_{65}$ are the two most critical residues required for DNA binding. This is consistent with the fact that the iodoacetamide-modified PapB (affecting the single Cys residue $Cys^{65}$) showed defective DNA binding.

The wt-PapB protein has a tendency to form large, insoluble aggregates, and previous studies have indicated that PapB can act as an oligomer and can protect regions as long as 30 to 70 nucleotides. However, both the even numbers of 9-bp repeats in the PapB binding site(s) and the results of binding saturation experiments suggested that PapB might act as a dimer or a tetramer *in vivo*[3]. The *in vivo* oligomerization studies suggested that wt-PapB could function as an oligomer *in vivo*. To identify the regions important for oligomerization, the conserved amino acid residues were mutated by alanine substitutions. By using the same oligomerization test system, it was found that PapB mutants with alanine substitutions at positions 35-36, 53-56, and 74-76 did not function like wt-PapB to replace the C-terminal oligomerization domain of the cI repressor and repressed the expression of the reporter genes. All the truncated PapB mutants showed the same phenotype, suggesting that the tertiary structure is required for oligomerization. In contrast, the DNA binding-defective PapB mutants in which $Arg_{61}$ or $Cys_{65}$ were mutated displayed similar oligomerization capability as that of wt-PapB. To further assess the different oligomerization states of wt and mutant PapB proteins, we performed *in vitro* cross-linking studies in the presence of cross-linker dimethyl suberimidate (DMS). Such cross-linking experiments showed that wt-PapB and DNA binding-defective mutants PapB(R61A) and PapB(C65A) indeed could form a kind of dimer in solution. However, the oligomerization defective mutants with alanine substitutions at positions 35-36, 53-56, and 74-76 did not form dimers in the presence of DMS. The results of the *in vivo* co-operative binding and the *in vitro* cross-linking tests were consistent with each other and pointed to the importance of these aa residues in the oligomerization of PapB.

All these oligomerization-defective mutants only retained weak DNA binding ability, which suggested that the protein interaction is important for PapB to bind cooperatively to the DNA. The transcriptional activation efficiency of either the DNA-binding or the oligomerization-defective mutants was much weaker than that of wt-PapB. Taken together, we conclude from these studies that both the DNA-binding and the oligomerization capabilities are required for PapB to fully function as an active transcriptional regulator.

## 4.    CONCLUSIONS

a)   Purified PapB protein was shown to recognize a motif including a 9-bp repeat sequence containing T/A triplets at a conserved position. PapB binding was affected by distamycin, and the results were consistent with the possibility that the binding to DNA occurred through minor groove interaction.

b)   The DNA binding saturation results and visualization of DNA-PapB complex by AFM suggested that PapB can bind DNA in an oligomeric fashion.

c)   Mutations altering $Arg_{61}$ or $Cys_{65}$ caused deficiency in DNA binding, indicating that these residues are critical for PapB binding to DNA. Alanine substitutions at positions 35-36, 53-56, and 74-76 resulted in mutants that were impaired in oligomerization.

d)   The transcriptional efficiency of all the mutants was clearly reduced as compared with that of wild-type PapB, indicating that both DNA binding and oligomerization are required for PapB as a transcriptional regulator.

## REFERENCES

1.  Båga, M., Göransson, M., Normark, S., and Uhlin, B.E., 1985, Transcriptional activation of a Pap pilus virulence operon from uropathogenic *Escherichia coli*. *EMBO J* **4**: 3887-3893.
2.  Forsman, K., Göransson, M., and Uhlin, B.E., 1989, Autoregulation and multiple DNA interactions by a transcriptional regulatory protein in *E. coli* pili biogenesis. *EMBO J* **8**: 1271-1277.
3.  Xia, Y., Forsnman, K., Jass J. and Uhlin, B.E., 1998, Oligomeric interaction of the PapB transcriptional regulator with the upstream activating region of pili adhesin gene promoters in *Escherichia coli*. *Mol. Microbiol.* **30**: 513-523.
4.  Xia, Y., and Uhlin, B.E., 1999, Mutational analysis of the PapB transcriptional regulator in *Escherichia coli*. **274**: 19723-19730.

# INTERACTION OF THE NUCLEOID-ASSOCIATED PROTEINS HHA AND H-NS TO MODULATE EXPRESSION OF THE HEMOLYSIN OPERON IN *ESCHERICHIA COLI*

[1] Antonio Juárez, [1]José M. Nieto, [1]Antoni Prenafeta, [1]Elisabet Miquelay, [2]Carlos Balsalobre, [3]Montserrat Carrascal and [1]Cristina Madrid
*[1]Departament de Microbiologia. Facultat de Biologia. Universitat de Barcelona, Spain
[2]Department of Microbiology. Umeå University, Sweden. [3]Espectrometría de Masas Estructural y Biológica. Departamento Bioanalítica Médica. IIBB, IDIBARS. CSIC, Spain*

## 1.     THE HHA PROTEIN FROM *E. COLI*

*Escherichia coli* Hha protein and *Yersinia enterocolitica* YmoA protein belong to a new class of modulators of bacterial gene expression[1]. Both are small basic proteins (molecular mass of about 8 kDa) and share extensive homology in their amino acid sequences (82% identity). YmoA protein participates in the temperature-dependent modulation of the expression of different virulence factors (the Yop proteins and the YadA adhesin) in *Y. enterocolitica*[2]. Hha protein is a temperature and osmolarity-dependent modulator of gene expression in *E. coli*[3,4,5]. Among others, the operon that encodes the toxin α-hemolysin (Hly) is modulated by Hha. Expression of the toxin is repressed when the osmolarity of the medium increases and, as well, when the temperature drops[6]. *hha* mutants partially alleviate this repression.

*hha/ymoA* mutants are pleiotropic: in addition to show alterations in the environmentally-dependent regulation of gene expression, they also present topological modifications of reporter plasmids[4] and increased frequency of transposition of IS elements[1,7]. These phenotypic properties are reminiscent of those of strains exhibiting abnormal levels of the well-characterized nucleoid-associated protein H-NS[8,9]. It was therefore suggested that Hha

*Genes and Proteins Underlying Microbial Urinary Tract Virulence*
Edited by L. Emödy *et al.*, Kluwer Academic/Plenum Publishers, 2000

127

and YmoA are as well nucleoid-associated proteins. For Hha, this has been confirmed by demonstrating that Hha binds in a concentration-dependent manner to DNA fragments that include regulatory sequences of the *hly* operon.

## 2.        HHA BINDS *IN VITRO* TO H-NS

To better understand the modulatory role of Hha, we decided to analyze if Hha interacts with other regulatory proteins. Purification of His-tagged proteins in non-denaturing conditions has been reported as a convenient method to detect protein-protein interactions. A His-tagged recombinant Hha protein (His-Hha) was purified by Immobilised-metal affinity chromatography by using the Nickel-nitriloacetic ($Ni^{2+}$-NTA) technology. A total cellular extract from an *E. coli* culture overexpressing His-Hha was bound to a $Ni^{2+}$-NTA agarose matrix. Cellular proteins not retained by the matrix were eluted by washing with a buffer containing a low imidazole concentration (50 mM). Proteins bound to the agarose resin were then eluted by increasing the imidazole concentration. Most of the recombinant protein eluted with 100 mM and 200 mM imidazole (Fig. 1A). A second protein, with an apparent mass of about 15 kDa coeluted with His-Hha. The sequence of the amino-terminal end of the protein copurifying with His-Hha matched exactly that of H-NS. When the His-Hha/H-NS complex was bound to the agarose matrix, it was possible to dissociate both proteins by adding KCl. Elution of H-NS was initially detected at 0.5M KCl and continued until 1M KCl (Fig. 1B).The need of high-salt conditions to elute H-NS suggests that this protein is tightly bound to Hha.

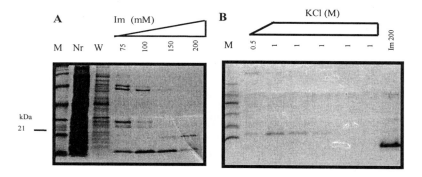

*Figure 1.* Copurification of His-Hha and H-NS. (A), Coomassie blue stained SDS-PAGE of fractions eluted with increasing concentrations of imidazole from the $Ni^{2+}$-NTA agarose resin, upon binding a cellular extract corresponding to a strain overexpressing His-Hha. M,

pre-stained broad-range molecular weight marker; Nr, cellular extract not retained by the resin; W, 50 mM imidazole wash; Im, fractions eluting at increasing concentrations of imidazole. The two bands eluted at 200 mM imidazole correspond to His-Hha and H-NS. (B) Elution of H-NS from the agarose-His-Hha matrix with washings starting at 0.5M KCl and continuing at 1M KCl. The last washing was performed with 200 mM imidazole and released His-Hha.

### 3.     BINDING OF HHA AND H-NS TO THE PROMOTER REGION OF THE *HLY* OPERON OF PLASMID PHLY152

It has been previously reported that H-NS also influences expression of the *hly* operon[10]. Both the *in vitro* interaction of Hha and H-NS and the fact that both proteins have been reported to influence expression of the *hly* operon suggested that an Hha-H-NS complex modulates hemolysin expression. To obtain further insight, we first tested if both proteins were able to interact with DNA generating nucleoprotein complexes different to those generated independently by each of them. Band shift assays were performed by using an about 500 bp DNA fragment covering the promoter region of the *hly* operon, and both H-NS and Hha proteins (Fig.2).

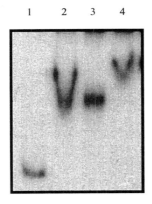

*Figure 2*. Binding of Hha and H-NS to a 549 bp DNA fragment corresponding to the promoter region of the *hly* operon of plasmid pHly152. Gel retardation using Hha, H-NS or a mixture of both proteins. Lane 1, free probe (0.2 ng); lane 2, H-NS added (0.15 µg); lane 3, Hha added (1,5 µg); lane 4, Hha and H-NS added.

When both proteins were added to the reaction mixture, the DNA-protein complex formed was different to those generated either by Hha or by H-NS. When Hha was incubated in the presence of the labelled DNA, a 10-fold excess of competitor DNA interfered with the interaction of the protein with the labelled probe. In contrast, the Hha-H-NS-labelled probe complex was still formed when a 100-fold  excess of competitor DNA was added. This suggests that the slow-migrating Hha-H-NS-DNA complex is not generated by Hha and H-NS independently interacting at different sites of the DNA molecule, but by a direct protein-protein-DNA interaction.

## 4.   HHA AND H-NS PARTICIPATE IN THE ENVIRONMENTAL MODULATION OF THE EXPRESSION OF THE *HLY* OPERON OF PLASMID PHLY152

To assign a modulatory role to the Hha-H-NS complex, we further used the model of the *hly* operon to assess its thermosmotic regulation in *hha*, *hns* and *hha hns* genetic backgrounds. The isogenic strains YK4122 (wt), YK4122H (*hha*), YK4124 (*hns*) and YK4124H (*hha hns*)[10] were used. To study hemolysin expression in the different genetic backgrounds, plasmid pHly152 was introduced by conjugation to each of the four strains. Hemolysin production was then measured in cells growing at different temperatures (25 and 37° C) or in media of different osmolarity (LB medium and LB medium containing 0.5M NaCl). To measure hemolysin production, the hemolytic activity in culture supernatants was evaluated (Table 1).  Both the *hha* and *hns* alleles partially derepressed hemolysin expression at high osmolarity and at low temperature. The double *hha hns* mutant showed the highest hemolysin production under all conditions tested, thus suggesting that the Hha-H-NS complex is mainly responsible for the thermoosmotic regulation of the *hly* operon of plasmid pHly152.

*Table 1.* Effect of *hha, hns* and *hha hns* mutations on the thermoosmotic regulation of  the *hly* operon of plasmid pHly152

| Strain | LB medium, 37° C[++] | Hemolytic activity [+] LB medium (0.5 M NaCl), 37° C[++] | LB medium, 25° C[++] |
|--------|------------------|------------------|------------------|
| YK4122 | 170 | 2 | 3 |
| YK4122H | 185 | 25 | 27 |
| YK4124 | 3,200 | 95 | 370 |
| YK4124H | 6,000 | 700 | 1,200 |

\*    hemolytic activity (units) was determined as described[6]
\*\*   Samples were collected at the exponential phase of growth ($OD_{600}$ = 0.4)

## 5.    CONCLUSION

Both the *in vitro* and *in vivo* data reported here strongly support the hypothesis that Hha and H-NS interact with DNA to generate a nucleoprotein complex that influences gene expression. The Hha-H-NS complex seems to be mainly responsible for the thermoosmotic modulation of the expression of the *hly* operon of plasmid pHly152. Binding sites for Hha and H-NS along the regulatory region of the *hly* operon, as well as the topological changes mediated by the interaction of both proteins with DNA, are currently being investigated.

## REFERENCES

1. Mikulskis, A.V. and Cornelis, G.R., 1994, A new class of proteins regulating gene expression in enterobacteria. *Mol. Microbiol.* 11: 77-86.
2. Cornelis, G.R., Sluiters, C., Delor, I., Gelb, D., Kaninga, K., Lambert de Rouvroit, C., Sory, M.P., Vanooteghem, J.C. and Michaelis, T., 1991, *ymoA*, a *Yersinia enterocolitica* chromosomal gene modulating the expression of virulence functions. *Mol.Microbiol.* 5: 1023-1034.
3. Nieto, J.M., Carmona, M., Bolland, S., Jubete, Y., De la Cruz, F. and Juárez, A., 1991, The *hha* gene modulates hemolysin expression in *Escherichia coli. Mol. Microbiol.* 5: 1285-1293.
4. Carmona, M., Balsalobre, C., Muñoa, F.J., Mouriño, M., Jubete, Y., De la Cruz, F. and Juárez, A., 1993, *Escherichia coli hha* mutants, DNA supercoiling and expression of the haemolysin genes from the recombinant plasmid pANN202-312. *Mol. Microbiol.* 9: 1011-1018.
5. Mouriño, M., Madrid, C., Balsalobre, C., Prenafeta, A., Muñoa, F.J., Blanco, J., Blanco, M., Blanco, J.E., and Juárez, A., 1996, The Hha protein as a modulator of the expression of virulence factors in *Escherichia coli. Inf. Immun.*64: 2881-2884.
6. Mouriño, M., Muñoa, F.J., Balsalobre, C., Díaz, P., Madrid, C. and Juárez, A., 1994, Environmental regulation of alpha-hemolysin expression in *Escherichia coli. Microb. Pathog.* 16: 249-259.
7. Balsalobre, C., Juárez, A., Madrid, C., Mouriño, M., Prenafeta, A. and Muñoa, F, 1996, Complementation of the *hha* mutation in *Escherichia coli* by the *ymoA* gene from *Yersinia enterocolitica*: dependence on the gene dosage. *Microbiology* 142: 1841-1846.
8. Atlung, T. and Ingmer, A., 1997, H-NS: a modulator of environmentally regulated gene expression. *Mol. Microbiol.* 24: 7-17.
9. Williams, R.M. and Rimsky, S. ,1997, Molecular aspects of the *E. coli* nucleoid protein H-NS: a central controller of gene regulatory networks. *FEMS Microbiol. Lett.* 156: 175-185.
10. Nieto, J.M., Mouriño, M., Balsalobre, C., Madrid, C., Prenafeta, A., Muñoa, F.J. and Juárez, A., 1997, Construction of a double *hha hns* mutant of *Escherichia coli*: effect on DNA supercoiling and α-hemolysin production. *FEMS Microbiol. Lett.* 155: 39-44.

# USE OF THE OMPS-DISPLAY– SYSTEM TO LOCALIZE THE RECEPTOR-BINDING REGION IN THE PAPG ADHESIN OF UROPATHOGENIC *ESCHERICHIA COLI*

Hannu Lång, Minna Mäki, Anssi Rantakari and Timo K. Korhonen
*Division of General Microbiology, Department of Biosciences, P.O. Box 56, FIN-00014, University of Helsinki*

## 1.     INTRODUCTION

In recent years there has been great interest in display of heterologous peptides on the surface of Gram-negative bacteria. This is generating intriguing opportunities for a number of applications including recombinant bacterial vaccine development and adhesin-receptor pair interaction studies. These applications would benefit from flexible display systems which can present the epitope of interest in functional form and can be used with epitopes of different sizes.

## 2.     THE LAMB FAMILY OF GLYCOPORINS

The LamB family of glycoporins contains trimeric outer membrane proteins responsible for the permeation of mono- di- and oligosaccharides across the bacterial outer membrane. Maltose-inducible glycoporins are present in many bacteria including *Escherichia coli*, *Salmonella typhimurium*, *Klebsiella pneumoniae*, *Aeromonas salmonicida*, *Vibrio cholerae* and *Yersinia enterocolitica*[1]. They constitute an interesting family of similarly folding proteins as their monomeric structure seem to contain 18

*Genes and Proteins Underlying Microbial Urinary Tract Virulence*
Edited by L. Emödy *et al.*, Kluwer Academic/Plenum Publishers, 2000

transmembrane β-sheets and 9 surface-accessible loops facing the outside world. The transmembrane β-sheets are very homologous among the LamB proteins but the surface loops differ considerably between members of the family.

## 3.     STRUCTURE OF OMPS

OmpS is the glycoporin of *V. cholerae*. The *ompS* gene has been cloned and sequenced[2]. Based on sequence similarity to other LamB proteins, a model of OmpS folding across the outer membrane was constructed[3] (Figure 1). This model helps us to identify the surface located loops. According to the model, OmpS contains 9 loops of which L1, L3 and L6 fold inside the OmpS β-barrel. L4, L5, L7, L8 and L9 could in principle be used to present foreign peptides on the bacterial cell surface by inserting the foreign epitope within the surface exposed loop. We developed an OmpS-expression plasmid –based system where L4 is utilized to express adhesive peptides in a functional form.

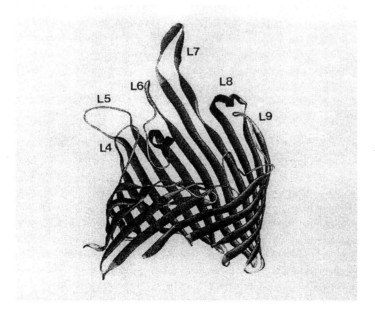

*Figure 1.* A model of the structure of OmpS monomer. Some of the surface-accessible loops are labelled.

## 4. PAPG IS THE ADHESIN OF P-FIMBRIAE

P-fimbriae –mediated adhesion of *E. coli* to the P blood group antigens present on host epithelium is dependent on the PapG protein that recognizes Galα1-4Gal containing globoseries receptors[4]. The PapG adhesin, known to exist in three tropism-determining classes, is located at the distal end of the P-fimbriae. It is important in the initial interaction between the pathogen and its host receptor, and can mediate induction of gene expression in *E. coli*[5]. The receptor-binding domain of PapG has been localized to the N-terminal half of the molecule using MalE-PapG fusion proteins[6].

## 5. APPLICATION OF OMPS-DISPLAY TO CHARACTERIZE RECEPTOR BINDING REGION OF PAPG

We have used the OmpS-display to localize the receptor binding epitope of a class II PapG adhesin[3]. DNA fragments covering the N-terminal half of PapG were cloned into surface accessible loop (L4) of OmpS. The *ompS-papG* hybrid genes were expressed in *E. coli* under a strong inducible promoter and the hybrid proteins were found to be localized to the cell surface. Binding to the receptor globoside was analyzed with erythrocyte agglutination, and binding of whole bacterial cells or membrane fractions of bacteria to immobilized globoside. Fragments of PapG encoding 52 or 186 amino acids from the N-terminal end of PapG were found to mediate binding to globoside. Deletion of 23 amino acids from the N-terminus of PapG did not affect binding, but deletion of 31 amino acids abolished it. A summary of the binding studies is presented in Table 1.

*Table 1.* Binding characteristics of *E. coli* strains producing OmpS-PapG hybrid proteins

| Strain | Globoside binding | | Insert |
|---|---|---|---|
| | Whole cells | Membrane fractions | |
| JT1 | - | - | Host strain |
| JT1(pPIL110-75) | +++ | +++ | P-fimbriated |
| JT1(pHLQ802) | - | - | OmpS |
| JT1(pHLQ12) | + | ++ | OmpSPapG(1-53) |
| JT1(pHLQ16) | ++ | ++ | OmpSPapG(1-186) |
| JT1(pHLQ34) | - | - | OmpSPapG(53-122) |
| JT1(pHLQ36) | - | - | OmpSPapG(53-186) |
| JT1(pHLQ96) | + | ++ | OmpSPapG(24-186) |
| JT1(pHLQ116) | - | - | OmpSPapG(32-186) |

+++ indicates very strong binding, + weak binding, - no binding

We raised antibodies against the purified hybrid protein containing 52 amino acids from PapG, and this antiserum recognized P-fimbriae and it partly inhibited binding of P-fimbriated *E. coli* to globoside in vitro.

## 6.    CONCLUSION

In conclusion, by using a display-system based on the OmpS glycoporin, we have localized a 30 amino acid region of PapG that is important in receptor binding.

We suggest that the OmpS-display -system offers an efficient tool to analyze ligand-receptor interactions. Coupling of adhesins to an outer membrane protein provides a means to transport them to the cell surface with a mechanism that is independent of their normal transport route. OmpS-display could be valuable when secreted components and contact-mediated signalling is characterized in bacteria.

## ACKNOWLEDGMENTS

This work was supported by grants from the Academy of Finland, the Technology development centre Finland and the University of Helsinki.

## REFERENCES

1.    Lång, H., and Ferenci, T., 1995, Sequence alignment and structural modelling of the LamB glycoporin family. *Biochem. Biophys. Res. Commun.* **208**: 927-934.

2.    Lång, H., and Palva, E.T., 1993, The *ompS* gene of *Vibrio cholerae* encodes a growth-phase-dependent maltoporin. *Mol. Microbiol.* **10**: 891-901.

3.    Lång, H., Mäki, M., Rantakari, A., and Korhonen, T.K., 1999, Characterization of adhesive epitopes with the OmpS-display –system. Submitted to *Eur. J. Biochem.*

4.    Strömberg, N., Marklund, B.-I., Lund, B., Ilver, D., Hamers, A., Gaastra, W., Karlsson, K.-A., and Normark, S., 1990, Host-specificity of uropathogenic *Escherichia coli* depends on differences in binding specificity to Gal1-4Gal containing isoreceptors. *EMBO J.* **9**: 2001-2010.

5.    Zhang, J.P., and Normark, S., 1996, Induction of gene expression in *Escherichia coli* after pilus-mediated adherence. *Science* **273**: 1234-1236.

6.    Haslam, D.B., Boren, T., Falk, P., Ilver, D., Chou, A., Xu, Z., and Normark, S., 1994, The amino-terminal domain of the P-pilus adhesin determines receptor specificity. *Mol. Microbiol.* **14**: 399-409.

# THE ROLE OF THE AirS TWO-COMPONENT SYSTEM IN UROPATHOGENIC *ESCHERICHIA COLI*

[1]Anna-Karin Pernestig, [1]Staffan J. Normark, [2]Dimitris Georgellis and [1]Öjar Melefors

*1: Microbiology and Tumorbiology Center, Karolinska Institutet, SE-171 77 Stockholm, Sweden:[2]Department of Microbiology and Molecular Genetics, Harvard Medical School, Boston, MA 02115, USA*

## 1.     INTRODUCTION

Uropathogenic *Escherichia coli* appear to sense contact with the uroepithelium. To find genes induced during this event, attachment of clinical isolate *DS17* or its isogenic mutant *DS17-8* lacking the P-pilus adhesin PapG, was followed by differential mRNA display. This identified the *airS* gene (Attachment and Iron Regulator Sensor, also known as *barA*); encoding a two-component sensor protein which had no known physiological function[1,2].

A typical two-component system consists of a sensor and a cognate regulator protein. External stimulation leads to auto-phosphorylation of the sensor, which relays the phosphate to the regulator, thus enabling transcriptional regulation of genes needed to adapt to the new environment[3]. The cognate regulator in the AirS two-component system has, so far, not been identified.

*Genes and Proteins Underlying Microbial Urinary Tract Virulence*
Edited by L. Emödy *et al.*, Kluwer Academic/Plenum Publishers, 2000

## 2.    RESULTS

In order to elucidate this regulatory system we first searched for open reading frames (ORFs) homologous to AirS in other bacterial species in the database using the BLASTP 2.0.7 program (National Institute of Health, Bethesda, USA). Sensor proteins exhibiting highest identity to AirS were ExpS (58 % identity) in Erwinia, and GacS (37 % identity) in Pseudomonas.

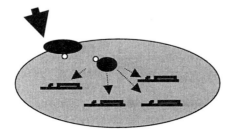

*Figure 1.* Prototype of a two-component system. A membranebound sensor protein phosphorylates a cytoplasmic regulator upon external stimulation, leading to transcriptional regulation of a set of genes.

The cognate regulators of these sensors are known; ExpA[4] and GacA5, respectively. A subsequent search for ORFs homologous to GacA and ExpA in the database identified a group of typical bacterial regulator proteins with high identity, including UvrY of *Escherichia coli*. This suggested that the *Escherichia coli* UvrY protein may be the cognate regulator protein to the AirS sensor (Table 1).

The *uvrY* gene derives its name from a linkage to the *uvrC* gene on a bicistronic transcript[6], an organisation that is conserved in the other listed bacterial species[4,5,7,8]. UvrC is involved in DNA repair, but mutations in *uvrY* have no specific effect on this system, and the real function of UvrY is not known[6].

*Table 1.* Two-component systems homologous to the putative AirS/UvrY system

| Organism | Regulator | Identity with UvrY | Sensor | Identity with AirS |
|---|---|---|---|---|
| *Salmonella* | SirA | 96 % | N.K. | - |
| *Erwinia* | ExpA | 82 % | ExpS | 58 % |
| *Pseudomonas* | GacA | 60 % | GacS | 37 % |
| *Vibrio* | VarA | 75 % | N.K. | - |

N.K.=not known

To experimentally probe the connection between AirS and UvrY, we decided to test if deletion, or over-expression, of the UvrY protein could affect the same phenotypes previously associated with the AirS protein.

Deletion of the *airS* gene was previously suggested to down-modulate the siderophore mediated iron uptake system. This was speculated to decrease growth in the urinary tract and the ability to cause infection[1].

Formation of siderophores can easily be detected by the Crome Azurol S (CAS) agar plate-assay[9]. CAS is a coloured iron complex which can be added to agar plates. Siderophores secreted from the bacterial colony will diffuse in the plate and chelate the iron from the dye complex, thereby releasing the free dye. This is accompanied by a colour change from blue to yellow. The production of siderophores can thus be quantified by measuring the radius of the yellow zone from the edge of the bacterial colony.

A *uvrY* gene inactivated by a chloramphenicol cassette, harboured in strain CS4923 (a kind gift of Dr. G. Moolenaar, University of Leiden)[6], was transduced to *Escherichia coli* K12 strain MC4100. The plasmid pCA9505 carrying the wild type *uvrY* gene[6] was transformed into the same strain, as overexpression of regulator proteins is known to substitute the effect of the sensor. Bacteria were grown in Luria Broth in the presence of the iron chelator desferrioxamine, in order to derepress the Fur-protein, which otherwise could repress the genes involved in siderophore formation. Cultures were grown until stationary phase, diluted in PBS and then plated on CAS containing agar plates, which were incubated at 30°C for two days, after which time the radius of the yellow zone was determined. The results clearly showed that the *uvrY* mutation causes a decrease in siderophore production, while overexpression of the UvrY-protein leads to an increase in siderophore production (Table 2).

There is a precedence in the literature that this group of two-component systems regulators can control the formation of siderophores. GacA, one of the homologous regulator proteins in *Pseudomonas* (Table 1), positively regulates the formation of siderophores in the pytopathogens, *Pseudomonas marginalis*[10] and *Pseudomonas viridiflava*[11]. It is not clear from these studies if the increase in siderophores depends on a direct induction of the biosynthetic genes or if the release of siderophores is affected.

Supported by this evidence we suggest that the AirS and UvrY proteins in *Escherichia coli* constitute a two-component system which is analogous to the GacS-GacA and ExpS-ExpA systems in *Pseudomonas* and *Erwinia*, respectively. The final conclusion will however await further biochemical and genetic evidence for this linkage.

All of the listed two-component regulators (Table 1) are known to control secreted factors which are involved in virulence. The *expS-expA* and *gacS-gacA* two-component systems in *Erwinia* and *Pseudomonas,* respectively, are the key regulators for secreted proteases, toxins and lipases which are central for the pathogenicity of these bacteria[4,5]. The *sirA* gene in *Salmonella typhimurium* controls the expression of *hilA*, which is a key factor controlling virulence genes on pathogenicity islands[12] whilst the *varA* gene in *Vibrio cholerae* regulates transcription of toxin genes[8]. The cognate sensor proteins have not been identified in these bacteria (Table 1).

*Table 2.* CAS agar assay

| Strain | Radius of the yellow halo (cm) ± s.d. |
|---|---|
| MC4100 | 1,65 ± 0,33 |
| MC4100 (uvrY°) | 0,83 ± 0,29 |
| MC4100/ pUvrY | 2,05 ± 0,16 |
| MC4100 (uvrY°)/pUvrY | 2,00 ± 0,41 |

## 3.   DISCUSSION

Iron is very important during bacterial colonisation and there is evidence that the urinary tract is an iron-limited environment. Even if chemical levels of iron in the urine may range from less than one micromolar up to 200 micromolar, most of this iron seems not to be bioavailable[13]. Uropathogenic bacteria isolated directly from urine of patients exhibit outer membrane protein profiles similar to the pattern observed in bacteria grown under iron limiting conditions, suggesting a strong induction of siderophore receptors[14,15].

While many *Escherichia coli* strains encode several different siderophores systems[16], it is not clear if this redundancy in iron uptake systems confers any advantage in the colonisation of the urinary tract. This contention is however supported by the fact that clinical isolates of *Escherichia coli* that produce the siderophore aerobactin grew faster in urine than isolates that did not produce aerobactin[17]. It is also noteworthy that *Escherichia coli* isolates from patients with urinary tract infections more often harbour the aerobactin system than other isolates[18-20]. It is also unclear if hemolysins produced by uropathogenic bacteria have a role in the iron homeostasis during infection.

In our search for genes controlled by the AirS two-component system, we will extend the study to clinical isolates from urinary tract infections. These strains seem to harbour large chromosomal segments (and plasmids) which are not found in K12 laboratory strains and which may well encode virulence genes under the control of this two-component system.

Physical adhesion to uroepithelial cells via AirS might not be the only cue involved in the adaptation to growth in the urinary tract. A recent report has concluded that several *Escherichia coli* genes are induced upon growth in urine as the result of deficiency for certain nutrients[21]. The identified genes encode proteins suggested to be needed for adaptation to changes in osmolarity, pH and lack of nutrients such as iron.

The elucidation of the regulatory systems which are activated during colonization of the urinary tract may well identify novel virulence factors. This could lead to new therapeutic approaches and the development of vaccines.

# REFERENCES

1. Zhang, J.P. and Normark, S., 1996, Induction of gene expression in *Escherichia coli* after pilus-mediated adherence. *Science* **273**: 1234-1236.
2. Nagasawa, S., Tokishita, S., Aiba, H:; and Mizuno; T., 1992, A novel sensor-regulator protein that belongs to the homologous family of signal-transduction proteins involved in adaptive responses in *Escherichia coli*. *Mol. Microbiol.* **6**: 799-807.
3. Parkinson, J.S., 1993, Signal transduction schemes of bacteria. *Cell* **73**: 857-8715.
4. Eriksson ,A.R.B., Andersson, R.A., Pirhonen, M., and Palva, E.T., 1998, Two-component regulators involved in the global control of virulence in *Erwinia carotovora* subsp. *carotovora*. *Mol. Plant-Micr. Interact.* **11**: 743-752.
5. Kitten, T., Kinscherf, T.G., McEvoy, J.L., and Willis, D.K., 1998, A newly identified regulator is required for virulence and toxin production in *Pseudomonas syringae*. Mol. Microbiol. **28**: 917-929.
6. Moolenaar, G.F., van Sluis, C.A., Backendorf, C., and van de Putte, P., 1987, Regulation of the *Escherichia coli* excision repair gene *uvrC*. Overlap between the *uvrC* structural gene and the region coding for a 24 kD protein. *Nucl. Acids Res.* **15**: 4273-4289.
7. Johnston, C., Pegues, D.A., Hueck, C.J., Lee, C.A., and Miller, S.I., 1996, Transcriptional activation of *Salmonella typhimurium* invasion genes by a member of the phosphorylated response-regulator superfamily. *Mol. Microbiol.* **22**: 715-727.
8. Wong, S.M., Carroll, P.A., Rahme, L.G., Ausubel, F.M., and Calderwood, S.B., 1998, Modulation of the ToxR regulon in *Vibrio cholerae* by a member of the family of response regulators. *Infect. Immun.* **66**: 5854-5861.
9. Schwyn, B., and Neilands, J.B., 1987, Universal chemical assay for detection and determination of siderophores. *Anal. Biochem.* **160**: 47-56.
10. Liao, C.H., McCallus, D.E., Fett, W.F., and Kang, G.Y., 1997, Identification of gene loci controlling pectate lyase production and soft-rot pathogenicity in *Pseudomonas marginalis*. *Can. J. Microbiology* **43**: 425-431.
11. Liao, C.H., McCallus, D.E., Wells, J.M., Tzean, S.S., and Kang, G.Y., 1996, The *repB* gene required for production of extracellular enzymes and fluorescent siderophores in *Pseudomonas viridiflava* is an analog of the *gacA* gene of *Pseudomona syringae*. *Can. J. Microbiology* **42**: 177-182.
12. Ahmer, B.M.M., van Reeuwijk, J., Watson, P.R., Wallis, T.S., and Heffron, F., 1999, *Salmonella* SirA is a global regulator of genes mediating enteropathogenesis. *Mol. Microbiol.* **31**: 971-982.
13. Weinberg, E.D., 1984, Iron withholding: A defence against infection and neoplasia. *Physiol. Rev.* **64**: 65-102.

14. Shand, G.H., Anwar, H., Kadurugamuwa, J., Brown, M.R.W., Silverman, S.H., and Melling, J., 1985, *In vivo* evidence that bacteria in urinary tract infection grow under iron restricted conditions. *Infect. Immun.* **48:** 35-39.

15. Robledo, J.A., Serrano, A., and Domingue, G.J., 1990, Outer membrane proteins of *E.coli* in the host-pathogen interaction in urinary tract infection. *J. of Urology* **143:** 386-391.

16. Braun, V., and Hantke, K., 1991, Genetics of bacterial transport. In *Handbook of microbal iron chelators* (G. Winkelmann, ed.), CRC Press, Boca Raton, pp. 107-138.

17. Montgomerie, J.Z., Bindereif, A., Neilands, J.B., Kalmanson, G.M., and Guze, L.B.. 1984, Association of hydroxamate siderophore (aerobactin) with *Escherichia coli* isolated from patients with bacteremia. *Infect. Immun.* **46:** 835-838.

18. Carbonetti, N.H., Boonchai, S., Parry, S.H., Väisänen-Rhen, V., Korhonen, T.K., and Williams, P.H., 1986, Aerobactin-mediated iron uptake by *Escherichia coli* isolates from extraintestinal infections. *Infect. Immun.* **51:** 966-968.

19. Ørskov, I., Svanborg-Edén, C., and Ørskov, F., 1988, Aerobactin production of serotyped *Escherichia coli* from urinary tract infections. *Med. Microbiol. Immunol.* **177:** 9-19.

20. Jacobson S.H., Hammarlind, M., Lidefeldt, K.J., Österberg, E., Tullus, K., and Brauner, A.,. 1988, Incidence of aerobactin positive *Escherichia coli* strains with symptomatic urinary tract infection. *Eur. J. Microbiol. Infect. Dis.* **7:** 630-634.

21. Russo T.A., Carlino, U.B., Mong, A., and Jodush, S.T., 1999, Identification of genes in an extraintestinal isolate of *Escerichia coli* with increased expression after exposure to human urine. *Infect. Immun.* **67:** 5306-5314.

# EXAMINATION OF REGULATORY CROSS-TALK BETWEEN THE DECAY ACCELERATING FACTOR-BINDING FIMBRIAL/AFIMBRIAL ADHESINS AND TYPE I FIMBRIAE

Nicola Holden, Claire Cotterill and David Gally
*Department of Veterinary Pathology, Royal (Dick) School of Veterinary Studies, University of Edinburgh, EH9 1QX.*

## 1.    INTRODUCTION

Bacterial adherence to host cells is often the initial step in infections caused by uropathogens such as *E. coli*. These organisms may carry the determinants for several fimbrial and afimbrial adhesins. However, since the expression of many adhesin gene clusters (which can be chromosomal or plasmid based) is phase variable, only a portion of the population may express a particular adhesin at a given time. Some of *E. coli* adhesins that have been associated with urinary tract infections include: type I, Pap pili and the Dr. family of adhesins (AFA-I, and AFA-III).

Previous work has shown that cross-talk can occur between some of the adhesin gene clusters, although differences have been demonstrated in the type of communication. Studies have indicated that expression of some adhesins leads to repression of others. For example, co-expression of both S fimbriae and type 1 fimbriae in a culture of strain 3040 occurred in only 3% of bacteria following growth for 35 hours at 37°C. The remainder of the culture contained 33% S fimbriate bacteria, 52% type 1 fimbriate bacteria

*Genes and Proteins Underlying Microbial Urinary Tract Virulence*
Edited by L. Emődy *et al.*, Kluwer Academic/Plenum Publishers, 2000

and 12 % were non-fimbriate[1]. A probable explanation for the above comes from recent studies showing that PapB reduces expression of type 1 fimbriae by repressing recombination carried out by FimB[2]. In contrast, studies with Prf and S fimbriae, have shown that the regulators PrfB and PrfI could complement, in part, for the loss of SfaB and SfaC, respectively. Moreover, the Prf regulators were required for efficient expression of S fimbriae[3]. This perhaps represents an example of co-operativity by which related adhesins could be co-expressed at the single cell level. This may allow consolidation of attachment to different host cell receptors. Alternatively, independent expression at the single cell level may be important to prevent interference and allow 'right time-right place' expression of relevant adhesins. Both of these factors relate to efficiency of expression from the perspective of the bacterium.

Sequence alignment of adhesin regulators show that many of the proteins fall into 2 categories, PapB-like and PapI-like proteins. Fig 1 shows an alignment of several of the PapB-like proteins. Regions of high homology are evident, especially in the central region of the sequences. The high level of homology indicates that these proteins play similar roles. Mutational analysis of PapB has indicated that the areas of the protein that most clearly affected DNA binding to the *pap* operon, or protein oligomerisation, are completely conserved in the PapB family (Fig 1)[4]. Differences in the amino termini of the PapB-like proteins suggest that this region may confer some specificity to the function of adhesin regulators. We are investigating members of the PapB family to determine whether differences in the proteins affect their ability to cross regulate type 1 fimbriae.

In this paper we have cloned the *papB* and *daaA* regulators into pBAD18 and compared the effects of their expression on phase switching of type 1 fimbriae.

## 2.        MATERIALS AND METHODS

### 2.1      Bacterial Strains

For all cloning work, the host strain *E. coli* AAEC185 was used[5]. For analysis of effect on type 1 fimbrial expression and phase switching, the following strains were used: *E. coli* K-12 MG1655 (wild type)[6], AAEC198A (*fimB⁺ fimE⁺ fimA-lacZYA*[7], AAEC370A (*fimB⁺ fimE fimA-lacZYA*[8].

```
PapB            --MAHHEVISRSGNAFLL--NIRESVLLPGSMSEMHFFLLIGISSIHSDRVILAMKDYLVGGHSRKEVCEKYQMN

PefB            MMLNRKDADYYLGKEIML-ARIRRGALIPAKVNEEHFWLLIGISSIHSEKIIQALRDYLVFGVSRKDVCERYEVN

FaeB            MKGGAMENRLSGQKGVFFSQRIKGHKLLPAELPEEKFWLLAEISPIRSEKVLYALRDYLVLGYERKEVCARYDVS

DaaA            ---------MRERYLHLA--DTPQGILMSGQVPEYQFWLLAEISPVHSEKVINALRDYLVMGYNRMEACGRHGVS

AfaA            ---------MRERYLYLA--DTPQGILMSGQVPEYQFWLLAEISPVHSEKVINALRDYLVMGYNRMEACGRHSVS

DaaA truncated       ----------------MSGQVPEYQFWLLAEISPVHSEKVINALRDYLVMGYNRMEACGRHGVS

FanB            MYIDNYLIMRKINMEETI-LSLTSYQLRPGKVDKKQFVLLIDVSSIRSYKVINALEDYFVNGKNRKEICDNHKIN


PapB            NGYFSTTLGRLIRLNALAARLAPYYTDESSAFD-----

PefB            NGYFSTSLNRLSRISQAAAQMVVYYS-----------

FaeB            SSYFSIALGRISHVNRVVYSLAPYYADPGNDFFDRPY-

DaaA            PGYFSGALKRFQRVSQTVYRLVPFYFPEAGHEVHRGE-

AfaA            PGYFSGALKRFQRVSQTVYRLVPFYFPEAGHEVHRGE-

DaaA truncated  PGYFSGALKRFQRVSQTVYRLVPFYFPEAGHEVHRGE-

FanB            QGYLSLKIRELQDISLRIYNISHCI------------
```

*Figure 1.* Optimal best-fit alignment of PapB-like proteins. Identical amino acids have been indicated in bold[9].

## 2.2 Plasmid Constructs

The *papB* and *daaA* genes were both PCR amplified and subsequently cloned into pBAD18 controlled by P$_{BAD}$, forming pBAD-*papB* and pBAD-*daaA*, respectively. pHGM88 plasmid, *papB* cloned into pACYC184, controlled by P$_{lac}$UV5, was a gift from B.E. Uhlin. pSSS9 contained the whole F1845 operon and pPAP5 contained the whole *pap* operon. The *daaA* gene was sequenced from the pBAD-*daaA*3', pSSS9 and pBAD-*daaA* plasmids, consecutively.

## 2.3 Switching Assays

Measurement of *fimB* switching (from OFF to ON) was carried out in strain AAEC370A *(fimA-lacZYA fimE)*, which was transformed with the plasmids of interest, described in Gally *et al*[10]. The results are presented as the switching frequency per cell per generation.

## 2.4 β–galactosidase Assays

The β-galactosidase assays were carried out essentially as described in Miller[11]. Strain AAEC198A *(fimA-lacZYA)* was transformed with the plasmids of interest. Inducing agents were added to the media after 3 hours of exponential growth.

## 2.5    Protein Hybridisation - Dot Blots

Strain MG1655 (type 1 positive) was transformed with plasmids of interest. The transformants were grown in static minimal MOPS media, (which contained the appropriate antibiotics and inducers) for 48 hours, at 37°C. AAEC185 (type 1 negative) was included as a negative control. The cells were collected onto Hybond N nitrocellulose filter using a Biorad DotBlot, which was incubated with monoclonal FimA antibody. Hybridisation to the FimA antibody was visualised using ECL chemiluminescent reagents.

## 3.    RESULTS

## 3.1    PapB Repressed the FimB OFF to ON Switching Frequency in AAEC370A

Switching by FimB was measured in strain AAEC370A (*fimA::lacZYA, fimE*). When PapB was overexpressed, either in pACYC184 or pBAD18 backgrounds, the FimB switching frequency was reduced by more than 2 orders of magnitude. In contrast, DaaA did not affect the frequency of FimB switching (Table 1).

## 3.2    Type 1 Fimbrial Expression is Repressed by *papB* in Static LB Medium

A dot blot (Fig 2) was carried out on bacteria that had been grown in static LB medium for 30 hours, at 37°C. The bacteria were harvested and incubated with monoclonal FimA antibody. FimA expression decreased more than 27-fold in the presence of *papB*. However, neither the complete version or the truncated version of *daaA* affected expression of type 1 fimbriae.

## 3.3    Revised Nucleic Acid Sequence of *daaA*

The *daaA* gene was sequenced, and revealed the presence a G/C insertion relative to the ribosome binding site (position 1108 – 1112) of the published sequence[12]. Consequently, the revised start codon is located 16 codons upstream of the originally proposed start site of *daaA*. (The same reading frame is used from the new start site). The new deduced amino acid sequence is 98% identical to that of the afimbrial adhesin regulator, AFAA-III, shown in Fig 1. The original sequence is also shown, referred to as DaaA truncated.

*Table 1.*   FimB switching in AAEC370

| Plasmid | FimB switching frequency (off to on) |
|---------|--------------------------------------|
| PGMH88 (*papB*) | $< 7 \times 10^{-5}$ [a] |
| Control vector | $2.53 \times 10^{-3}$ +/- 0.68 |
| PBAD-*papB* | $< 7 \times 10^{-5}$ [a] |
| PBAD-*daaA* | $2.8 \times 10^{-3}$ +/- 0.48 |
| PBAD-*daaA* truncated | $1.56 \times 10^{-3}$ +/- 0.08 |
| Control vector | $2.06 \times 10^{-3-}$ +/- 0.1 |

a – no colonies were recovered in the on phase

## 3.4     PapB Reduces *fimA::lacZYA* Expression in AAEC198A

β–galactosidase activity was monitored in strain AAEC198A, which contained a transcriptional fusion of *fimA::lacZYA*. In the presence of PapB, *fimA* expression was reduced by approximately 50%, when *papB* was cloned into the pACYC184 background, i.e. pHGM88. The DaaA regulator appeared to have no effect on *fimA* expression (Table 2).

*Table 2.* Expression of *fimA*, assessed from β-galactosidase activity, in AAEC198A

| Plasmid | Expt.1 LB | Expt.2 LB | Expt.3 MOPS |
|---------|-----------|-----------|-------------|
| PGMH88 | 91 +/- 4 | 88 +/-4 | 290 +/-1 |
| Control Vector | 145 +/-3 | 121 +/-13 | 564 +/-18 |

| Plasmid | Expt.1 LB | Expt.2 LB |
|---------|-----------|-----------|
| PBAD-*daaA* | 341 +/-5 | 378 +/-6 |
| Control Vector | 332 +/- 13 | 285 +/-6 |

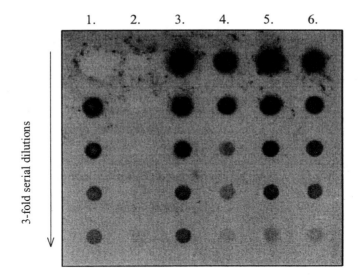

*Figure 2.* Dot blot showing type 1 fimbriae expression in MG1655. 1 MG1655 positive control. 2 AA185 negative control. 3 pBAD vector. 4 pBAD-*papB*. 5 pBAD-*daaA*. 6 pBAD-*daaA* truncated

## 4.      CONCLUSION

Several studies have shown that cross-regulation occurs between adhesin gene clusters in *E. coli*, although differences in the type of cross talk have been demonstrated. Our findings confirmed the repression effect of *papB* on FimB switching[2]. In this study we demonstrate that the PapB homologue, DaaA, did not repress type 1 fimbriae expression. Mutational analyses of the PapB protein have indicated that amino acids involved in DNA binding and oligomerisation are present in the highly conserved domains of the PapB family[4]. However, significant differences in the PapB family occur at the amino terminal of the proteins, and it is possible that this region is important for functions of the proteins that vary between the family members. For example, the ability to cross regulate between adhesin gene clusters. This remains to be tested.

The finding that members of the PapB family differ in their ability to inhibit type 1 fimbrial expression raises interesting questions concerning co-ordination of adhesin production at the single cell level. Why would it be an advantage for Pap and S fimbriae to prevent type 1 fimbriae from being produced simultaneously? Why is this likely not to be the case for F1845, AFA-I and AFA-III or do alternative mechanisms of cross talk exist?

We are currently addressing these and other questions about the co-ordinate expression of adhesin gene clusters in *E. coli* at the single cell level.

## 5. SUMMARY

- The revised sequence of DaaA means that the protein is 98% identical to the afimbrial adhesin regulator AFAA-III.
- While PapB repressed FimB OFF to ON switching in strain AAEC370A, this was not the case for DaaA.
- PapB, but not DaaA, reduced the level of expression of type 1 fimbriae, in static LB media.
- Attention is now focused on the amino terminus of the PapB protein as the possible domain involved in cross talk with type 1 fimbriae.

## ACKNOWLEDGEMENT

This study was supported by the British Biotechnology and Science Research Council. Thank you to Yan Xia and Professor B.E. Uhlin for their support and for providing reagents.

## REFERENCES

1. Norwicki, B., Rhen, M., Vaisanen-Rhen, V., Pere, A., Korhonen., T.K., 1985, Kinetics of phase variation between S and type 1 fimbriae of *Escherichia coli*. *FEMS Microbiol. Lett.* **28:** 237 – 242.
2. Xia, Y, Gally, D., Forsman, K., Ulhin, B.E., Manuscript in preparation.
3. Morschhäuser, J., Vetter, V., Emődy, L., Hacker, J., 1994, Adhesin regulatory genes within large, unstable DNA regions of pathogenic *Escherichia coli*: cross-talk between different adhesin gene clusters. *Mol Microbiol.* **11:** 555 – 566.
4. Xia, Y., Uhlin, B., E., 1999, Mutational analysis of the PapB transcriptional regulator in *Escherichia coli J. Biol. Chem.* **274:** 19723 – 19730.
5. Blomfield, I.C., Mcclain, M.S., Eisenstein, B.I., 1991, Type-1 fimbriae mutants of Escherichia-coli K12 - characterization of recognized afimbriate strains and construction of new fim deletion mutants. *Mol. Microbiol.* **5:** 1439 – 1445.
6. Guyer, M.S., Reed, R.R., Steitz, J.A., Low, K.B., (1981, Identification of a sex-factor-affinity site in *E. coli* as gamma delta. *Cold Spring Harb. Symp. Quant. Biol.* **45:** 135 – 140.
7. Blomfield, I.C., Mcclain, M.S., Princ, J.A., Calie, P.J., Eisenstein, B.I., 1991, Type I fimbriation and fimE mutants of Escherichia coli K-12. *J. Bacteriol.* **173:** 5298 – 5307.

8. Blomfield, I.C., Vaughn, V., Rest, R.F., Eisenstein, B.I., 1991, Allelic exchange in Escherichia coli using the Bacillus subtilis sacB gene and a temperature sensitive pSC101 replicon. *Mol. Microbiol.* **5:** 1447 – 1457.

9. Altschul, S.F., Carroll, R.J., and Lipman, D.J., 1989, Weights for data related by a tree. J. Mol.. Biol. **207:** 647-653.

10. Gally, D.L., Bogan, J.A., Eisenstein, B.I., Blomfield, I.C., 1993, Environmental regulation of the *fim* switch controlling type 1 fimbrial phase variation in *Escherichia coli* K-12: effects of temperature and media. *J. Bacteriol.* **175:** 6186 – 6193.

11. Miller, J.H., 1972, *Experiments in molecular genetics.* Cold Spring Harbor, New York.

12. Bilge, S.S., Apostol, J.M., Fullner, K.J., Moseley,S.L., 1993,Transcriptional organization of the F1845 fimbrial adhesin determinant of *Escherichia coli. Mol. Biol.* **6:** 993-100.

# MODULATION OF THE POLYSACCHARIDE INTERCELLULAR ADHESIN (PIA) EXPRESSION IN BIOFILM FORMING *STAPHYLOCOCCUS EPIDERMIDIS*

*Analysis of Genetic Mechanisms*

[1]Wilma Ziebuhr, [1]Isabel Lößner, [1]Shwan Rachid, [1]Katja Dietrich, [2]Friedrich Götz, and [1]Jörg Hacker

[1]*Institut für Molekulare Infektionsbiologie, Röntgenring 11, 97070 Würzburg, Germany*
[2]*Mikrobielle Genetik, Waldhäuser Str. 70/8, 72076 Tübingen, Germany*

## 1.    INTRODUCTION

*Staphylococcus epidermidis* is a major pathogen in nosocomial infections especially in immunocompromised patients[1]. The majority of *S. epidermidis* infections are associated with the use of indwelling medical devices and it is suggested that the ability of *S. epidermidis* to generate biofilms on smooth surfaces contributes significantly to the pathogenesis of polymer associated infections. Recently, essential mechanisms of biofilm formation in *S. epidermidis* and *S. aureus* have been elucidated on the genetic and biochemical level. Thus, biofilm formation was found to depend on the presence and the expression of the *ica*ADBC gene cluster which is involved in the production of an extracellular polysaccharide adhesin (PIA)[2,3,4] . The PIA mediates the contact of the bacterial cells to each other and bacteria become embedded in this slimy matrix during the accumulative phase of biofilm formation[4]. The *ica* operon was found to be widespread in *S. epidermidis* multiresistant isolates causing polymer-associated infections and its expression was shown to undergo strong phenotypic variation[5]. This work summarizes genetic mechanisms which contribute to an altered *ica*

*Genes and Proteins Underlying Microbial Urinary Tract Virulence*
Edited by L. Emödy *et al.*, Kluwer Academic/Plenum Publishers, 2000

151

expression and subsequently to a varying biofilm production in pathogenic
*S. epidermidis*.

## 2.        GENETIC MECHANISMS OF ALTERED *ICA*-EXPRESSION

### 2.1      Phase Variation of Biofilm Formation is Mediated by the Insertion and Precise Excision of the Naturally Occurring Insertion Sequence IS*256* into the *ica*-operon

Upon subcultivation of biofilm-forming strains, biofilm-negative
variants occur in a frequency of $10^{-6}$. After repeated passages these variants
shift back to the biofilm-forming phenotype of the parent strains (Fig 1).

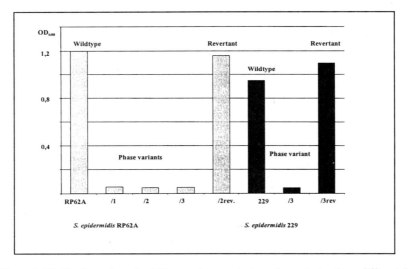

*Figure 1.* Biofilm formation of wild types, phase variants, and revertants of two different *S. epidermidis* strains.

In a substantial part of the variants the mobile genetic element IS*256* was
found to be inserted in different sites of the *ica* gene cluster, causing the
inactivation of these genes and leading to a subsequent impaired PIA
production[6]. In each case a target site duplication of 8 base pairs was

created. In the revertant strains nucleotide sequence analyses of the *ica* genes revealed that the IS*256* element had been precisely excised, including the duplicated 8-bp target site and the wild type *ica* sequence was found to be completly restored. Southern analysis of chromosomal DNA with an IS*256*-specific gene probe revealed that IS*256* resides in multiple copies on the chromosome of the *S. epidermidis* isolates investigated. In all biofilm-negative variants additional IS*256*-specific fragments were observed. Also, in case of the revertants the hybridization patterns differed clearly from those of the wild type strains.

Interestingly, the majority of IS*256* insertions occured closely clustered within the *icaC* gene which seems to represent a preferred insertion site of the element (Fig 2).

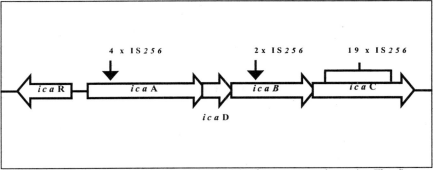

*Figure 2.* Number and insertion sites of IS*256* in the *ica* gene cluster in. The figure summarizes data obtained from the analyses of different *S. epidermidis* isolates and illustrates that the majority of IS insertions occur in the *icaC* gene which might represent a hot spot for IS*256* insertions.

## 2.2     Loss of PIA Production by Large Chromosomal Deletions

In the course of our studies biofilm negative variants were observed that did not revert to the biofilm forming phenotype of the wild type. Analysis of these variants revealed that the PIA negative phenotype was caused by the complete loss of the *ica* gene cluster (Ziebuhr *et al.*, unpublished). Chromosomal *ica* deletions were detected in different clinical isolates and comprised DNA-fragments of approximately 150 kb in size. They also resulted in impaired IS*256* hybridization patterns of the mutants in comparison to their corresponding wild type strains. The deletion frequency was found to range from $10^{-7}$ to $10^{-8}$ in different isolates. This value is much lower than the frequency determined previously for the insertion of the IS*256* element into the *ica*-operon which is $10^{-6}$. Currently, the large chromosomal DNA-fragments are investigated by nucleotide sequencing. The intention of this work is the identification of the flanking DNA regions of the deleted fragments which might give advices on the underlying deletion mechanism.

## 2.3     Loss    of    PIA    Production    by    Chromosomal Rearrangements

Although staphylococcal infections preferentially cause acute diseases, bacterial persistence and relapsing infections are a common clinical problem[7]. The molecular basis of this phenomenon is not clear, however, staphylococci are known to have the capacity to change phenotypic features very rapidly[8,9,10,11]. It is assumed that this phenotypic variability might reflect the flexibility of the staphylococcal genome.

We have isolated five multiresistant *S. epidermidis* isolates from different courses of a recurrent polymer-associated infection. Three *S. epidermidis* strains were obtained before and during an antibiotic therapy and, two further strains were isolated after the therapy and a relapse of the infection. All strains were analyzed with regard to biofilm production and antibiotic susceptibility. *S. epidermidis* 1-3 were found to produce biofilms on polystyrene tissue culture plates, whereas strains *S. epidermidis* 4 and 5 were biofilm negative. The five isolates exhibited identical antibiotic resistance pattern, except that in the strains from the recurrent infection resistance to rifampicin and increased minimal inhibitory concentrations to aminoglycoside antibiotics had emerged.

DNA-fingerprinting by PFGE indicated the clonal origin of all isolates (Fig 3). However, some DNA-rearrangements and differences in the IS*256*-specific hybridization pattern (data not shown) could be identified in the isolates *S. epidermidis* 4 and 5 from the relapsing infection (Fig 3, lanes 4, and 5). Although the *ica* gene cluster was not directly involved, the rearrangements led to altered biofilm formation and increased expression of aminoglycoside resistance traits by an unknown mechanism. This observation highlights that variation of biofilm expression obviously occurs *in vivo* and can be accompanied by complex reorganizations of the staphylococcal genome. It is tempting to speculate that these processes are favoured by the selective pressure of antibiotics. However, more experimental work is needed to investigate the molecular mechanisms in more detail.

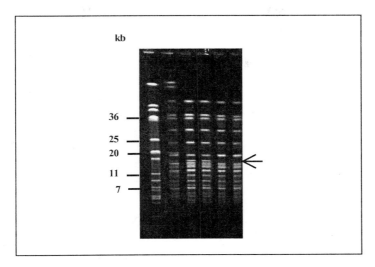

*Figure 3.* Analysis of *Sma*I-restricted genomic DNA by pulsed field gel electrophoresis of the *S. epidermdis* isolates of two infection courses. Lanes 1, 2, 3: *S. epidermidis* 1-3; lanes 4 and 5: *S. epidermidis* 4 and 5; M: Molecular weight standard. The differing DNA fragments are marked by an arrowhead.

## 3.     DISCUSSION

Numerous pathogens, which are common sources of persistent and recurrent infections, e.g. *Pseudomonas aeruginosa*, *E. coli*, Streptococci as well as Staphylococci, have been shown to generate biofilms[12]. In a sense, bacteria organized in biofilms can be considered to resemble multicellular organisms and this point of view is supported by the fact that bacterial cells in biofilms considerably differ from their planctonic counterparts in terms of metabolic activity, gene expression and an inherent higher resistance to antibiotics[13]. In the course of an infection caused by biofilm-forming bacteria planctonic cells, which obviously cannot efficiently be eliminated by host defense mechanisms, are currently released from the sessile population. In this respect, it has been hypothesized that, additionally to mechanic detachment, specific genetic programs might exist which abolish the extracellular matrix substance expression[14]. However, these genetic mechanisms are not well characterized and only poorly understood.

We have analyzed the varying biofilm expression in the nosocomial pathogen *S. epidermidis* and, so far, we have identified three mechanisms which contribute to biofilm detachment. These processes include phase variation of the *ica* expression, large chromosomal deletions, and DNA-rearrangements. Interestingly, in all of these processes IS*256* seems to be involved. Preliminary epidemiological investigations on the distribution of IS*256* in biofilm forming *S. epidermidis* isolates suggest a strong correlation between the presence of the *ica* gene cluster and the IS element (Ziebuhr *et al.*, unpublished). Insertion sequence elements are known to contribute to the flexibility of the bacterial genome and they play an important role in microevolution[15,16]. However, they are also involved in the variation of gene expression. Thus, IS elements have the capacity to cause irreversible inactivation of genes by random or site-specific transposition and, many elements control neighboring gene expression by the creation of hybrid promoters or by the exhibition of polar effects. In addition to simple transposition, IS elements can also give rise to complex DNA rearrangements including deletions, inversions, gene amplifications and the fusion of two DNA molecules by cointegrate formation[15]. At the present stage of experimental work it is tempting to speculate that the action of IS*256* is the driving force in the variation of biofilm expression in *S. epidermidis*. However, it is also likely that other mechanisms do exist which influence this process as well.

Finally, in addition to the detachment from sessile biofilms, the complete loss of biofilm synthesis could also have other biological consequences. For example, it is conceivable that this mechanism contributes to the evasion of the host immune response. However, it remains yet to be investigated to what extent the varying biofilm production contributes to the pathogenesis of polymer-associated *S. epidermidis* infections.

## ACKNOWLEDGEMENTS

The authors' work is supported by the BMBF (grant no. 01KI9608), the Paul-Ehrlich-Gesellschaft for Chemotherapy, the Deutsche Forschungs-gemeinschaft (Graduiertenkolleg Infektiologie) and the Fond der Chemischen Industrie.

## REFERENCES

1.  Rupp, M.E. and Archer, G.L., 1994, Coagulase-negative staphylococci: pathogens associated with medical progress. *Clin. Infect. Dis.* **19:** 231-243.
2.  Heilmann, C., Schweitzer, O., Gerke, C., Vanittanakom, N., Mack, D. and Götz, F., 1996, Molecular basis of intercellular adhesion in the biofilm-forming Staphylococcus epidermidis. *Mol. Microbiol.* **20:** 1083-1091.

3. Gerke, C., Kraft, A., Süssmuth, R., Schweitzer, O. and Götz, F., 1998, Characterization of the N-acetylglucosaminyltransferase activity involved in the biosynthesis of the Staphylococcus epidermidis polysaccharide intercellular adhesin. *J. Biol. Chem.* **273:** 18586-18593.

4. Mack, D., Fischer, W., Krokotsch, A., Leopold, K., Hartmann, R., Egge, H. and Laufs, R., 1996, The intercellular adhesin involved in biofilm accumulation of Staphylococcus epidermidis is a linear beta-1,6-linked glucosaminoglycan: purification and structural analysis. *J. Bacteriol.* **178:** 175-183.

5. Ziebuhr, W., Heilmann, C., Götz, F., Meyer, P., Wilms, K., Straube, E. and Hacker, J., 1997, Detection of the intercellular adhesion gene cluster (ica) and phase variation in Staphylococcus epidermidis blood culture strains and mucosal isolates. *Infect. Immun.* **65:** 890-896.

6. Ziebuhr, W., Krimmer, V., Rachid, S., Lößner, I., Götz, F. and Hacker, J., 1999, A novel mechanism of phase variation of virulence in Staphylococcus epidermidis: evidence for control of the polysaccharide intercellular adhesin synthesis by alternating insertion and excision of the insertion sequence element IS256. *Mol. Microbiol.* **32:** 345-356.

7. Proctor, R.A., van Langevelde, P., Kristjansson, M., Maslow, J.N. and Arbeit, R.D., 1995, Persistent and relapsing infections associated with small-colony variants of Staphylococcus aureus. *Clin. Infect. Dis.* **20:** 95-102.

8. Deighton, M., Pearson, S., Capstick, J., Spelman, D. and Borland, R., 1992, Phenotypic variation of Staphylococcus epidermidis isolated from a patient with native valve endocarditis. *J. Clin. Microbiol.* **30:** 2385-2390.

9. Christensen, G.D., Baddour, L.M. and Simpson, W.A., 1987, Phenotypic variation of Staphylococcus epidermidis slime production in vitro and in vivo. *Infect. Immun.* **55:** 2870-2877.

10. Christensen, G.D., Baddour, L.M., Madison, B.M., Parisi, J.T., Abraham, S.N., Hasty, D.L., Lowrance, J.H., Josephs, J.A. and Simpson, W.A., 1990, Colonial morphology of staphylococci on Memphis agar: phase variation of slime production, resistance to beta-lactam antibiotics, and virulence. *J. Infect. Dis.* **161:** 1153-1169.

11. Mempel, M., Feucht, H., Ziebuhr, W., Endres, M., Laufs, R. and Grüter, L., 1994, Lack of mecA transcription in slime-negative phase variants of methicillin-resistant Staphylococcus epidermidis. *Antimicrob. Agents Chemother.* **38:** 1251-1255.

12. Costerton, J.W., Stewart, P.S. and Greenberg, E.P., 1999, Bacterial biofilms: a common cause of persistent infections. *Science* **284:** 1318-1322.

13. Shapiro, J.A., 1998, Thinking about bacterial populations as multicellular organisms. *Ann. Rev. Microbiol.* **52:** 81-104.

14. Costerton, J.W., Lewandowski, Z., Caldwell, D.E., Korber, D.R. and Lappin-Scott, H.M., 1995, Microbial biofilms. *Ann. Rev. Microbiol.* **49:** 711-745.

15. Arber, W., 1993, Evolution of prokaryotic genomes. *Gene.* **135:** 49-56.

16. Mahillon, J. and Chandler, M., 1998, Insertion sequences. *Microbiol. Mol. Biol. Rev.* **62:** 725-774.

# INDUCTION OF *STAPHYLOCOCCUS EPIDERMIDIS* BIOFILM FORMATION BY ENVIRONMENTAL FACTORS: THE POSSIBLE INVOLVEMENT OF THE ALTERNATIVE TRANSCRIPTION FACTOR SIGB

Shwan Rachid, Seunghak Cho, Knut Ohlsen, Jörg Hacker, and Wilma Ziebuhr
*Institut für Molekulare Infektionsbiologie der Universität Würzburg, Röntgenring 11, D-97070 Würzburg, Germany*

## 1.    INTRODUCTION

*Staphylococcus epidermidis* is a major cause of nosocomial infections associated with the use of indwelling medical devices[1]. Chronic infection of a prosthetic implant can serve as a septic focus that can lead to osteomyelitis, acute sepsis, and death, especially in immunocompromised patients[2]. The ability of *S. epidermidis* to generate thick biofilms on smooth polymer surfaces is regarded as the crucial step in the pathogenesis of these infections. It is associated with the production of a polysaccharide intercellular adhesin (PIA). The PIA represents a linear β-1,6-linked glucosaminoglycan and the bacteria become embedded in this slimy extracellular matrix during the accumulative phase of biofilm formation[3]. The enzymes involved in the PIA synthesis are encoded by the *ica*ADBC operon which was found to be widespread in *S. epidermidis* clinical isolates [4,5,6]. The expression of this operon undergoes strong intrastrain variation and the investigation of the varying *ica*-expression revealed that this phenomenon is based on different genetic mechanisms including phase variation, *ica*-deletions and large chromosomal rearrangements [6,7]. In this work we give evidence that *S. epidermidis* biofilm expression can also be

*Genes and Proteins Underlying Microbial Urinary Tract Virulence*
Edited by L. Emödy *et al.*, Kluwer Academic/Plenum Publishers, 2000

159

influenced by environmental factors. Preliminary data on regulatory pathways of the *ica* expression suggest that the alternative transcription factor sigB might be involved in the *S. epidermidis* biofilm regulation.

## 2.     THE EFFECT OF ENVIRONMENTAL FACTORS ON THE ICA EXPRESSION

For these studies we used the biofilm-forming clinical isolate *S. epidermidis* 215 which was obtained from a catheter-related septicemia from a immunocompromised patient. Biofilm formation was determined quantitatively by optical density measurement of the bacteria on polystyrene tissue culture plates[8].

A preculture was diluted 1:200 in trypticase soy broth, and 0.2-ml aliquots were placed into the wells of a tissue culture plate. Plates were incubated 18 hours at 37 °C. Following washing of the wells the adhereing bacteria were stained with crystal violet and the density of the biofilm was measured by using an ELISA reader at 570 nm. The influence of different concentrations of sodiumdodecyl sulfate (SDS), urea, ethanol, and $H_2O_2$ on the biofilm production was studied. High expression of biofilm was detected by addition of 0,005 and 0,01 per cent SDS to the growth medium. The biofilm production was 20-fold higher in comparison to the control. (Fig 1, 2). Likewise, the addition of 0,007-0,5% urea increased the biofilm expression 8-fold (Fig 3). Incubation of the bacteria with ethanol or $H_2O_2$ in concentrations ranging from 0,015- 3 per cent and 0,0015 - 0,0125 per cent, respectively, also induced the expression of the biofilm in *S. epidermidis* 215 (Fig 4, 5).

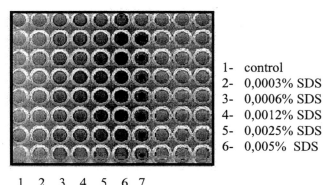

1-  control
2-  0,0003% SDS
3-  0,0006% SDS
4-  0,0012% SDS
5-  0,0025% SDS
6-  0,005% SDS

1   2   3   4   5   6   7

*Figure 1.* Effect of different concentrations of sodiumdodecyl sulfate (SDS) on the *S. epidermidis* 215 biofilm formation on a polystyrene tissue culture plate.

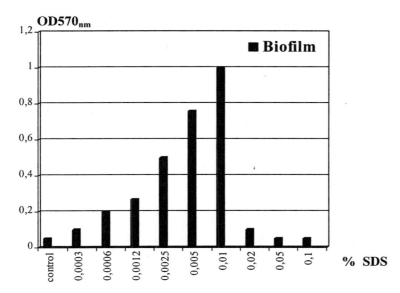

*Figure 2.* Effect of different concentrations of SDS on the biofilm production in *S. epidermidis* 215.

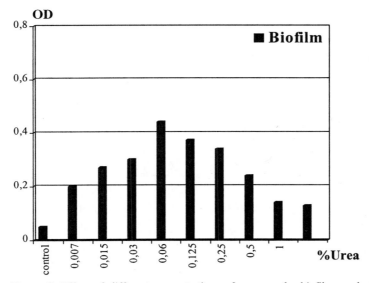

*Figure 3.* Effect of different concentrations of urea on the biofilm production in S. epidermidis 215.

*Shwan Rachid et al.*

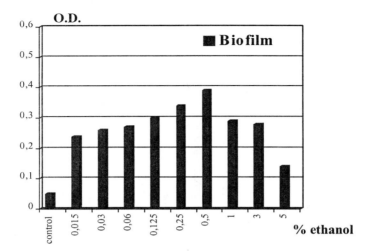

*Figure 4.* Effect of ethanol on the biofilm production in *S. epidermidis* 215.

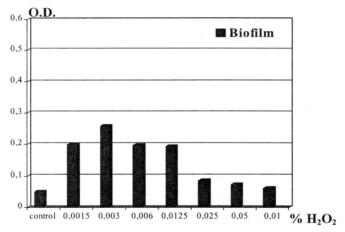

*Figure 5.* Effect of different concentrations of $H_2O_2$ on the biofilm production in *S.epidermidis* 215.

## 3. IDENTIFICATION OF THE ALTERNATIVE TRANSCRIPTION FACTOR *SIG*B IN *S. EPIDERMIDIS*

The survival of bacteria in different environments depends on their ability to response to a wide range of changing external conditions. Sigma factors are likely to play an important role in the bacterial adaptive response[9,10]. In several pathogenic species alternative transcription factors (e. g. $\sigma^B$) are involved in the expression of virulence associated genes[11].

Recently, in *Staphylococcus aureus* an alternative sigma factor with strong amino acid sequence similarities to the *sig*B gene of *Bacillus subtilis* was identified[12]. Characterization of this factor elucidated its role in the expression of stationary phase genes, heat shock, stress response, and the regulation of virulence genes[13,14,15].

We use a *sig*B specific DNA probe from *S. aureus* in Southern hybridization experiments and identified the corresponding gene locus in *S. epidermidis*. We have tested a range of *S. epidermidis* strains obtained from infections as well as saprophytic isolates from the mucosa. All strains hybridized specifically with the *sig*B gene probe. Additionally, the *sig*B operon was PCR-amplified from *S. epidermidis* by using the corresponding *S. aureus* specific primers. Direct nucleotide sequencing of the PCR products revealed strong sequence similarities both on the nucleotide and amino acid level.

In order to elucidate the possible involvement of the sigB factor in the regulation of biofilm expression in *S. epidermidis* we investigated the $\sigma^B$ expression under conditions which are known to induce the *ica* expression. For this purpose we used again *S. epidermidis* 215 and a second isolate, *S. epidermidis* 567, which was obtained from a catheter-associated urinary tract infection. Northern blot analysis of the *sig*B transcription by using a [32]P-labelled gene probe revealed that the operon is expressed in the stationary growth phase (Fig. 6, lanes 1, 2, 3, and 4), and upon osmotic stress by addition of 3, 4, and 5 per cent sodium chloride to the growth medium (Fig 6, lanes 5-10) in both *S. epidermidis* strains.

## 4. DISCUSSION

Staphylococci represent a substantial part of the healthy skin and mucosal microflora. However, in the last decades especially the coagulase-negative species emerged as a common cause of nosocomial infections. The ability to generate biofilms on polymer surfaces has now been recognized as the major mechanism in the *S. epidermidis* pathogenesis. While the molecular

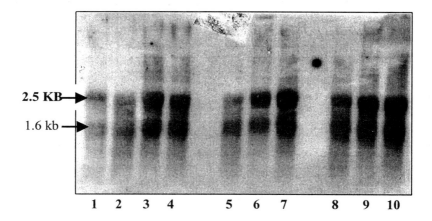

Fig. 6. Northern analysis of the *sig*B expression during different phases of the bacterial growth. Lane 1, lag phase; lane 2, logarithmic phase; lane 3, stationary phase; lane 4 late stationary phase. Lane 5, 6 and 7 logarithmic phase under the influence of 3, 4 and 5 per cent NaCl in *S. epidermidis* 215. Lane 8, 9 and 10 logarithmic phase under the influence of 3, 4 and 5 per cent NaCl in *S. epidermidis* 567 .

mechanisms of staphylococcal biofilm synthesis have been elucidated on the genetic and biochemical level, our knowledge on the regulation of this important virulence factor is still limited. Our results suggest that biofilm formation in *S. epidermidis* is strongly influenced by external signals. Thus, we demonstrate that biofilm formation is enhanced under conditions that are toxic for the bacterial cell (e. g. high osmolarity, influence of detergents, urea, and ethanol or oxidative stress by hydrogene superoxide). Although these factors act on different metabolic pathways or cell structures, they all resulted in a clear increase of biofilm production. Our data are consistent with observations made in many other bacteria (e. g. *Pseudomonas aeruginosa* or *E. coli*), where biofilm formation is also induced by environmental stress[2,16]. It is suggested that the multicellular organization in biofilms is a crucial mechanism for bacteria to withstand unfavourable external conditions[17,18]. Thus, bacteria in biofilms are protected from the host immune response or antibiotics. Thereby, biofilms do not only act as a mechanical or diffusion barrier. Their protective effect is also due to varying gene expression patterns of biofilm forming bacteria in comparison to planctonic cells[16]. The induction of biofilm formation by external factors, especially by detergents or ethanol which are common constituents of disinfectants, might explain the high survival rate of Staphylococci in the hospital environment.

Alternative sigma factors of the RNA polymerase complex are known to be involved in the regulation of gene expression in many bacteria[9,10]. Extensive studies in *B. subtilis*, *E. coli*, *P. aeruginosa* and *S. aureus* give evidence that the stress response of the bacterial cell is controlled by alternative transcription factors. They function as global regulators which also influence the expression of many virulence-associated genes, including biofilm formation[19]. Our data obtained in *S. epidermidis* suggest that also in this organism the generation of biofilms might be associated with the expression of the alternative transcription factor sigB. Thus, Northern blot analysis revealed that the sigB transcription is induced under external stress conditions. The same conditions were shown to induce the formation of biofilms in *S. epidermidis*. Therefore, we speculate that the *ica* genes might be directly or indirectly controlled by sigB. In order to substantiate our assumption, we currently create a *sig*B knock-out mutant which will give more information on the role of this factor in the *S. epidermidis* pathogenesis.

## ACKNOWLEDGEMENT

The authors' work is supported by the BMBF (grant no. 01KI9608), the Deutsche Forschungsgemeinschaft (Graduiertenkolleg Infektiologie) and the Fond der Chemischen Industrie.

## REFERENCES

1. Rupp, M.E. and Archer, G.L., 1994, Coagulase-negative staphylococci: pathogens associated with medical progress. *Clin. Infect. Dis.* **19**: 231-43.
2. Costerton, J.W., Stewart, P.S. and Greenberg, E.P., 1999, Bacterial biofilms: a common cause of persistent infections. *Science* **284**: 1318-22.
3. Mack, D., Fischer, W., Krokotsch, A., Leopold, K., Hartmann, R., Egge, H. and Laufs, R., 1996, The intercellular adhesin involved in biofilm accumulation of Staphylococcus epidermidis is a linear beta-1,6-linked glucosaminoglycan: purification and structural analysis. *J. Bacteriol.* **178**: 175-83.
4. Gerke, C., Kraft, A., Süssmuth, R., Schweitzer, O. and Götz, F., 1998, Characterization of the N-acetylglucosaminyltransferase activity involved in the biosynthesis of the Staphylococcus epidermidis polysaccharide intercellular adhesin. *J. Biol. Chem.* **273**: 18586-93.
5. Heilmann, C., Schweitzer, O., Gerke, C., Vanittanakom, N., Mack, D. and Götz, F., 1996, Molecular basis of intercellular adhesion in the biofilm-forming Staphylococcus epidermidis. *Mol. Microbiol.* **20**: 1083-91.

6.  Ziebuhr, W., Heilmann, C., Götz, F., Meyer, P., Wilms, K., Straube, E. and Hacker, J., 1997, Detection of the intercellular adhesion gene cluster (ica) and phase variation in Staphylococcus epidermidis blood culture strains and mucosal isolates. *Infect. Immun.* **65:** 890-6.

7.  Ziebuhr, W., Krimmer, V., Rachid, S., Lößner, I., Götz, F. and Hacker, J., 1999, A novel mechanism of phase variation of virulence in Staphylococcus epidermidis: evidence for control of the polysaccharide intercellular adhesin synthesis by alternating insertion and excision of the insertion sequence element IS256. *Mol. Microbiol.* **32:** 345-356.

8.  Christensen, G.D., Simpson, W.A., Younger, J.J., Baddour, L.M., Barrett, F.F., Melton, D.M. and Beachey, E.H., 1985, Adherence of coagulase-negative staphylococci to plastic tissue culture plates: a quantitative model for the adherence of staphylococci to medical devices. *J. Clin. Microbiol.* **22:** 996-1006.

9.  Hecker, M., Schumann, W. and Völker, U., 1996, Heat-shock and general stress response in Bacillus subtilis. *Mol. Microbiol.* **19:** 417-28.

10. Hecker, M. and Völker, U., 1998, Non-specific, general and multiple stress resistance of growth- restricted Bacillus subtilis cells by the expression of the sigmaB regulon. *Mol. Microbiol.* **29:** 1129-36.

11. Mekalanos, J.J., 1992, Environmental signals controlling expression of virulence determinants in bacteria. *J. Bacteriol.* **174:** 1-7.

12. Wu, S., de Lencastre, H. and Tomasz, A., 1996, Sigma-B, a putative operon encoding alternate sigma factor of Staphylococcus aureus RNA polymerase: molecular cloning and DNA sequencing. *J. Bacteriol.* **178:** 6036-42.

13. Deora, R. and Misra, T.K., 1996, Characterization of the primary sigma factor of Staphylococcus aureus. *J. Biol. Chem.* **271:** 21828-34.

14. Clements, M.O. and Foster, S.J., 1999, Stress resistance in Staphylococcus aureus. *Trends Microbiol.* **7:** 458-62.

15. Kullik, I., Giachino, P. and Fuchs, T., 1998, Deletion of the alternative sigma factor sigmaB in Staphylococcus aureus reveals its function as a global regulator of virulence genes. *J. Bacteriol.* **180:** 4814-20.

16. Costerton, J.W., Lewandowski, Z., Caldwell, D.E., Korber, D.R. and Lappin-Scott, H.M., 1995, Microbial biofilms. *Ann. Rev. Microbiol.* **49:** 711-45.

17. Shapiro, J.A., 1998, Thinking about bacterial populations as multicellular organisms. *Ann. Rev. Microbiol.* **52:** 81-104.

18. Smith, T., 1998, United they withstand. *Nat. Med.* **4:** 1243.

19. Brown, M.R. and Barker, J., 1999, Unexplored reservoirs of pathogenic bacteria: protozoa and biofilms. *Trends Microbiol.* **7:** 46-50.

# EXPRESSION OF VIRULENCE GENES IN *CANDIDA ALBICANS*

[1]Peter Staib, [2]Marianne Kretschmar, [2]Thomas Nichterlein, [1]Gerwald Köhler and [1]Joachim Morschhäuser
[1]*Zentrum für Infektionsforschung, Universität Würzburg, Röntgenring 11, Würzburg, Germany;*
[2]*Institut für Medizinische Mikrobiologie und Hygiene, Klinikum der Stadt Mannheim, Mannheim, Germany*

## 1.      INTRODUCTION

In comparison to infections caused by protozoal, bacterial and viral pathogens, fungi have played only a minor role as human pathogens in the history of mankind because they generally exhibit only little pathogenic potential and are usually held in check in healthy people by a high natural immunity against them. However, this situation has changed dramatically during the last decades, due to the increasing number of immunosuppressed patients[1]. One factor contributing to this situation is the AIDS pandemic. Almost all AIDS patients suffer from mucosal *Candida* infections at least once during the course of the disease and are at a high risk for life-threatening cryptococcal meningitis. On the other hand, the progress in medical technology that prolonged the life-expectancy of patients with severe underlying diseases, for example cancer patients or organ transplant recipients, has also led to a growing population of severely immunosuppressed people. In addition, the use of intravenous catheters and broad-spectrum antibiotics are also risk factors for systemic fungal infections. Opportunistic fungal infections are now a significant cause of morbidity and mortality in immunocompromised patients. Among the most important human fungal pathogens are species of the genus *Candida*, especially *C. albicans*[2].

*Genes and Proteins Underlying Microbial Urinary Tract Virulence*
Edited by L. Emődy *et al.*, Kluwer Academic/Plenum Publishers, 2000

## 2.     VIRULENCE CHARACTERISTICS OF
   *C. ALBICANS*

*Candida* species are not highly virulent microorganisms, instead, they are ubiquitous human commensals, primarily residing in the gastrointestinal tract without causing any harm. Especially *C. albicans* readily colonizes host epithelia and is probably harboured by most individuals at some stage in their lives. As an essentially opportunistic pathogen *C. albicans* needs an immunocompromised host to do more than just colonize the epithelial surface. In hosts with defects in cell-mediated immunity it commonly causes superficial infections of mucosae, skin and nails but rarely penetrates beyond such sites to invade into deeper tissue. Disseminated infections predominantly occur in severely immunocompromised, neutropenic patients, for example organ transplant recipients or cancer patients. Yet, since *C. albicans* is by far the most frequent yeast species causing infections in such debilitated patients, it is conceivable that it must possess traits that make this species better adapted than others to overcome the residual host barriers and cause disease[3].

### 2.1     Adherence to Host Tissues

Adhesion to host tissues generally is a prerequisite for colonization of the host by infecting microorganisms. The adhesion of different *Candida* species to host tissue correlates with their relative virulence, *C. albicans* adhering far better than other *Candida* species or the apathogenic yeast *Saccharomyces cerevisiae* to epithelial and endothelial cells as well as to extracellular matrix proteins[4]. In addition, differences in relative virulence have also been observed in *C. albicans* strains with differing degrees of adherence, and spontaneous mutants defective in adherence to buccal epithelial cells are less virulent in animal models than the parent strain.

As *C. albicans* adheres to many different types of host surfaces, it probably also possesses a broad panel of adherence factors. Various adherence mechanisms have been described. A lectin-like interaction of *C. albicans* surface proteins with fucosyl or N-acetyl-glucosamine containing glycosides on epithelial cells seems to be involved in binding to mucosal surfaces, whereas protein-protein interactions have been implicated in adherence to endothelial cells and extracellular matrix proteins[5]. Several genes encoding putative adhesins have recently been cloned. The *ALS* gene family encodes *C. albicans* cell surface proteins, and expression of the *ALS1* gene in *S. cerevisiae* confers adherence to epithelial and endothelial cells upon this normally non-adherent yeast[6,7]. *HWP1* codes for a hyphae-specific surface protein that serves as a substrate for mammalian transglutaminases and is necessary for stable attachment to human buccal epithelial cells[8]. The *INT1* gene encodes an integrin-like protein necessary for adhesion to epithelial cells. In addition, *INT1* is also necessary for hyphae formation, thus providing a linkage between two *C. albicans* virulence factors[9].

## 2.2 Hyphae Formation

One outstanding characteristic of *C. albicans* is its ability to switch from the budding yeast form to mycelial growth. Although many other *Candida* species are able to grow in chains of largely elongated cells called pseudohyphae, *C. albicans* and the recently described new species *C. dubliniensis* are the only ones that form true hyphae[10]. For a long time it was a widely held view that the yeast form is representative of the commensal stage of *C. albicans* colonizing epithelial surfaces whereas hyphae are the pathogenic, invasive form (Fig 1).

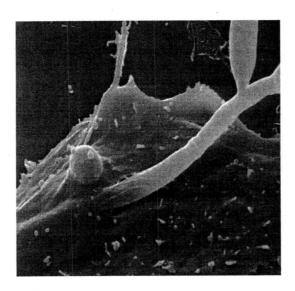

*Figure 1.* Scanning electron micrograph of *C. albicans* hyphae invading into a human endothelial cell.

However, histopathological observations demonstrate that both yeasts and hyphae are found in infected tissue and sometimes *C. albicans* yeasts invade tissue without any hyphae formation. Therefore, it is certainly not correct to consider the mycelial form as the exclusive virulent form of *C. albicans*; rather it seems to be the ability to switch between the two growth forms that is necessary to establish infection. Hyphae adhere more strongly to host surfaces than yeast cells and may also be better adapted for tissue invasion, whereas dissemination through the bloodstream to other organs might be more readily accomplished by the smaller yeasts. In this respect it is interesting that both mutants unable to form hyphae as well as mutants derepressed for mycelial growth are avirulent[11,12].

## 2.3    Phenotypic Switching

The yeast-hyphae transition is not the only morphological switch *C. albicans* is able to perform. The fungus can also undergo spontaneous or induced reversible switching between different types of cells which is easily detected by a characteristic appearance of the corresponding colonies on agar plates[13]. Many *C. albicans* strains have their own repertoire of switch phenotypes, the best characterized system being the white-opaque switching of strain WO-1. Switching to a different cell type involves changes in antigenicity, drug resistance and expression of virulence factors and may therefore be a prerequisite for the adaptation to different host niches or the evasion of host defense mechanisms[14].

## 2.4    Secretion of Hydrolytic Enzymes

*C. albicans* produces secreted hydrolytic enzymes like phospholipases and proteinases. The ability of *C. albicans* to secrete aspartic proteinases has been known for a long time[15] and linked to virulence by many investigators since the proteolytic activity of different *Candida* species is correlated with their relative virulence[16] and since *C. albicans* strains with the highest proteinase production are also the most virulent in different experimental infection models[17,18]. Possible roles of the secreted aspartic proteinases in pathogenicity may include the supply with nitrogen[15], the degradation of tissue barriers during invasion[19,20], the evasion of host defense mechanisms[21,22], or adhesion[23]. During the last years it became evident that *C. albicans* possesses a family of at least ten genes, *SAP1-10*, encoding aspartic proteinases[24,25]. Mutants in which single or multiple *SAP* genes are disrupted display reduced virulence in animal models of candidiasis[26,27,28]. The individual members of the *SAP* gene family are differentially regulated *in vitro*[29,30,31], suggesting that they are also induced in different host niches during infection.

## 3. *CANDIDA ALBICANS* VIRULENCE GENE EXPRESSION DURING INFECTION

Instead of single dominant virulence factors, the high adaptability of *C. albicans* to different host niches is probably one of the main characteristics that makes this species one of the most successful human fungal pathogens. This adaptation is reflected by the expression of different adhesins for the colonization of various host tissues, the yeast-hyphae transition, and the phenotypic switching between different cell types, including the expression of phase-specific genes. The fact that *C. albicans* possesses families of related genes encoding specific virulence factors, like the *SAP* gene family, suggests that the fungus has evolved mechanisms to adapt to host microenvironments by the production of isoenzymes with specific functions at various stages of an infection. Correspondingly, regulatory mechanisms must have evolved to guarantee the expression of individual virulence genes in the appropriate niche by specific host signals. The identification of gene expression patterns at various stages of the infectious process would therefore allow a better understanding of fungus-host interactions.

### 3.1 Development of an *in vivo* Expression Technology for *Candida albicans*

For bacterial pathogens, genetic reporter systems have been developed to detect the expression of a gene during infection[32]. One of these *in vivo* expression technologies (IVET) that uses site-specific recombination as a reporter of gene activation is especially suitable to detect the induction of genes that are only transiently activated at a certain stage of an infection[33]. We have adapted this system to analyze the expression of *C. albicans* virulence genes *in vivo* during infection of its host. For this purpose, the gene encoding the site-specific recombinase FLP from *S. cerevisiae* was placed under control of the *SAP2* gene and integrated into the genome of a *C. albicans* strain containing a marker that was flanked by direct repeats of the FLP recognition sequences. Induction of the *SAP2* promoter results in the production of the recombinase enzyme which in turn catalyzes the excision of the marker from the genome, leading to its irreversible loss from the cell and all its progeny. Using this reporter system, a previous gene activation in a cell during infection can be detected later, after its reisolation from an infected animal and the analysis of its progeny for the presence or absence of the marker (Fig 2).

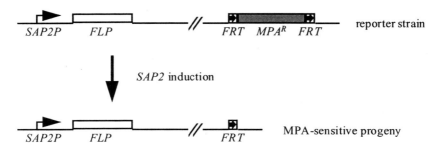

*Figure 2.* Use of FLP-mediated genetic recombination as a heritable marker of gene activation.

To establish this *in vivo* expression technology for *C. albicans*, the *FLP* gene had to be genetically engineered by changing the CUG codons, which would be mistranslated in *C. albicans* as serine instead of leucine[34], into UUG codons, resulting in the functional expression of the FLP recombinase. As a deletable marker we used a mutated form of the *C. albicans IMH3* gene conferring resistance against the specific inhibitor mycophenolic acid[35]. A reporter strain carrying the deletable $MPA^R$ marker and the *SAP2P-FLP* fusion did not exhibit FLP activity during growth in rich or minimal medium containing low molecular weight nitrogen sources, conditions under which the *SAP2* gene is normally repressed. In contrast, in a medium that contains proteins as the sole nitrogen source the *SAP2* gene is expressed, and *SAP2* activation during growth of the reporter strain in this medium could be monitored by the appearance of MPA-sensitive colonies after spreading the cells on suitable indicator plates[36].

## 3.2    Stage-Specific Virulence Gene Activation by Host Signals

After the reliability of the reporter system had been confirmed *in vitro*, we used the reporter strain containing the *SAP2P-FLP* fusion in various experimental models of candidiasis to analyze the expression of the *SAP2* gene at different stages of the infection process. In a model of oesophageal infection in mice in which *C. albicans* invades into the epithelium but does not disseminate hematogeneously into deep organs, significant *SAP2* expression was not detected at any time point, indicating that activation of the *SAP2* gene was not necessary for infection of the oesophageal epithelium. In contrast, in two mouse models of disseminated candidiasis in which the animals were infected either intraperitoneally or intravenously, a strong induction of the *SAP* gene occurred at late stages of systemic infection, after spread of the fungus into deep organs, but not before dissemination (Fig 3). These results suggest that the Sap2 proteinase has some function after the establishment of *C. albicans* in deep tissue, in which it is specifically activated by host signals, but that other proteinases might be needed during epithelial infection and invasion.

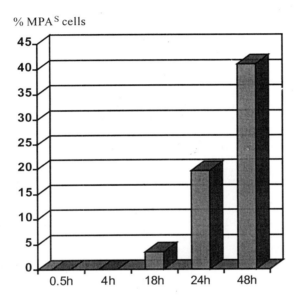

*Figure 3.* Expression of the *SAP2* gene at various stages after intraperitoneal infection of mice.

## 4.     CONCLUSION

The analysis of virulence gene expression patterns during infection gives insights into regulatory adaptation mechanisms of microbial pathogens in various host niches. The establishment of an *in vivo* expression technology for *C. albicans* allows us to investigate at which stage of an infection virulence genes might play a role in the host-pathogen interaction and will, therefore enhance our understanding of fungal pathogenicity.

## ACKNOWLEDGMENTS

The work in our laboratory was supported by the Bundesministerium für Bildung, Wissenschaft, Forschung und Technologie (BMBF grant O1 K1 8906-0 and the Deutsche Forschungsgemeinschaft (DFG grant MO 846/1-1). Peter Staib is the recipient of a grant from the Studienstiftung des deutschen Volkes.

## REFERENCES

1.   Sternberg, S., 1994, The emerging fungal threat. *Science* **266:** 1632-1634.
2.   Odds, F.C., 1988, *Candida* and candidosis: a review and bibliography. Bailliere Tindall, London.
3.   Odds, F.C., 1994, *Candida* species and virulence. ASM News **60:** 313-318.
4.   Calderone, R.A., and Braun, P.C., 1991, Adherence and receptor relationships in *Candida albicans. Microbiol. Rev.* **55:** 1-20.
5.   Calderone, R.A., 1993, Recognition between *Candida albicans* and host cells. *Trends Microbiol.* **1:** 55-58.
6.   Hoyer, L.L., Payne, T.L., and Hecht, J.E., 1998, Identification of *Candida albicans ALS2* and *ALS4* and localization of Als proteins to the fungal cell surface. *J. Bacteriol.* **180:** 5334-5343.
7.   Fu, Y., Rieg, G., Fonzi, W.A., Belanger, P.H., Edwards Jr, J.E., and Filler, S.G., 1998, Expression of the *Candida albicans* gene *ALS1* in *Saccharomyces cerevisiae* induces adherence to endothelial and epithelial cells. *Infect. Immun.* **66:** 1783-1786.
8.   Staab, J.F., Bradway, S.D., Fidel, P.L., and Sundstrom, P., 1999, Adhesive and mammalian transglutaminase substrate properties of *Candida albicans* Hwp1. *Science* **283:** 1535-1538.
9.   Gale, C.A., Bendel, C.M., McClellan, M., Hauser, M., Becker, J.M., Berman, J., and Hostetter, M., 1998, Linkage of adhesion, filamentous growth, and virulence in *Candida albicans* to a single gene, *INT1. Science*, **279:** 1355-1358.
10.  Sullivan, D.J., Westerneng, T J., Haynes, K.A., Bennett, D.E., and Coleman, D.C., 1995, *Candida dubliniensis* sp. nov.: phenotypic and molecular characterization of a novel species associated with oral candidosis in HIV-infected individuals. *Microbiology* **141:** 1507-1521.
11.  Lo, H.-J., Köhler, J.R., DiDomenico, B., Loebenberg, B., Cacciapuoti, A., and Fink, G.R., 1997, Nonfilamentous *C. albicans* mutants are avirulent. *Cell,* **90:** 939-949.
12.  Csank, C., Makris, C., Meloche, S., Schröppel, K., Röllinghoff, M., Dignard, D., Thomay, D.Y., and Whiteway, M., 1997, Derepressed hyphal growth and reduced virulence in a VH1 family-related protein phosphatase mutant of the human pathogen *Candida albicans. Mol. Cell. Biol.* **8:** 2539-2551.
13.  Soll, D.R., Morrow, B., and Srikantha, T., 1993, High-frequency phenotypic switching in *Candida albicans. Trends Genet.* **9:** 61-65.
14.  Soll, D.R., 1997, Gene regulation during high-frequency switching in *Candida albicans. Microbiology* **143:** 279-288.
15.  Staib, F., 1965, Serum-proteins as nitrogen source for yeast-like fungi. *Sabouraudia,* **4:** 187-193.

16. Odds, F.C., 1985, *Candida albicans* proteinase as a virulence factor in the pathogenesis of *Candida* infections. Zbl. Bakt. Hyg. **260:** 539-542.

17. Kondoh, Y, Shimizu, K., and Tanaka, J., 1987, Proteinase production and pathogenicity of *Candida albicans* II. Virulence for mice of *C. albicans* strains with different proteinase activity. *Microbiol. Immunol.* **31:** 1061-1069.

18. Cassone, A., De Bernardis, F., Mondello, F., Ceddia, T., and Agatensi, L., 1987, Evidence for a correlation between proteinase secretion and vulvovaginal candidosis. *J. Infect. Dis.* **156:** 777-783.

19. Colina, A.R., Aumont, F., Deslauriers, N., Belhumeur, P., and de Repentigny, L., 1996, Evidence for degradation of gastrointestinal mucin by *Candida albicans* secretory aspartyl proteinase. *Infect Immun* **64:** 4514-4519.

20. Morschhäuser, J., Virkola, R., Korhonen, T.K., and Hacker, J., 1997, Degradation of human subendothelial extracellular matrix by proteinase-secreting *Candida albicans*. *FEMS Microbiol Lett* **153:** 349-355.

21. Rüchel, R., 1986 Cleavage of immunoglobulins by pathogenic yeasts of the genus *Candida*. *Microbiol Sci* **36:** 316-319.

22. Kaminishi, H., Miyaguchi, H., Tamaki, T., Suenaga, N., Hisamatsu, M., Mihashi, I., Matsumoto, H., Maeda, H., and Hagihara Y., 1995, Degradation of humoral host defense by *Candida albicans* proteinase. *Infect Immun* **63:** 984-988.

23. Ray, T.L., and Payne, C.D., 1988, Scanning electron microscopy of epidermal adherence and cavitation in murine candidiasis: a role for *Candida* acid proteinase. *Infect. Immun.* **56:** 1942-1949.

24. Monod, M., Togni, G., Hube, B., and Sanglard, D., 1994, Multiplicity of genes encoding secreted aspartic proteinases in *Candida* species. *Mol Microbiol* **13:** 357-368.

25. Monod, M., Hube, B., Hess, D., and Sanglard, D., 1998, Differential regulation of *SAP8* and *SAP9*, which encode two new members of the secreted aspartic proteinase family in *Candida albicans*. *Microbiology* **144:** 2731-2737.

26. Hube, B., Sanglard, D., Odds, F.C., Hess, D., Monod, M., Schäfer, W., Brown, A.J.P., and Gow, N.A.R., 1997, Disruption of each of the secreted aspartyl proteinase genes *SAP1*, *SAP2*, and *SAP3* of *Candida albicans* attenuates virulence. *Infect Immun* **65:** 3529-3538.

27. Sanglard, D., Hube, B., Monod, M., Odds, F.C., and Gow, N.A.R., 1997, A triple deletion of the secreted aspartyl proteinase genes *SAP4, SAP5*, and *SAP6* of *Candida albicans* causes attenuated virulence. *Infect. Immun.* **65:** 3539-3546.

28. De Bernardis, F., Arancia, S., Morelli, L., Hube, B., Sanglard, D., Schäfer, W., and Cassone, A., 1999, Evidence that members of the secretory aspartyl proteinase gene family, in particular *SAP2*, are virulence factors for *Candida* vaginitis. *J. Infect. Dis.* **179:** 201-208.

29. Hube, B., Monod, M., Schofield, D.A., Brown, A.J.P., and Gow, N.A.R., 1994, Expression of seven members of the gene family encoding secretory aspartyl proteinases in *Candida albicans*. *Mol Microbiol* **14:** 87-99.

30. White, T., and Agabian, N., 1995, *Candida albicans* secreted aspartyl proteinases: Isoenzyme pattern is determined by cell type, and levels are determined by environmental factors. *J Bacteriol* **177:** 5215-5221.

31. Schaller, M., Schäfer, W., Korting, H.C., and Hube, B., 1998, Differential expression of secreted aspartyl proteinases in a model of human oral candidosis and in patient samples from the oral cavity. *Mol Microbiol* **29:** 605-615.

32. Heithoff, D.M., Conner, C.P., and Mahan, M.J., 1997, Dissecting the biology of a pathogen during infection. *Trends Microbiol.* **5:** 509-513.

33. Camilli, A, Beattie, D.T., and Mekalanos, J.J., 1994, Use of genetic recombination as a reporter of gene expression. *Proc Natl Acad Sci USA* **91**: 2634-2638.
34. Santos, M.A., Ueda, T., Watanabe, K., and Tuite, M., 1997, The non-standard genetic code of *Candida* spp.: an evolving genetic code or a novel mechanism for adaptation? *Mol Microbiol* **26**: 423-431.
35. Köhler, G.A., White, T.C., and Agabian, N., 1997, Overexpression of a cloned IMP dehydrogenase gene of *Candida albicans* confers resistance to the specific inhibitor mycophenolic acid. *J Bacteriol* **179**: 2331-2338.
36. Staib, P., Kretschmar, M., Nichterlein, T., Köhler, G., Michel, S., Hof, H., Hacker, J., and Morschhäuser, J., 1999, Host-induced, stage-specific virulence gene activation in *Candida albicans* during infection. *Mol. Microbiol.* **32**: 533-546.

# EFFECT OF SPONTANEOUS AND INDUCED MUTATIONS ON OUTER MEMBRANE PROTEINS AND LIPOPOLYSACCHARIDES OF *PROTEUS PENNERI* STRAIN 357

[1]Ildikó Kustos, [2]Vilmos Tóth, [3]Ferenc Kilár, [1]Béla Kocsis, [1]Levente Emődy
[1]*Department of Medical Microbiology and Immunology,* [2]*Department of Stomatology,* [3]*Central Research Laboratory, UniversityMedical School of Pécs, Hungary*

## 1.     INTRODUCTION

In 1982 the name *Proteus penneri* was proposed for a group of bacteria previously known as indol negative *Proteus vulgaris*, or *P. vulgaris* biogroup 1[1]. They are opportunistic pathogens eliciting infections mainly in the urinary tract, particularly in patients with pre-disposing conditions.

Several virulence factors have already been known to be produced by *P. penneri* strains, e.g. IgA protease, haemagglutinating fimbriae, urease, haemolysins[2], outer membrane proteins (OMP), lipopolysaccharides (LPS).

In this study the OMP and LPS profiles of the wild type of *P. penneri* strain 357, and its two isogenic mutants ( a transposon-, and a spontaneous mutant variant) were analysed together with a set of conventional bacteriological virulence assays.

The bacterial surface and its components play an important role in the interaction of bacteria by the host cells. Knowledge of these structure might give insight into the pathogenesis of infectious bacteria.

OMPs of these genetic variants were analysed by a new and modern method, capillary electrophoresis (CE). This is a fast, and reproducible method, which requires very low sample and buffer consumption. Furthermore it can be automated, and provides quantitative data.

*Genes and Proteins Underlying Microbial Urinary Tract Virulence*
Edited by L. Emődy *et al.*, Kluwer Academic/Plenum Publishers, 2000

The aim of the present study was to analyse how the cell surface components of the genetic variants of *P. penneri* strain 357 relate to one another, and to examine if the electrophoretic analysis of OMPs and LPS has additional diagnostic value or may explain pathogenetic findings.

## 2.        MATERIALS AND METHODS

### 2.1        Bacterial Strains

Wild type of *P. penneri* strain 357 was isolated in our laboratory. The non-haemolytic transposon mutant was constructed with the help of *E. coli* DB5243 kanamycin transposon donor strain obtained from D. Berg (Dept. Mol. Microbiol., Washington University, St. Louis, USA). The *P. penneri* strain 357 stored in stock agar for at least two years was chosen for unfolding spontaneous non-haemolytic mutants.

### 2.2        Examination of Outer Membrane Proteins

Whole membrane fraction was isolated by lyzozyme treatment and sonication, and OMPs were prepared by sucrose gradient ultracentrifugation[3]. Capillary electrophoretic analysis of the OMPs was performed with a Biofocus 3000 CE System in a 24 cm long, 50 μm ID uncoated capillary. Experimental conditions have been described previously[3].

### 2.3        Analysis of Lipopolysaccharides

LPS was extracted from bacterial cells by the hot aqueous-phenol procedure[4]. SDS-PAGE was performed in a Laemmli discontinuous system, in 4 % stacking gel and 15 % separating gel. Gels were silver stained by the method of Tsai and Frasch[5].

### 2.4        Virulence Assays

Cytotoxicity of bacterial cells was examined on HEp-2, HeLa and Vero cells[6], *in vivo* virulence was examined by lung toxicity assay, and ip. and iv. injection of mice as described elsewhere[7].

# 3.     RESULTS

## 3.1     Outer Membrane Protein Profiles

The OMP patterns obtained by CE can be seen in Fig 1. The OMP profiles of each variants were dominated by two major proteins, with molecular weights 39 and 43 kDa, respectively. In the wild type of *P. penneri* 357 the relative percentage of the two proteins was 60 to 40 %, while in both mutants 45 to 55 %.

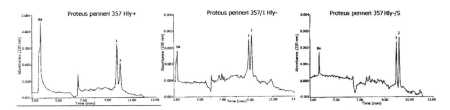

*Figure 1.* Capillary electrophoretic outer membrane protein profiles of the wild type of *P. penneri* 357 (Hly+), and its transposon –(357/1 Hly-) and spontaneous mutants (357 Hly-/S).

## 3.2     Lipopolysaccharide Patterns

The LPS of the wild type of *P. penneri* 357 showed typical ladder pattern in the silver stained gel, characteristic for "S" bacteria, while both mutants possessed only a few bands in the low molecular weight region, characteristic for "R" forms of bacteria (data not shown).

## 3.3     Virulence Tests

As shown in Table 1. $10^5$ germs of the wild type strain elicited a marked cytotoxic effect on all the three cell lines applied. On the contrary $10^8$ or more bacteria were needed to evoke the same effect when the cell cultures were infected with either of the mutant strains.

In the mouse assays - as shown by both the lethal doses and the death rates - the haemolytic wild type strain proved to be more virulent than its non-haemolytic spontaneous or transposon mutants. The differences in the death rates between the wild type strain and the mutants were highly significant as to their intravenous lethality and lung toxicity ($p < 0.001$).

Table 1. *In vitro* and *in vivo* virulence of *P. penneri* 357 and its non-haemolytic mutants

| Cell line | Wild type | In vitro assays Transposon mutant | Spontaneous mutant |
|---|---|---|---|
| HeLa | $10^5$ | $>10^8$ | Non toxic |
| Vero | $10^5$ | $>10^8$ | $>10^8$ |
| HEp-2 | $10^6$ | $>10^8$ | Non toxic |
| | | In vivo assays | |
| Mouse i.p. $LD_{50}$ | $4.7 \times 10^7$ | $>5 \times 10^8$ | $4.3 \times 10^8$ |
| Mouse i.v. $LD_{50}$ | $2.2 \times 10^8$ | $>5 \times 10^8$ | $>5 \times 10^8$ |
| Mouse i.v. lethality | 20/20 | 0/20 | 0/20 |
| Mouse lung toxicity | 10/10 | 0/10 | 0/10 |

Figures for cytotoxicity and $LD_{50}$ values represent bacterial cells eliciting 50 % effect
Figures for mouse i.v. lethality and lung toxicity show the ratios of animals died/infected

## 4.    CONCLUSIONS

Capillary electrophoresis was suitable for the comparative analysis of the OMPs of the wild type and mutant variants of *P. penneri* strain 357. The patterns were reproducible and characteristic for the different genetic types examined. OMP patterns of the two mutants showed significant changes compared to the wild type. Examination of the LPS molecules showed also altered patterns in the mutants (S-R mutation). One part of alterations in OMP profiles might be explained by the specific interaction of OMP and LPS components; the proper trimerisation and function of porin proteins requires specific LPS structure[8]. Beside that the mutants showed neither toxicity *in vitro*, nor pathogenicity *in vivo* in the virulence assays.

So the electrophoretic characterisation of both OMP and LPS composition can significantly improve the sensitivity of classical methods extensively used to identify and characterise bacterial strains.

## REFERENCES

1. Krajden, S., Fuksa, M., Petrea, C., Crisp, L., and Penner, J.L., 1987, Expanded Clinical Spectrum of Infections Caused by *Proteus penneri*, *J. Clin. Microbiol.* **25**: 578-579
2. Senior, B.W., 1993, The production of HlyA toxin by *Proteus penneri* strains, *J. Med. Microbiol.* **39**: 282-289.
3. Kustos, I., Kocsis, B., Kerepesi, I., and Kilar, F., 1998, Protein profile characterization of bacterial lysates by capillary electrophoresis, *Electrophoresis* **19**: 2324-2330.
4. Westphal, O., Lüderitz, O., Bister, F., 1952, Über die Extraktion von Bakterien mit Phenol-Wasser, *Z. Naturforsch.* **7b**: 148-155.
5. Tsai, C.-M., and Frasch, C.E., 1982, A sensitive silver stain for detecting lipopolysaccharides in polyacrylamide gels, *Anal. Biochem.* **119**: 115-119.

6. Brown, E.J., Griffin, D.E., Rothman, S.W., and Doctor, B.P., 1982, Purification and biological characterization of Shiga toxin from *Shigella dysenteriae* 1. *Infect. Immun.* **36:** 996-1005.
7. Emődy, L., Vörös, S., and Pál, T., 1982, Alpha-haemolysin, a possible virulence factor in *Proteus morganii. FEMS Microbiol. Lett.* **13:** 329-331.
8. Nurminen, M., Hirvas, L., and Vaara, M., 1997, The outer membrane of lipid A-deficient *Escherichia coli* mutant LH530 has reduced levels of OmpF and leaks periplasmic enzymes, *Microbiology* **143:** 1533-1537.

# ROLE OF BACTERIAL LECTINS IN URINARY TRACT INFECTIONS
*Molecular Mechanisms for Diversification of Bacterial Surface Lectins*

[1]Itzhak Ofek, [2]David L. Hasty, [3]Soman N. Abraham, and [4]Nathan Sharon
*[1]Department of Human Microbiology, Tel-Aviv University, Tel-Aviv 69978, Israel: [2]Department of Anatomy and Neurobiology, University of Tennessee, Memphis, and VA Medical Center Memphis TN 38163: [3]Departments of Pathology and Microbiology, Duke University, Durham, NC 27710: [4]Department of Membrane Research and Biophysics, The Weizmann Institute of Science, Rehovot 76100, Israel*

## 1.    INTRODUCTION

Since lectins were first implicated in mediating adhesion of *E.coli* to animal cells[1], many bacteria were found to produce lectins that bind to carbohydrate moieties of glycoproteins and glycolipids on the surface of the host cells[2].   In most cases, the lectins produced are expressed on the bacterial surface.  The best studied lectin-producing bacteria are those that colonize animal tissues,. The role of surface lectins in mediating adhesion of bacteria to animal tissue is well-established, but under some circumstances an intracellular lectin may also participate in the adhesion process.    For example, periplasmic lectins released from lysing *Pseudomonas aeruginosa* can form bridges between the remaining pseudomonas and target tissue[3]. Virtually all animal tissue colonizers produce one or more lectins/adhesins, but recently it was found that bacteria that colonize inanimate or animate substrata in the environment also use lectins for binding For example, *Vibrio furnissi*  binds to a glycocalyx-containing inanimate substratum[4], and *Vibrio shiloi* colonizes coral by binding via a galactose specific lectin[5].

*Genes and Proteins Underlying Microbial Urinary Tract Virulence*
Edited by L. Emődy *et al.*, Kluwer Academic/Plenum Publishers, 2000          183

The bacterial lectins are generally classified according to the structure of the carbohydrates they recognize. Their specificity is usually defined as the simplest carbohydrate structure (usually a monosaccharide) that best inhibits the lectin-mediated adhesion. This are referred to as the primary sugar specificity of the lectin (Table 1). Within lectins possessing the same primary sugar specificity, differences in the binding of different oligosaccharides is often observed. This are referred to as the fine sugar specificity. The determination of the fine sugar specificity of a bacterial lectin is usually based on two different types of assays In one assay, the concentration of various derivatives of the primary sugar inhibitor resulting in 50% inhibition of adhesion (i.e. $IC_{50}$) is established for the various isolates.     In the other assay, the magnitude of adhesion to various glycoproteins that contain the primary sugar in different contexts is quantified.

*Table 1.* Inter- and intraspecies diversity in the primary and fine sugar specificities of enterobacterial fimbrial lectins.

| Type of Diversity | Group and Species | Primary Specificity | Fine Specificity |
|---|---|---|---|
| Interspecies | Enterobacteria | | |
| | *E. coli* (T1F) | Mannoside | pNPα Man >>Man |
| | *K. pneumoniae* (T1F) | Mannoside | pNPα Man > Man |
| | *S. typhimurium* (T1F) | Mannoside | Man > pNPα Man |
| Intraspecies | E. coli | | |
| | UPEC (T1F) | Mannoside | Man = Man3 |
| | Fecal EC (T1F) | Mannoside | Man3 >> Man |
| | UPEC (PF-G1) | Galα4Gal | GbO3 |
| | UPEC (PF-G2) | Galα4Gal | GbO4 |
| | UPEC (PF-G3) | Galα4Gal | GbO5 |

UPEC = uropathogenic E. coli; T1F = type 1 fimbriae; pNPα-Man = paranitrophenylα mannoside; Man = mannose; Man3= Manα3Manα6Man; PF = P fimbriae; G1, G2, G3 = PapG adhesin subclasses; GbO3=Galα4Galβ4GlcβCer; GbO4= GalNAcα2Galα4Galβ4GlcβCer; GbO5= GalNAcα2GalNacα2Galα4Galβ4GlcβCer[6]. GalNAc = N-acetylgalactosamine; Gal = galactose; Glc = glucose. Data adopted from Ofek & Sharon 1990[7]; Hasty and Sokurenko 2000[8]

In the following, we will focus on a particular class of bacterial lectins to better illustrate the potential biological effects of the diversification of the fine sugar specificity found within a given family of lectins.   This class of lectins is expressed on the bacterial surface in the form of fimbriae and mediate the adhesion of many enterobacterial species to animal tissue including the urinary tract.

## 2. STRUCTURAL FEATURES OF FIMBRIAL LECTINS OF ENTEROBACTERIA

Enterobacterial fimbriae share a number of common features[2]. They are all encoded by complex operons and have genes for regulatory proteins, a periplasmic chaperone, an outer membrane assembly platform and major as well as minor structural subunits. In most cases, the lectin subunits are minor components of the fimbrial superstructure. These lectin subunits are complexed with other minor and/or major subunits, which comprise the fimbrial, shaft and are situated at the fimbrial tip to be optimally positioned to mediate interaction with host cells. It has been thought that the lectin subunit contains two separate domains, one for saccharide binding in the amino terminal region and one for polymerization with shaft subunits in the carboxy terminal region[9,10]. Recent crystallographic studies has confirmed this prediction[11].

The primary sugar specificities of a number of enterobacterial fimbrial adhesins have been characterized (for review, see Ofek and Doyle, 1994[2]). Structure-function studies of the fine sugar specificity of enterobacterial lectins have only been carried out in detail for two types of fimbriae, type 1 fimbriae of several enterobacteria and P fimbriae of *E. coli* (Table 1). In this brief review, we will focus only on the type 1 fimbrial lectins. Type 1 fimbriae share a common primary sugar specificity, mannose, but vary in their fine sugar specificities. There is diversity between different species (interspecies) as well as between different isolates of the same species (intraspecies) (Table 1). Two molecular mechanisms have been suggested to account for this diversity. One mechanism involves the association between the FimH adhesin and one or more subunits of the fimbrial shaft (i.e. FimA, FimF and/or FimG). This mechanism has been shown to account for the interspecies diversities observed[12,13].

Another mechanism involves allelic variations of the *fimH* gene of *E. coli* which has been shown to account for intraspecies diversity in binding among type 1 fimbriated *E.coli*[14,15]. In the following, we will briefly describe the molecular basis underlying these two mechanisms for diversity of fine sugar specificity and will discuss the impact of this variation on tissue tropism of the lectin bearing bacteria.

### 3.     THE INFLUENCE OF TYPE I FIMBRIAL SHAFTS ON THE FINE SUGAR SPECIFICITY OF ENTEROBACTERIAL FIMH

Using different aromatic mannosides to inhibit type 1 fimbriae-mediated binding interactions, distinct differences in the $IC_{50}$s were noted between *E. coli*, *K. pneumoniae* and *S. Typhimurium*[7,16]. Evidence that the fimbrial subunits of the shaft that presents the FimH adhesin at the fimbrial tip (i.e. FimA, FimF and/or FimG) influence the fine sugar specificity of this lectin was first described for the type 1 fimbriae of *K. pneumoniae* and *E. coli*[12]. When the genes encoding the fimbrial shaft and the fimbrial adhesin were swapped between these species, it became apparent that one or more components of the fimbrial shaft influences the fine sugar specificity of fimbriae from each species. For example, the relative inhibitory activity of aromatic mannosides was 3-4 fold greater as compared to aliphatic ones (e.g. Methyl αMan) for a recombinant strain expressing *E. coli* shaft and *K. pneumoniae* FimH as compared to a recombinant strain expressing *K. pneumoniae* shaft and FimH. Conversely, the relative inhibitory activity of a recombinant strain expressing the *K. pneumoniae* shaft and *E. coli* FimH was 5-6 times less than that for a recombinant strain expressing *E. coli* shaft and FimH. These results are consistent with the high degree of identity in the carboxy-terminal regions of *E. coli* and *K. pneumoniae* FimH that associate with the shaft (GenBank[TM] accession number L19338).

In contrast to the high degree of homology between *E. coli* FimH and *K. pneumoniae* FimH, there is limited sequence homology between these proteins and the FimH of *S. typhimurium*[13]. To determine whether the marked difference in the fine sugar specificity between *S. typhimurium* FimH (FimH[S]) and *E. coli* FimH (FimH[E]) in affinity for aromatic mannosides (Table 1) is due to the primary structure of fim H or to the FimH-presenting shaft , a chimeric FimH was constructed[13]. This fusion protein consisted of the amino terminus of *E. coli* FimH (FimH[E]) which contain the carobohydrate binding domain and the carboxy terminus of *S. typhimurium* FimH (FimH[S]) which contain the region that associates with the fimbrial shaft. When this FimH[E/S] fusion was expressed in a recombinant strain and presented on *S. typhimurium* type 1 fimbrial shaft, the recombinant strain bound aromatic mannosides with an anffinity similar to that of FimH[s] (Abraham et al., unpublished observations). The data taken together support the concept that the affinity of FimH of enterobacteria toward aromatic mannosides is significantly influenced by the fimbrial shaft proteins.

## 4. ALLELIC VARIATION OF FIMH AMONG *E. COLI* STRAINS

Naturally occurring phenotypic variants of the FimH protein have recently been recognized[17,18]. These alleles are 99% conserved among the *E. coli* strains varying by as little as one amino acid substitution within the amino terminal region of the FimH molecule in most of the strains studied. Because this region contains the mannose-binding site, as discussed above, it was reasoned that at least some of these alleles may exhibit differences in their fine sugar specificity. In fact, all *E. coli fimH* alleles studied to date encode subunits that mediate high levels of binding to tri-mannose structures ($Man_3$= $Man\alpha3Man\alpha6Man$), but binding to mannose ($Man_1$) residues among the FimH alleles can differ up to 15-fold[19].

To exclude the possibility that the association of the FimH alleles with the fimbrial shaft may have been responsible for the differences in fine sugar specificity observed, recombinant strains were constructed to express the same fimbrial shaft but different FimH genes derived from natural isolates. The results showed a remarkable correlation between the recombinant and wild strains in their $Man_1$ to $Man_3$ binding ratios. Because at least one of the subunits of the fimbrial shaft, FimA, exhibits wide antigenic variations between different strains[2], it is unlikely that the differences in the fine sugar specificity in each of these cases is due to association of FimH with the shaft. These adhesive variations of the FimH alleles, therefore, appear to be due primarily to structural differences in FimH that affect receptor-specificity of the lectin[18,19].

Because mannooligosaccharides are naturally presented as glycoproteins on animal cell surfaces, a battery of glycoproteins was tested for their ability to serve as effective ligands for type 1 fimbriae-mediated adhesion[19]. *E.coli* that carried the Fim H alleles that were classified as $Man_1$ binders exhibited a distinctly different pattern of adhesion to the panel of glycoproteins than did bacteria carrying the $Man_3$ FimH allele. For example, $Man_1$ binding allelic variants bound well to mannan and RNAse B, whereas $Man_3$ binding allelic variants bound well only to RNAse B. The binding of each of these allelic variants to the various ligands was inhibited by the simple sugar, mannose, suggesting that the differences in adhesion patterns reflected differences in the fine sugar specificity.

## 5. BIOLOGICAL CONSEQUENCES OF INTERSPECIES AND INTRASPECIES VARIATION IN FIMH BINDING

As a first approach to investigating the contribution of the observed differences in fine sugar specificity to the infectivity of the bacteria, studies on type 1 fimbriae-mediated adhesion to various animal cells were caried out. The interspecies differences between *E. coli*, *K. pneumoniae* and *S. typhimurium* were reflected in their relative binding affinity to mouse uroepithelial and enterocyte cell lines (Table 2). While *E. coli* bound several fold better to uroepithelial cells than to enterocytes, *S. typhimurium* bound in a reversed manner. The binding pattern of *K. pneumoniae* was similar to that of *E. coli*, but the differences in binding to uroepithelial cells and enterocytes were much less pronouced. Recombinant strains were used to test the effect of the fimbrial shaft on this binding. When *E. coli* FimH was expressed on the *S. typhimurium* fimbrial shaft, the resultant recombinant strain bound to cells in a *S. typhimurium*-like pattern. Furthermore, when *fimH* genes of the three enterobacterial species were fused with a maltose-binding protein (MBP) gene, blots of the soluble fusion proteins bound intact uroepithelial and enterocyte cells equally well (Abraham et al., unpublished observations). All of these cell-binding activities were inhibited by similar concentrations of mannose, suggesting that the magnitude of differences in adhesion reflected differences in the fine sugar specificity. Collectively, these data suggest that interspecies differences in type 1 fimbriae-mediated binding to various animal cell types may be influenced by the fimbrial shaft on which the FimH is borne.

Intraspecies differences in adhesion to mannose-containing glycoprotein were reflected in the binding of wild-type and recombinant strains to various cell lines. For example, $Man_1$ binding FimH variants bound to uroepithelial cell lines to a much greater degree than did tri-mannose-only-binding FimH variants (Table 2). However, the two FimH variants bound to buccal epithelial cells in an equivalent manner[14]. As in all other cases, binding was equally inhibited by mannose.

The differences in fine sugar specificities of FimH alleles and in binding to animal cells were observed to result in marked differences in bladder

*Table 2.* Binding traits of FimH lectins that diverge in their fine sugar specificity

| Type of Diversity | Species or Strain | Fine Sugar Specificity | Relative Adhesion To Animal Cells |
|---|---|---|---|
| Interspecies | *E. coli* (T1F) | pNPα Man >>Man | Uro[a]>>Entero |
| | *K. pneumoniae* (T1F) | pNPα Man > Man | Uro[a] > Entero |
| | *S. typhimurium* (T1F) | Man > pNPα Man | Entero > Uro[a] |
| | *E. coli* (FimH[E/S]/FShaft[s]) | Man > pNPα Man | Entero > Uro |
| Intraspecies | *E. coli* | | |
| | UPEC | $Man_1$ = $Man_3$ | Buccal>>Uro[b] |
| | Fecal | $Man_3$>> $Man_1$ | Buccal=Uro[b] |

For designations of fine sugar specificity, see Table 1. Uro[a]=mouse uroepithelial cell line MM45T.BL, from ATCC; Entero=mouse enterocyte cell line SI-H10, from ATCC (adapted from Thankavel et al., 1999[13]; Abraham et al., unpublished observations). Buccal = epithelial cells scrapped from the buccal mucosa of healthy volunteers; Uro[b]=J82 human uroepithelial cell line, from ATCC (adapted from Sokurenko et al., 1997[19]).

colonization by *E. coli*. The $Man_1$ binding FimH variants that bound 15-fold more effectively to uroepithelial cell lines also colonized mouse bladders in 15-fold higher numbers[14].

## 6. CONCLUSIONS

The remarkable diversity in the fine sugar specificty of the type 1 fimbrial lectins clearly illustrates the concept that functional diversity of fimbrial lectins plays an important role in tissue tropism and infectivity. Lack of awareness of this diversity contributed significantly to relatively slow realization of the importance of type 1 fimbriae in determining bacterial tissue tropism and infectivity. Duguid's early studies (reviewed in Dugiud and Old, 1980[20]) implied that such diversity existed because he noted that although guinea pig erythrocytes were agglutinated by all type 1 fimbriated enterobacterial strains agglutination of erythrocytes of other animals varied between different enterobacterial species and even within the same enterobacterial species. Later, this concept was extended by the realization that it was the presentation of the mannooligosaccharide receptors on particular erythrocytes that resulted in apparent strain differences[21]. The ability to dissect the molecular mechanisms of binding interactions by genetic approaches has not only shown that the diversity is more complex than originally appreciated, but also that it has important consequences for tissue infectivity. In fact, it has recently been postulated that the intraspecies diversity in fine sugar speficity exhibited by the allelic variants of *E. coli* FimH represents an important evolutionary mechanism for pathoadaptive mutation[15]. Further studies of the interspecies differences in the fine sugar specificity of type 1 fimbriae may lead to a better understanding of the relative infectivity of *E. coli, K. pneumoniae* and *S. typhimurium* isolates and possibly those of other enterobacterial species too.

The diversity in the fine sugar specificity of bacterial lectins is clearly not limited to type 1 fimbriae. There are at least three classes of the PapG adhesin expressed on E.coli, and differences in the receptor specificity lead to differences not only in their tissue tropism, but also their host tropism[22]. The diversity is probably also not limited to the sugar binding capacity of these bacterial adhesins. For example, some allelic variants of *E. coli* FimH bind to non-glycosylated peptide moieties of fibronectin and collagen, still in a mannose-inhibitable manner[23,24]. Peptide binding specificity of a lectin has also been noted for Concanavalin A, a plant lectin[25,26]. Eventually, the crystallization of the FimH lectins with saccharide receptor moieties in the presence and absence of the fimbrial shaft should uravel the molecular basis for the fine sugar specificity. Initial crystallization analysis of an uropathogenic *E. coli* FimH in the presence of its chaperone revealed much information about the overall structure of the two-domain molecule[11]. However, co-crystallization of FimH with classic inhbitors of bacterial adhesion mediated by type 1 fimbriae has not yet been performed.

It is now recognized that most pathogens utilize lectins as adhesins in their binding to host cells[2]. This is undoubtedly due primarily to the virtually infinite variability of animal cell oligosaccharide structures[27]. Given the large number of enterobacterial lectins/adhesins with distinct primary sugar specificities and the expected additional diversities based on fine sugar specificity, further studies will hopefully reveal an underlying principle for the role of lectin mediated-adhesion in bacterial pathogenicity.

## ACKNOWLEDGMENTS

The work from our laboratories was supported by grants from the National Institutes of Health [AI-35678 and DK-50814 (SNA); AI42886 (DLH)], the Department of Veteran's Affairs (DLH).

## REFERENCES

1. Ofek, I., Mirelman, D., and Sharon, N., 1977, Adherence of *Escherichia coli* to human mucosal cells mediated by mannose receptors. *Nature* **265**: 623-625.

2. Ofek, I. and R. J. Doyle, 1994, *Bacterial Adhesion to Cells and Tissues*, Chapman & Hall, New York, NY.

3. Wentworth, J. S., F. E. Austin, N. Barger, N. Gilboa-Garber, C. A. Paterson, and R. J. Doyle, 1991, Cytoplasmic lectins contribute to the adhesion of *Pseudomonas aeruginosa*. *Biofouling* 4: 99-104.

4. Yu , C., A. M. Lee, and S. Roseman, 1987, The sugar-specific adhesion/deadhesion apparatus of the marine bacterium *Vibrio furnissi* is a sensorium that continuously monitors nutriend levels in the environment. *Biochem. Biophys. Res. Commun.* 149: 86-92.

5. Rosenberg, E., Y. Ben-Haim, A. Toren, E. Banim, A. Kushmaro, M. Fine, and Y. Loya, 1999, Effects of temperature on bacterial bleaching of corals. In .Microbial Ecology and Infectious Diseases (E. Rosenberg, ed). ASM Press, Washington D.C. pp242-254.

6. Strömberg, N., P. G. Nyholm, I. Pascher, and S. Normark, 1991, Saccharide orientation at the cell surface affects glycolipid receptor function. *Proc. Natl. Acad. Sci. USA* 88: 9340-9344.

7. Ofek, I. and N. Sharon, 1990, Adhesins as lectins: Specificity and role in infection. In *Bacterial Capsules and Adhesins: Facts and Principles. Current Topics in Microbiology and Immunology.* (K. Jann and B. Jann, eds.), Springer-Verlag, Berlin Heideberg, Vol. 151, 91-113.

8. Hasty, D. L. and E. V. Sokurenko, 2000, FimH, an adaptable adhesin. In *Glycomicrobiology.* (R. J. Doyle, ed.), Plenum Press, Inc. London. In press.

9. Hultgren, S. J., F. Lindberg, G. Magnusson, J. Kihlberg, J. M. Tennant and S. Normark, 1989, The PapG adhesin of uropathogenic *Escherichia coli* contains separate regions for receptor binding and for the incorporation into the pilus. *Proc. Natl. Acad. Sci.* USA 86: 4357-4361.

10. Klemm, P., and Krogfeld, K.A., 1994, Type 1 fimbriae of *Escherichia coli*. In: Fimbriae, adhesion, genetics, biogenesis and vaccins.. P. Klemm, ed. pp. 9-26. CRC press, Boca Raton, Fla.

11. Choudhury, D., A. Thompson, V. Stojanoff, S. Langermann, J. Pinkner, S. J. Hultgren and S. D. Knight, 1999, X-ray structure of the FimC-FimH chaperone-adhesin complex from uropathogenic Escherichia coli. *Science* 285: 1061-1066.

12. Madison, B., I. Ofek, S. Clegg, and S. N. Abraham, 1994, The type 1 fimbrial shafts of *Escherichia coli* and *Klebsiella pneumoniae* influence the sugar specificity of their FimH adhesins. *Infect. Immun.* 62: 843-848.

13. Thankavel, K., A. H. Shah, M. S. Cohen, T. Ikeda, R. G. Lorenz, R. Curtiss III, and S. N. Abraham, 1999, Molecular basis for the enterocyte tropism exhibited by *Salmonella typhimurium* type 1 fimbriae. *J. Biol. Chem.* 274: 5797-5809.

14. Sokurenko, E. V., V. Chesnokova, D. E. Dykhuizen, I. Ofek, X.-R. Wu, K. A. Krogfelt, C. Struve, M. A. Schembri and D. L. Hasty, 1998, Pathogenic adaptation of *Escherichia coli* by natural variation of the FimH adhesin. *Proc. Natl. Acad. Sci. USA* 95: 8922-8926.

15. Sokurenko, E. V., D. L. Hasty and D. E. Dykhuizen, 1999, Pathoadaptive mutations: gene loss and variation in bacterial pathogens. *Trends Microbiol.* 7: 191-195.

16. Firon, N., I. Ofek and N. Sharon, 1983, Carbohydrate specificity of the surface lectins of *Escherichia coli, Klebsiella pneumoniae,* and *Salmonella typhimurium.* *Carbohydr. Res.* 120: 235-249.

17. Sokurenko, E.V., H.S. Courtney, D. E. Ohman, P. Klemm, and D. L. Hasty, 1994, FimH family of type 1 fimbrial adhesins: Functional heterogeneity due to minor sequence variations among *fimH* genes. *J. Bact.* 176: 748-755.

18. Sokurenko, E.V., H. S. Courtney, J. Maslow, A. Siitonen, and D. L. Hasty, 1995, Quantitative differences in adhesiveness of type 1 fimbriated *Escherichia coli* due to structural differences in *fimH* genes. *J. Bact.* 177: 3680-3686.
19. Sokurenko, E. V., V. Chesnokova, R. J. Doyle and D. L. Hasty, 1997, Diversity of the *Escherichia coli* type 1 fimbrial lectin. Differential binding to mannosides and uroepithelial cells. *J. Biol. Chem.* 272: 17880-17886.
20. Duguid, J.P., and Old, D.C., 1980, Adhesive properties of *Enterobacteriaceae* In *Bacterial adherence (Receptors and recogition).* (E.H. Beachey, ed.). Chapman and Hall, London, pp. 187-217
21. Ofek I., J. Goldhar, Y. Eshdat, and N. Sharon , 1982, The importance of mannose specific adhesins (lectins) in infections caused by *Escherichia coli Scand. J. Infect. Dis. Suppl.* 33:61-67.
22. Strömberg, N., B.-I. Marklund, B. Lund, D. Ilver, A. Hamers, W. Gaastra, K.-A. Karlsson, and S. Normark, 1990, Host-specificity of uropathogenic *Escherichia coli* depends on differences in binding specificity to Gal_1-4Gal-containing isoreceptors, *EMBO J.* 9: 2001-2010
23. Sokurenko, E. V., H. S. Courtney, S. N. Abraham, P. Klemm, and D. L. Hasty, 1992, Functional heterogeneity of type 1 fimbriae of *Escherichia coli, Infect. Immun.* 60: 4709-4719.
24. Pouttu, R., T. Puustinen, R. Virkola, J. Hacker, P. Klemm, and T. K. Korhonen, 1999, Amino acid residue Ala-62 in the FimH fimbrial adhesin is critical for the adhesiveness of meningitis-associated *Escherichia coli* to collagens. *Mol. Microbiol.* 31: 1747-1757.
25. Barondes, S. H., 1988, Bifunctional properties of lectins: lectins redefined, *Trends Biochem. Sci.* 13: 480-482.
26. Kaur KJ, Khurana S, Salunke DM. (1997). Topological analysis of the functional mimicry between a peptide and a carbohydrate moiety. J. Biol. Chem. 272::5539-5543
27. Varki, A., 1993, Biological roles of oligosaccharides: all of the theories are correct. Glycobiology 3: 97-130.

# ADHERENCE OF ENTERIC BACTERIA ONTO THE MAMMALIAN EXTRACELLULAR MATRIX
*Test-tube Artefact or a Virulence Function?*

Timo K.Korhonen
*Division of General Microbiology, Department of Biosciences, University of Helsinki, Finland*

## 1.     INTRODUCTION

The pathogenesis of bacterial infection results from a complex series of interactions that often involve a molecular recognition between the invading bacterium and the host. For decades, bacterial attachment to host epithelial surfaces has been recognized as an important virulence property of bacterial pathogens. Adherence to epithelial surfaces of the host is thought to protect the bacteria against mechanical defences, such as removal from epithelial surfaces by urine flow in the urinary tract, peristalsis in the intestine, as well as coughing and saliva secretion in the respiratory tract. Recent studies have indicated that pathogenic bacteria frequently adhere to the mammalian extracellular matrix (ECM) underlaying epithelial or endothelial surfaces. This chapter summarizes what is presently known about the mechanisms and functions of enterobacterial interactions with the mammalian ECM. For more comprehensive reviews, the reader is referred to references 1 and 2.

*Genes and Proteins Underlying Microbial Urinary Tract Virulence*
Edited by L. Emödy *et al.*, Kluwer Academic/Plenum Publishers, 2000

*Table 1.* Enterobacterial ECM-binding proteins

| Bacterial species | Adhesin | ECM target | Reference |
|---|---|---|---|
| Escherichia coli | FimH lectin of the type-1 fimbriae | High-mannose chains of laminin | 3 |
| | CB-FimH | Collagens | 4 |
| | MF-FimH | N-terminus of fibronectin | 5 |
| | SfaS lectin of the S fimbriae | Sialyl-oligosaccharide chains of laminin and cellular fibronectin | 6,7 |
| | DraE minor protein of the Dr fimbriae | 7S domain of type IV collagen | 8 |
| | CsgA protein of curli | Fibronectin | 9 |
| | GafD minor protein of the G fimbriae | GlcNAc-containing oligosaccharides of laminin | 10 |
| | PapE and PapF minor proteins of the P fimbriae | N-terminus of fibronectin | 11 |
| Yersinia enterocolitica | YadA | Collagens, laminin, fibronectin | 12,13 |
| Yersinia pestis | Surface protease Pla | Laminin | 14 |
| Salmonella typhimurium | Outer membrane proteins Rck and PagC | Laminin | 15 |
| Klebsiella | MrkD$_p$ adhesin of the type 3 fimbriae | Type V collagen | 16 |
| | MrkD$_c$ | Type IV and V collagens | 17 |

## 2.     ENTEROBACTERIAL ADHERENCE TO ECM: MULTIPLE MECHANISMS

To date, several molecular interactions of enteric bacteria with the ECM have been characterized; these are listed in Table 1. The interactions differ in regard of the bacterial surface protein involved, the ECM target, as well as the target specificity. Fimbriae are the major class of enterobacterial ECM-binding proteins, the mechanisms of their interactions with the ECM are based either on a protein-carbohydrate interaction or on a protein-protein interaction. Most enterobacterial isolates express the mannoside-binding type-1 fimbria, which bind to the high-mannose chains of laminin of basement membranes (BM). The common occurrence of the type-1 fimbriae in enterobacterial species means that majority of *Escherichia coli* and *Salmonella* isolates have the capacity to bind to BM. Laminin is a highly glycosylated BM protein with several differing carbohydrate chains[18] and also recognized by the S fimbriae of meningitis-associated *E. coli*, which bind to terminal sialylα2-3 galactosides. Terminal sialylα2-3 galactosides also occur in human cellular fibronectin that also is reconized by the SfaS lectin of the S fimbriae[7]. The role in ECM-binding of the fimbrial minor components, or the lectin proteins, has been inferred from studies using specific knock-out mutants, and in a few cases, by expressing the lectin protein in a fusion form.

Somewhat suprisingly, many of the fimbriae-ECM interactions are based on a protein-protein interaction. The P fimbriae of uropathogenic *E. coli* bind to the carbohydrate-free N-terminus of fibronectin via the PapG and PapE minor proteins[11]. The P fimbriae bind to the globoseries of glycolipids on human epithelial and endothelial cells via the PapG component[19], and it thus appears that the P fimbriae are multifunctional adhesive complexes with different components binding to epithelial and on the other hand to ECM receptors. Recent studies have indicated that the mannoside-binding lectin FimH of the type-1 fimbriae is subjected to minor structural variability and that certain FimH variants bind to ECM proteins, such as collagens or fibronectin [4,5]. These interactions are inhibitable with mannosides, although the target proteins or peptides are devoid of them. The phenomenom has been explained by conformational changes in FimH that are induced by mannoside-binding and prevent fibronectin- or collagen-binding. Similar sequence variability affecting ECM-binding apparently occurs also in the MrkD fimbrial adhesin subunit of the type-3 fimbriae of *Klebsiella*.

YadA is a polymeric, S-layer-like protein covering the surface of *Yersinia enterocolitica* and expressing a variety of ECM interactions. The protein has a high affinity to various collagen types, a poorer binding capacity to laminin, and a low-affinity binding to fibronectin[12,13].

Mutagenesis of specific regions in YadA[12,13] as well as heterologous expression of YadA fragments by the flagella display[20] have indicated that at least the laminin- and collagen-binding are distinguishable properties.

The third class of ECM-binding proteins in enteric bacteria consists of outer membrane proteins. Pla is a surface protease of *Yersinia pestis* and responsible for the invasive character of plaque[21]. Pla is a proteolytic activator of plasminogen and cleaves it to plasmin, a potent broad-spectrum serine protease. Pla also is a laminin-specific adhesin, and we have hypothetized that a virulence function of Pla is to direct plasmin activity onto laminin in BMs that is sensitive to plasmin proteolysis. Recently Rck and PagC, which are virulence-plasmid- encoded outer membrane proteins of *Salmonella typhimurium*, were reported to bind to laminin. The adhesive functions of Pla, Rck, and PagC have been only recently described, and it can be assumed that more species of ECM-adhesive outer membrnae proteins will be detected in near future.

The enterobacterial ECM-binding proteins differ in their target specificity, and it is obvious that the conformation of the ECM target also is important for the interaction. Some of the interactions are highly specific, e.g. the plasmid-encoded $MrkD_p$ adhesin of the type-3 fimbriae binds to the immobilized comformation of type V collagen but not to other collagen types or to solubilized type V collagen[14]. The receptor site within the type IV collagen molecule for the DraE fimbrial adhesin has been mapped to the N-terminal 7S domain[8], which is involved in cross-linking of the collagen network in BMs. On the other hand, YadA and CB-FimH recognize multiple collagen types.


## 3.       ...BUT FEW PATHOGENETIC FUNCTIONS

Most of the ECM-interactions listed in Table 1 have also been observed in frozen tissue of human or animal tissue or by using extracted BM or ECM. The binding of the Dr fimbriae to type IV collagen in glomerular mesangium has been demonstrated *in vivo* in rats injected with purified Dr fimbriae[22]. The Dr fimbriue are deposited in the renal glomeruli, where BM is exposed to circulation, and the deposition is specifically inhibited by solubilized type IV collagen. It thus seems safe to conclude that fimbriae-ECM interactions represent true tissue-adherence mechanisms. However, given the high number of the identified ECM-enterobacteria interactions, it is somewhat disturbing that we know so little of the functional or pathogenetic significance of these interactions. Table 2 gives a summary of putative pathogenetic functions of enteric bacteria-ECM interactions.

Adherence to collagens by the YadA protein is needed for the virulence of *Y. enterocolitica* and the spread of the bacteria from the intestine into circulation, liver, and spleen[12,13]. This is the only case where enterobacterial virulence has been specifically attributed to ECM-adherence. YadA has multiple functions and interactions with the host, but introduction into wild type strains of mutations specifcially abolishing collagen-binding dramatically lowers the bacterial virulence. It is not known which stage of the invasive process the mutations affect, and consequently the precise function of the collagen-adherence is not known.

Traditionally, adherence to ECM has been thought to promote bacterial colonization at damaged tissue sites, such as wounds. This may hold for opportunistic uropathogens such as *Proteus* and *Klebsiella*. These bacteria express ECM-adhesins but lack efficient epithelium-binding adhesins, and rarely cause urinary tract infections in otherwise healthy individuals. On the other hand, these bacteria are associated with catheter-associated infections, which easily involve tissue damage by the indwelling catheter.

ECM-adherence has recently been indicated in the invasion of epithelial cells by Gram-postive bacteria [23]. The invasion is triggered by recognition of

*Table 2.* Putative virulence functions of enterobacterial ECM-binding proteins

| Bacterial species | Adhesion property and biological function | Reference |
|---|---|---|
| *Yersinia enterocolitica* | Adherence to collagens needed for bacterial virulence as well as for bacterial spread from the intestine into circulation and liver and spleen | 12,13 |
| *Klebsiella* | Adherence to damaged tissue sites in the urinary tract and the lung | 16,17 |
| *Shigella dysentriae* | Adherence to fibronectin, laminin or type IV collagen stimulates release from the bacterial surface of Ipa proteins needed in bacterial invasion into Caco-2 cells | 24 |
| *Yersinia pestis* | Adherence to laminin potentiates plasmin-mediated damage of BM and bacterial penetration through reconstituted BM | 12 |

bacterium-bound fibronectin by β1 integrins on the epithelial surface. Fibronectin-binding proteins on the Gram-positive bacteria are needed for the process. This invasion mechanism has not been reported for a Gram-negative bacterium yet. However, *Shigella dysentriae* invades intestinal epithelium from the basolateral side of the target cells, and bacterial adherence to ECM proteins stimulates release from the bacterial surface of Ipa proteins that are crucial in the invasion process [24].

An intriguing function for ECM-adherence in enteric bacteria is in bacterial spread through tissue barriers formed by BM and ECMs. Pla of *Y. pestis* is needed for the bacterial invasion from the subcutaneous site into circulation, the protein does not affect virulence in intravenously infected animals[21]. Pla is a protease that activates plasminogen but also is a laminin-specific adhesin. Pla does not cleave laminin directly but requires presence of plasminogen for the activity. We presented evidence in favor of the hypothesis that adherence to BM and plasmin formation on adherent bacteria lead to damage of laminin and BM function, which results in enhanced bacterial penetration through a reconstituted BM[12]. The hypothesis indicates similarity in the behaviour of invasive bacteria and metastatic tumor cells, hence the term "bacterial metastasis".

## 4.    CONCLUSIONS

The common occurrence of ECM-binding proteins in enteric bacteria supports the notion that ECM-adherence has an ecological and/or pathogenetic role in the life style of enteric pathogens. Indeed, we have few cases where the ECM-adherence has been shown to take place *in vivo* and on the other hand to potentiate bacterial virulence and spread within the host. Enterobacterial adhesion to ECM also is involved in bacterial invasion into epithelial cells, and it is likely that new functions will be detected as the ECM-binding proteins are better characterized. It is notable that enterobacterial adhesins appear to be multifunctional: they express multiple adhesive characteristics or have nonadhesive functions as well, such as proteolytic activity. An intriguing possibility is the role of ECM-adherence in bacterial metastasis across BMs. Many of the enterobacterial ECM-binding proteins also function as plasminogen receptors (fimbriae) or plasminogen activators (Pla) and enhance conversion of plasminogen into active plasmin that can be targeted at BM through bacterial adherence. This has been demonstrated *in vitro* to potentiate bacterial penetration through reconstituted BM[14,25], but the *in vivo* evidence is lacking. These findings, however, give evidence for a multifunctional nature of enterobacterial adhesion proteins.

# REFERENCES

1. Westerlund, B., and Korhonen, T.K., 1993, Bacterial proteins binding to the mammalian extracellular matrix. *Mol. Microbiol..* **9:** 687-694.
2. Patti, J.M., Allen, B.L., and Hook, M., 1994. MSCRAMM-mediated adherence of microorganisms to host tissues. *Ann. Rev. Microbiol.* **48:** 585-617.
3. Kukkonen, M., Raunio, T., Virkola, R., Lähteenmäki, K., Mäkelä, P.H., Klemm, P. Clegg, S., and Korhonen, T.K., 1993, Basement membrane carbohydrate as a target for bacterial adhesion: binding of type 1 fimbria of *Salmonella enterica* and *Escherichia coli* to laminin. *Mol. Microbiol.* **7:** 229-237.
4. Pouttu, R., Puustinen, T., Virkola, R., Hacker, J., Klemm, P., and Korhonen, T.K., 1999, Amino-acid residue Ala-62 in the FimH fimbrial adhesin is critical for the adhesiveness of meningitis-associated *Escherichia coli* to collagens. *Mol. Microbiol.* **31:** 1747-1757.
5. Sokurenko, E.V., Courtney, H.S., Ohman, D.E., Klemm, P., and Hasty, D., 1994, FimH family of type 1 fimbrial adhesins: functional heterogeneity due to minor sequence variations among *fimH* genes. *J. Bacteriol.* **176:** 748-755.
6. Virkola, R., Parkkinen, J., J. hacker, and Korhonen, T.K., 1993, Sialyloligosaccharide chains of laminin as an extracellular matrix target for S fimbriae of *Escherichia coli*. *Infect. Immun.* **61:** 4480-4484.
7. Sarén, A., Virkola, R., hacker, J., and Korhonen, T.K., 1999, The cellular form of human fibronectin as an adhesion target for the S fimbriae of meningitis-associated *Escherichia coli*. *Infect. Immun.* **67:**2671-2676.
8. Westerlund, B., Kuusela, P., Risteli, J., Risteli, L., Vartio, T., Rauvala, H., Virkola, R., and Korhonen, T.K., 1989, The O75X adhesin of uropathogenic *Escherichia coli* is a type IV collagen-binding protein. *Mol. Microbiol.* **3:** 329-337.
9. Olsen, A., Jonsson, A., and Normark, S., 1989, Fibronectin-binding mediated by a novel class of surface organelles in *Escherichia coli*. *Nature* **338:** 652-655.
10. Saarela, S., Westerlund-Wikström, B., Rhen, M., and Korhonen, T.K., 1996, The GafD protein of the G /F17) fimbrial complex confers adhesiveness of *Escherichia coli* to laminin. *Infect. Immun.* **64:** 2857-2860.
11. Westerlund, B., van Die, I., Kramer, C., Kuusela, P., Holthöfer, H., Tarkkanen, A.-M., Virkola, R., Riegman, N., Bergmans, H., Hoekstra, W., and Korhonen, T.K., 1991, Multifunctional nature of P fimbriae of uropathogenic *Escherichia coli*: mutations in *fsoE* and *fsoF* influence fimbrial binding to renal tubui and immobilized fibronectin. *Mol. Microbiol.* **5:** 2965-2975.
12. Tamm, A., Tarkkanen, A.-M., Korhonen, T.K., Kuusela, P., Toivanen, P., and Skurnik, M., 1993, Hydrophobic dimains affect the collagen-binding specificity and surface polymerization as well as the virulence potential of the Yada protein of *Yersinia enterocolitica*. *Mol. Microbiol.* **10:** 995-1011.
13. Roggenkamp, A., Neuberger, H.-R., Flugel, A., Schmoll, T., and Heesemann, J., 1995, Substitution of two histidine residues in YadA protein of *Yersinia enterocolitica* abrogates collagen binding, cell adherence and mouse virulence. *Mol. Microbiol.* **16:** 1207-1219.
14. Lähteenmäki, K., Virkola, R., Sarén, A., Emödy, L., and Korhonen, T.K., 1998, Expression of plasminogen activator Pla of *Yersinia pestis* enhances bacterial attachment to the mammalian extracellular matrix. *Infect. Immun.* **66:** 5755-5762.
15. Crago, A.M., and Koronakis, V., 1999, Binding of extracellular matrix laminin to *Escherichia coli* expressing the *Salmonella* outer membrane proteins Rck and PagC. *FEMS Microbiol. Lett.* **176:** 495-501.

16. Tarkkanen, A.-M., Allen, B.L., Westerlund, B., Holthöfer, H., Kuusela, P., Risteli, L., Clegg, S., and Korhonen, T.K., 1990, Type V collagen as the target for type-3 fimbriae, enterobacterial adherence organelles. *Mol. Microbiol.* **4:**1353-1361.

17. Schurtz Sebghati, T.A., Korhonen, T.K., Hornick, D.B., and Clegg, S. 1998. Characterization of the type 3 fimbrial adhesins of *Klebsiella* strains. Infect. Immun. **66:** 2887-2894.

18. Arumugan, R.G., Hsieh, T.C., Tanzer, M.L., and Laine, R.A., 1986, Structures of the asparagine-linked sugar chains of laminin. *Biochem. Biophys. Acta* **883:** 112-126.

19. Kuehn, M.J., Heuser, S., Normark, S., and Hultgren, S., 1992, P pili of uropathogenic *Escherichia coli* are composite fibres with distinct fibrillar adhesive tips. *Nature* **356:**2 52-255.

20. Westerlund-Wikström, B., Tanskanen, J., Virkola, R., Hacker, J., Lindberg, M., Skurnik, M., and Korhonen, T.K., 1997, Functional expression of adhesive peptides as fusions to *Escherichia coli* flagellin. *Prot. Engin.* **10:** 1319-1326.

21. Sodeinde, O.A., Subrahmanyam, V.B.K., Stark, K., Quan, T., Rao, Y., and Goguen, J.D., 1992, A surface protease and the invasive character of plague. Science **258:** 1004-1007.

22. Miettinen, A., Westerlund, B., Tarkkanen, A.-M., Törnroth, T., Ljunberg, P., Renkonen, O.-V., and Korhonen, T.K., 1993, Binding of bacterial adhesins to rat glomerular mesangium *in vivo*. *Kidney Int*. **43:** 592-600.

23. Sinha, B., Francois, P.P., Nüsse, O., Foti, M., hartford, O.M., Vaudaux, P., Foster, T., Lew, D.P., Herrman, P., and Krause, K.-H., 1999, Fibronectin-binding protein acts as *Staphylococcus aureus* invasin via fibronectin bridging to integrin $\alpha_5\beta_1$. . **1:**101-117.

24. Watarai, M., Tobe, T., Yoshikawa, M., and Sasakawa, C., 1995, Contact of *Shigella* with host cells triggers release of Ipa invasins and is an essential function of invasiveness. *EMBO J.* **14:** 2461-2470.

25. Lähteenmäki, K., Virkola, R., Pouttu, R., Kuusela, P., Kukkonen, M., and Korhonen, T.K., 1998, bacterial plasminogen receptors: in-vitro evidence for a role in degradation of the mammalian extracellular matrix. *Infect. Immun.* **63:** 3659-3664.

# INTERRELATIONSHIP BETWEEN VIRULENCE PROPERTIES OF UROPATHOGENIC *E. COLI* AND BLOOD GROUP PHENOTYPE OF PATIENTS WITH CHRONIC URINARY TRACT INFECTION

Reinhard Fünfstück, Niels Jacobsohn, Günter Stein
*Department of Internal Medicine IVFriedrich-Schiller-University of Jena, D-07740 Jena, Erlanger Allee 101, Germany*

## 1. INTRODUCTION

Urinary tract infections (UTI) rank among the most common infectious diseases. For the development of an infection, pathogenicity and virulence of the infective agent are of importance as well as the efficacy of local and systemic immunologic and non-immuno-logic defence mechanisms of the human organism. The interaction of these different factors determines the course of the disease and characterizes the clinical picture of an infection.

In the pathogenesis of UTI, the attachment of microorganisms to mucosal surfaces of the urinary tract is of great importance. In the process of bacterial cytoadherence, infectious agents interfere with specific molecules on epithelial cells[1,2]. Bacteria possess small surface-projecting organellae known as pili or fimbriae. These structures enable the organisms to attach to specific receptors on uroepithelial cells. *E. coli* expresses an array of adhesive structures, including P-, S-, Dr- and type 1- fimbriae. These structures as well as other virulence properties of microorganisms are encoded by chromosomal gene clusters.

P-fimbriae, for instance, recognize $Gal\alpha 1$-$4Gal\beta$ and $GalNA\beta$-$3Gal\alpha 1$-$4Gal\beta$ as receptors, which contain oligosaccharide sequences in the

*Genes and Proteins Underlying Microbial Urinary Tract Virulence*
Edited by L. Emödy *et al.*, Kluwer Academic/Plenum Publishers, 2000

201

globoseries of glycolipids[3]. The molecules are antigens of the P- and ABO-blood group system.

A predisposition to UTI and to other infectious diseases is associated with the expression of $P_1$ as well as the presence of ABO-blood group antigen on the cells of the boundary layer and with the secretor status[4,5]. The frequency of the $P_1$-blood group phenotype is increased among children with recurrent pyelonephritis[6].

Bacteria may adapt to the host-specific situation, with chromosomal genes and plasmids enabling the uropathogenic microorganisms to express different fimbriae and other virulence properties to invade as well as to persist and survive in the host.

In this study, a possible interrelationship between the blood group phenotype and the virulence characteristics of microorganisms in patients with chronic non-obstructive UTI was analyzed.

## 2.         PATIENTS AND METHODS

### 2.1      Patients

In 53 women (mean age $42 \pm 12$ years) with chronic non-obstructive pyelonephritis, *E. coli* strains were examined. All patients suffering from an acute UTI were examined micro-biologically. Subsequent investigations of the patients did not provide any clinical or biochemical clues to an acute infection. The diagnosis was established on the basis of clinical history as well as clinical, laboratory and radiological findings (renal scarring, caliceal clubbing and blunting). In all patients, a vesicoureteral reflux, an obstruction due to concrements or a metabolic disorder (diabetes mellitus, hyperuricemia) were ruled out. In no case was urinary tract infection associated with glomerulonephritis or a gynecological disease. No immunocompromised host was included.

In all cases, significant bacteriuria by *E. coli* ($>10^5$ colonies/ml urine) was found in midstream urine samples.

### 2.2      Methods

*Determination of Disease Activity:* the inflammatory parameters erythrocyte sedimentation rate, leukocyte count, $\alpha_2$-globulin fraction, C-reactive protein, leukocyturia and erythro-cyturia were determined.

*Microbiological Investigations:* a total of 144 *E. coli* strains was studied over a period of 3 years. On average, 2.8 ± 1.6 germ analyses were carried out for each patient.

*Bacteria:* the bacterial examination included bacterial count, species identification, and antibiotic susceptibility determination according to Edwards and Ewing[7].

*Hemolysin:* the hemolytic activity of the bacterial strains was determined as described by Springer and Goebel[8]. The amount of hemoglobin released was identified spectrophoto-metrically at 420 nm and served as a quantitative measure of the hemolytic activity of the strains.

*Fimbriae (mannose-resistant hemagglutination):* hemagglutination was tested using a slide agglutination test[9]. Washed red blood cells (group A) obtained from humans, cattle and guinea pigs were used in a 5% solution, and 0.1 M mannose was added at a ratio of 1:4. The strain to be studied was incubated on CFA agar for 24 h. Several colonies were suspended in a drop of red blood cell suspension without adding D-mannose. The presence of P-fimbriae and of type F 7 to 14-fimbriae was recorded in cases where agglutination of human group A erythrocytes without agglutination with erythrocytes from cattle or guinea pigs occurred, often in the presence of D-mannose.

*Hydroxamate/aerobactin:* the production of aerobactin was measured according to Stuart et al.[10] and Wittig et al[11], an E. coli K 12 strain LG 1622 serving as the indicator strain. This bioassay is 1.000 times more sensitive than chemical analysis.

*K 1-antigen:* the detection of K 1-antigen was carried out by means of K 1-specific phages[12]. Confluent or semiconfluent lysis by K 1-phages was regarded as documenting K 1-antigen.

*Blood group assays:* the ABO-phenotype was determined by macroscopic hemagglutination performed with a drop of erythrocyte suspension and two drops of anti-A and anti-B (BIOTEST AG, Germany) in separate tubes. The $P_1$-antigen was analyzed by incubating one drop of erythrocyte suspension with two drops of anti-$P_1$ serum (BIOTEST AG, Germany) at 4 °C for 30 min. The Lewis phenotyping was performed by incubating one drop of 4% erythrocyte suspension with two drops of anti-Le(a) and anti-Le(b) serum (ORTHO DIAGNOSTIC SYSTEM, USA) in separate tubes at room temperature for 30 min. Macroscopic hemagglutination was assessed after test tubes had been centrifuged at 3400 rpm for 15 sec.

*Statistical analysis:* after calculating the frequency distributions of the statistical testing, the exact two-tailed Fisher test was performed. In order to test the dependence between qualitative features, Pearson's $X^2$-method and methods of logistic regression and discrimination were employed.

## 3.    RESULTS

## 3.1    Patients

In the first stage of investigation, all patients were suffering an acute episode of an upper urinary tract infection indicated by symptoms like dysuria, pollakisuria, flank pain and rise in temperature above 38 °C. For the treatment of pyelonephritis, ampicillin, gentamicin, sulfameracin/ trimethoprim, ciprofloxacin or ofloxacine were administered. During the following microscopical investigations no signs of clinically acute disease were observed in all patients. The laboratory data of the patient group are presented in Table 1.

*Table 1.*  Characteristics of the patient group (n = 53)

| Criteria | Acute episode of pyelonephritis | Asymptomatic Stage |
|---|---|---|
| *Duration of UTI* | 11,9 ± 9,5 years | |
| *Symptoms:* | | |
| Dysuria | + | - |
| Pollakisuria | + | - |
| Flank pain | + | - |
| Rise in temperature (above 38°C) | + | - |
| *Laboratory findings:* | | |
| Blood sedimentation rate (mm) | 19.7 ± 5.8 | 10.4 ± 9.4 |
| Leucocytes (Gpt/l) | 10.8 ± 1.9 | 6.4 ± 1.9 |
| $\alpha_2$-globulin | 0.12 ± 0.03 | 0.08 ± 0.02 |
| C-reactive protein (pos.) | 100 % | 8 % |
| Creatinin (µmol/l) | 104.7 ± 20.1 | 98.2 ± 12.7 |
| Leucocyturia | 53 (100 %) | 6 (11 %) |
| Erythrocyturia | 12 (22 %) | - |
| Bacteriuria | 53 (100 %) | 53 (100 %) |

In all patients, the ABO-, $P_1$- and Lewis-blood group statuses were investigated. It was remarkable that the proportion of persons with B-phenotype was around 23% in the patient group. Generally, the incidence of this feature in the German population is 14.5%[13]. $P_1$-antigen was found in 76% of patients, which corresponds to the frequency of $P_1$-antigen presence in the population. Individuals with $P_1$-antigen are more predisposed to an adherence with P-fimbriated microorganisms. In comparison with $P_1$-antigen-negative individuals, $P_1$-antigen-positive persons have a longer disease history and suffer more frequently from symptomatic infectious events as well as destructive renal changes. These findings are summarized in Figure 1.

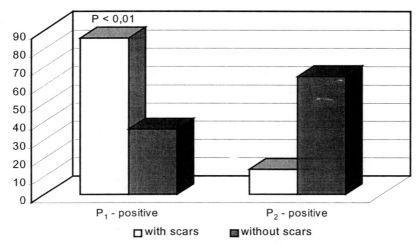

*Figure 1.* $P_1$-blood group antigen distribution and detection of renal scarring in urogram and sonogram

*Table 2.* Incidence of virulence properties in *E. coli* in 53 patients with an acute episode of non-obstructive pyelonephritis

| Virulence property | Rate of incidence |
|---|---|
| Hemolysin formation | 26 (49 %) |
| Fimbriae (mannose-resistant hemaglutination) | 26 (49 %) |
| Hydroxamate/aerobactin | 25 (47 %) |
| K 1-antigen | 9 (17 %) |

The Le(a)-antigen was detected in 82% and the Le(b)-phenotype could be observed in 18% of patients. The frequency of the ABO-, $P_1$- and Lewis-antigen in the patients with the urinary tract infection showed no statistically significant differences when compared to the distribution of the blood group phenotypes in the general population[4,13].

## 3.2　Microorganisms

Incidence of virulence properties in the acute episode: the virulence factors of *E. coli* strains were demonstrated to varying degrees. Hemolysin formation (n = 26/49%), mannose-resistant hemagglutination/fimbriae (n = 26/49%) and the ability to produce hydroxamate/ aerobactin (n = 25/47%) were detected most frequently. The expression of K 1-antigen (n = 9/17%) was seen less frequently. The frequency distribution is displayed in Table 2.

Distribution of virulence properties over a period of 3 years: during a 3-year period, 144 E. coli strains were analyzed in all patients. The properties of hydroxamate/aerobactin (n = 47/33%) and mannose-resistant hemagglutination (n = 44/31%) were detected most frequently. The ability to form hemolysin (n = 38/27%) and the expression of K 1-antigen (n = 12/8%) were found in a minority of the bacterial strains. There is a statistical relationship (probability of error: 5%) between the ability of hemolysin formation and the property of mannose-resistant hemagglutination (evidence of fimbriae) as well as the ability of hydroxamate production and K 1-antigen expression.

Analysis during the 3-year period showed a striking decrease in the virulence of the microorganisms during their persistence in the urogenital tract. In particular, the loss of hemolysin expression was statistically significant (p = 0.05). The incidence of virulence properties of 144 E. coli strains over a 3-year follow-up period is demonstrated in Figure 2.

## 3.3　Interrelationship Between Blood Group Phenotype and Virulence Properties of Microorganisms

A correlation between the existence of specific molecules on the epithelial surfaces and the expression of typical virulence markers for uropathogenic strains was detected for single blood group phenotypes only. Virulent *E. coli* strains were rarely found in $P_1$-antigen-positive persons. In contrast to this finding, in patients without an $P_1$-antigen, microorganisms with a concomitant ability of hemolysin formation and of mannose-resistant hemagglutination (fimbriae) were found significantly more often (p = 0.05) than in P-positive cases. The probability of this association was even higher

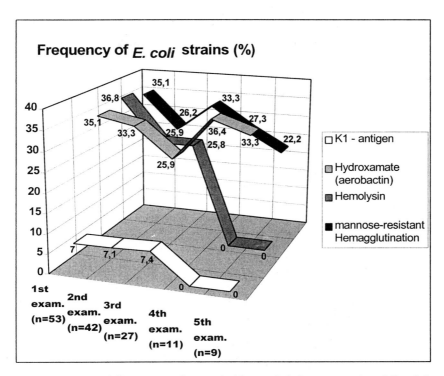

*Figure 2.* Long-term follow-up over 3 years: incidence of virulence properties of *E. coli* in patients with non-obstructive urinary tract infections without clinical symptom

| VIRULENCE OF *E. COLI* | HOST BLOOD GROUP | | |
|---|---|---|---|
| *Hly + mrH* ▲ | *P1-antigen:* | ‒ | *p = 0.05* |
| *Hly + mrH* ▲▲ | *B-antigen:* | + | *p = 0.008* |
| *K 1-antigen* ▲ | *Le(a+):* | + | *p = 0.05* |

(Results of 144 *E. coli* from 53 patients)

*Figure 3.* Tendencies of an association between blood group phenotypes and virulence properties of uropathogenic microorganisms

in patients with a simultaneous appearance of the B-antigen (p = 0.001*). E. coli* strains with K 1-antigen were found significantly more often in patients with the Lewis(a) sign. A summary of the associations between host-specific genetic factors and virulence properties of uropathogenic *E. coli* strains is shown in Fig 3.

## 4.    DISCUSSION

A bacterial infection is preceded by overcoming the multiple natural host defense mechanisms by the microorganisms. A pathogenic bacterial strain must be able to interfere with the host physiology in several ways, to survive in the host evironment, to attach to and multiply on the body surface and to resist the defense mechanisms. Uropathogenic bacterial strains seem to fulfil these requirements[14,15,16]. Depending on the immunological and non-immunological defense mechanisms of the host, microorganisms are able to adapt their virulence by producing special markers. These properties of pathogenic bacteria are encoded by chromosomal and plasmid genes[17,18].

Potential virulence properties include O- and K-antigens, the capacity of fimbria or pili to adhere to cells of the epithelial layer as well as the ability to form hemolysin or hydroxamate (aerobactin)[19,20]. Microorganisms causing an acute infection are particularly characterized by their ability to adhere to the uroepithelial cells (mannose-resistant hemagglutination) and to form hemolysin. In contrast to Löffler et al.[21] and Elo[22], who described this property in 90% of the E. coli strains from patients with pyelonephritis, this investigation demonstrates the property of mannose-resistant hemagglutination in 49% of the acute episodes and in 31% of cases without a symptomatic disease. Hemolysin was more frequent in strains isolated from acute infections (Table 2). This factor appears to be a prerequisite for bacterial invasion of the host. With a prolonged persistence of microorganisms in the urinary tract, a significant loss of the ability to produce hemolysin was found (p = 0.05). In the course of time, strains with two ore more virulence properties became rarer. Microorganisms are able to change their virulence profile, depending on the host situation[23,24].

Adherence of the infecting bacteria is a nesessary prerequisite to the development of UTI. Bacterial surface proteins, like fimbriae or pili, interfere with specific receptors of vaginal and uroepithelial cells[25]. Individuals with a $P_1$-antigen are more predisposed to an adherence with P-fimbriated microorganisms (mannose-resistant hemagglutination positive strains). The epidemiological studies of Hooton et al.[25], Kinane et al.[27] or J. Sheinfeld et al.[28] have demonstrated that women with a history of recurrent urinary tract infection are three to four times more frequently non-secretors of ABO-blood groups antigens than women without such a history. The antigens of ABO-blood groups are present in two forms: as an alcohol-soluble element in the tissue of all subjects and as a water-soluble element in most body fluids and organs of secretors. The Lewis-antigens $Le^a$ and $Le^b$ are biochemically related to the ABO group. The ABO- and Lewis-antigen profiles of cells are the result of a complex interaction among the structural loci of ABO and Le[4]. The expression of $P_1$-phenotype is attributed to the structure of $\alpha$-D-Gal(1-4)-ß-D-Gal which is known to bind to uropathogenic bacteria. The composition of glyco-sphingolipids and glycoprotein receptors is determind by the activity of glycosyltransferases, the expression of which are is under genetic control[25]. A correlation between virulence properties of infecting microorganisms and the structure of receptor molecules on the uroepithelium is interesting from the pathogenetic point of view. Only few data are available on the above suject. Lomberg et al.[29] showed that the non-secretor phenotype was significantly linked with the occurence of renal scarring. In contrast to these findings, Lurie et al.[4] could not demonstrate an association of ABO-, Lewis- or P-blood group phenotypes with recurrent pelvic inflammatory disease. Both studies gave no information on the virulence profile of infecting agents. Plos et al.[30] have shown that $P_1$-individuals have an increased tendency to carry P-fimbriated *E. coli* strains in the fecal flora compared to individuals of the $P_2$-blood group. In this study, virulent strains possessing the hemolysin marker were rarely found in $P_1$-antigen-positive patients. In contrast to this finding, microorganisms with properties of mannose-resistant hemagglutina-tion (fimbriae) and hemolysin formation were found more frequently in $P_1$-antigen-negative individuals. These persons express a smaller amount of receptors for P-fimbriated *E. coli*, so that for infecting strains the attachment to and the passage through the boundary layer seem to be more difficult. It could be concluded that the existence of $P_1$-antigen may be a gap in the protective mechanisms and might be an indicator for an increased susceptibility to UTI. Under these circumstances, infecting bacteria do not need to express a variety of different virulence factors to invade the host. For the blood group B-antigen, and especially for B-secretors, a protective effect by galactose-containing surface molecules can be postulated, because these molecules are without binding affinities for *E. coli* strains[31,32]. In these patients, an increased virulence of the infective microorganisms along with an increased ability to form hemolysin and an increased expression of fimbriae appears to be explicable to overcome this situation. *E. coli* strains with K 1-antigen were significantly more often found in patients with the Lewis(a+) phenotype. Bacteria equipped with capsular antigens are more resistant to bactericidal effects of the host organisms[12]. As IgA and IgG levels are increased in Lewis(a+) and in non-secretors, according to investigations by Blackwell et al.[33], the presence of K-antigen in microorganisms is likely to be a protective mechanisms for host-specific defense reactions.

The association between blood group antigens and secretor status and the virulence of uropathogenic bacteria represents one interesting aspect of urinary tract infection. A better understanding of these interrelations may result in a better diagnostic strategy, especially in cases with recurrent urinary tract infections. Further studies are required to characterize the relationship to other local defense systems, to disease activity and frequency of infective episodes.

## 5.    CONCLUSION

The ABO- and Lewis-antigens located at the cells of the epithelial boundary layer of the human organism represent a natural protective mechanism against the invasive efforts of pathogens. However, antigen structures on the uroepithelial cells, such as the glycosphingo-lipids of the P-blood group system, serve as receptors for adhesion. In dependence on this situation, microorganisms are able to express virulence factors at different degrees.

In 53 patients, ABO-, $P_1$- and Lewis-blood group phenotypes as well as the secretor status were investigated in terms of virulence properties of *E. coli* strains and the degree of bacterial adherence to uroepithelial cells. Pathogenicity was determined in 144 *E. coli* strains over three years. Patients with $P_1$-antigens (n = 40/76%) had fewer microorganisms with the ability to produce hemolysin and mannose-resistant hemagglutination than persons without P-antigen. This difference was statistically significant (p = 0.05) and greater in patients with blood group B (n = 13/23%), especially in B-secretors (n = 9/16%; p < 0.0005). *E coli* strains with K 1-antigen were significantly more often found in patients with Lewis(a+).

The phenotypic expression of virulence properties of *E. coli* is very likely to be determined by host-specific factors, such as the antigens $P_1$ and B as well as the Lewis-blood group phenotype.

## ACKNOWLEDGMENTS

The bacterial examinations (bacterial count, differentiation) were performed at the Insitute of Medical Microbiology of the University of Jena.

# REFERENCES

1.  Kunin, C.M., 1994, Urinary tract infections in femals. *Clin. Infect. Dis.* **18**: 1 – 12.
2.  Svanborg-Eden, C., Hagberg, L., Hanson, L.A., Hult, S., Hult, R., Jodal, U., Leffler, H., Lomberg, H., and Straube, E., 1993, Bacterial adherence - a pathogenic mechanism in urinary tract infections caused in *Escherichia coli. Prog. Allergy* **33**: 175 – 188.
3.  Johnson, J.R., 1991, Virulence factors in *Escherichia coli* urinary tract infections. *Clin. Microbiol. Rev.* **4**: 80 – 128.
4.  Lurie, S., Sigler, E., and Fenakel, K., 1991, The ABO, Lewis or P blood group phenotypes are not associated with recurrent pelvic inflammatory disease. *Gyn. Obstet. Invest.* **31**: 158 – 160.
5.  Lomberg, H., Cedergren, B., Leffler, H., Nilsson, B., Carlstrom, A.S., and Svanborg-Eden, C., 1986, Influence of blood groups on the availability of receptors for attachment of uropathogenic *Escherichia coli. Infect. Immun.* **51**: 919 – 926.
6.  Lomberg, H., Hanson, L.A., Jacobsson, B., Jodal, U., Leffler, H., and Svanborg-Eden, C., 1983, Correlation of P blood group, vesicoureteral reflux, and bacterial attachment in patients with recurrent pyelonephritis. *N. Engl. J. Med.* **308**: 1189 – 1192.
7.  Edwards, R.P., and Ewing, W.H., 1962, Indentification of *Enterobacteriaceae*. Progress Publishing Co., Minneapolis
8.  Springer, W., and Goebel, W., 1980, Synthesis and secretion of hemolysin *by Escherichia coli. J. Bacteriol.* **144**: 53 – 59.
9.  Evans, D.J., Evans, D.G., Young, L.S., and Pit, I., 1980, Hemagglutination typing of *E. coli*: Definition of serum hemagglutination types. *J. Clin. Microbiol.* **12**: 235 – 242.
10. Stuart, S.J., Greenwood, K.R., and Luke, R.K.J., 1982, Iron-suppressible production of hydroxamate by *E. coli* isolates. *Infect. Immun.* **36**: 870 – 873.
11. Wittig, W., Prager, R., Tietze, E., Seltmann, G., and Tschäpe, H., 1988, Aerobactin-positive *Escherichia coli* as causative agents of extraintestinal infections among animals. *Arch. Exp. Vet. Med.* **42**: 211 – 219.
12. Nimmich, W., Naumann, G., Budde, E., and Straube, E., 1980, K-Antigen, Adhärenzfaktor, Dulcitol-Abbau und Hämolysinbildung bei *E. coli*-R-Stämmen aus Urin. *Zentralbl. Bakteriol. Mikrobiol. Hyg. [A]* **247**: 35 – 42.
13. Prokop, O., and Göhler, G., 1986, Die menschlichen Blutgruppen. Fischer, 5. Aufl., Jena.
14. Mühldorfer, I,m and Hacker, J., 1999, Pathogenitätscharakteristika potentieller Infektionserreger im Urogenitaltrakt. *Nieren- und Hochdruckk.* **3**: 8 – 84.
15. Johnson, J.R., 1991, Virulence factors in *Escherichia coli* urinary tract infection. *Clin. Microbiol. Rev.* **4**: 80 – 128.
16. Mobley, H.L.T., Island, M.D., and Massad, G., 1994, Virulence determinants of uropathogenic *Escherichia coli* and *Proteus mirabilis. Kidney Int.* **47 (Suppl.)**: 129 – 136.
17. Mühldorfer, I., and Hacker, J., 1994, Genetic aspects of Escherichia coli virulence. *Microb. Pathogen.* **16**: 171 – 181.
18. Ludwig, A., and Goebel, W., 1991, Genetic determinants of cytolytic to×ins from gram-negative bacteria*In Sourcebook of Bacterial Protein Toxins.* ( J.E. Alouf and J.H. Freer, eds.) Academic Press, London, pp. 117 – 146.
19. Fünfstück, R. ,Tschäpe, H., Stein, G., Vollandt, R., and Schneider, S., 1989, Virulence of *Escherichia coli* strains in relation to their hemolysin formation, mannose-resistant hemagglutination, hydroxamate production, K 1-antigen and the plasmid profile in patients with chronic pyelonephritis. *Clin. Nephrol.* **4**: 178 – 184.

20.   Foxman, B., Zhang, L., Palin, K., Tallman, P., and Marrs, C.F., 1995, Bacterial
      virulence characteristics *of Escherichia coli* isolates from first-time urinary tract
      infection. *J. Infect. Dis.* **171:** 1514 – 1521.
21.   Leffler, H., and Svanborg-Eden, C., 1981, Glycolipid receptors for uropathogenic *E.
      coli* binding to human erythrocytes and uroepithelial cells. Globoseries glycolipid
      versus other receptors. *Infect. Immun.* **34:** 920 – 929.
22..  Elo, J., 1991, Mikrobiologische Aspekte in der Pathogenese der Pyelonephritis. In
      *Harnwegsinfektion* (G. Stein. and R. Fünfstück, R eds), pmi-Verlag, Frankfurt/Main,
      pp. 11 – 13.
23.   Russo, T.A., Stapleton, A., Wenderoth, S., Hooton, T.M., and Stamm, W.E., 1995,
      Chromosomal restriction fragment length polymorphism analysis of *Escherichia coli*
      strains causing recurrent urinary tract infections in young women. *J. Infect. Dis.* **172:**
      440–445.
24.   Savoia, D., Millesmo, M., and Fontana, G., 1994, Evaluation of virulence factors and
      the adhesive capability of *Escherichia coli* strains. *Microbio.* **80:** 73 – 81.
25.   Stapleton, A., and Stamm, W.E., 1997, Prevention of urinary tract infection. *Infect. Dis.
      Clin. North. Am.* **3:** 719 – 733.
26.   Hooton, T.M., Roberts, P.L., and Stamm, W.E., 1994, Effects of recent sexual activity
      and use of a diaphragma on the vaginal microflora. *Clin. Infect. Dis.* **19:** 274 – 278.
27.   Kinane, D.F., Blackwell, C.C., Brettle, R.P., Weir, D.M. Winstanley, F.P., and Elton,
      R.A., 1982, ABO blood group, secretor state, and susceptibility to recurrent urinary
      tract infection in women. *Br. Med. J. Clin. Res. Ed.* **285:** (6334), 7 – 9.
28.   Sheinfeld, .J., Schaeffer, A.J., and Cordon-Cardo, C., 1989, Association of the Lewis
      blood-group phenotype with recurrent urinary tract infection in women. *N. Engl. J.
      Med.* **320:** 773 – 777.
29.   Lomberg, H., Hellström, M., Jodal, U., and Svanborg-Eden, C., 1989, Secretor state and
      renal scarring in girls with recurrent pyelonephritis. *FEMS Microbiol. Immunol.* **1:** 371
      – 376.
30.   Plos, K., Connel, H., Jodal, U., Marklund, B-I., Märild, S., Wettergren, B., and
      Svanborg, C., 1995, Intestinal carriage of P-fimbriated *Escherichia coli* and the
      susceptibility to urinary tract infection in yound children. *J. Infect. Dis.* **171:** 625 – 631.
31.   Blackwell, C.C., 1989, The role of ABO blood groups and secretor status in host
      defences. *FEMS Microbiol. Immunol.* **1:** 341 – 349.
32.   Jacobsohn, N., 1997, Thesis *Erreger-Wirt-Beziehung bei chronischer Pyelonephritis
      unter besonderer Berücksichtigung des ABO-, P- und des Lewis-Blutgruppensystems
      sowie des Sekretorstatus.* University of Jena.
33.   Blackwell, C.C., May, S.J., Brettle, R.P., Mac Callum, O.J., and Weir, D.M., 1987,
      Secretor state and immunglobulin levels among women with recurrent urinary tract
      infections. *J. Clin. Lab. Immunol.* **22:** 133 – 137.

# GLYCOLIPID RECEPTORS OF F1C FIMBRIAL ADHESIN OF UROPATHOGENIC *ESCHERICHIA COLI*

A. Salam Khan and Jörg Hacker

*Institut für Molekulare Infektionsbiologie der Universität Würzburg, Röntgenring 11, D-97070 Würzburg, Germany*

## 1.    INTRODUCTION

One of the indispensable steps in several infections caused by *Escherichia coli* and other gram-negative bacteria is their specific adherence to host cell surface carbohydrates linked to glycoproteins or to glycolipids[1,2,3,4,5].

Urinary tract infections (UTI) in humans are strongly associated with *E.coli* producing P-, type 1, S- and F1C- fimbriae. P fimbriae are defined by the ability to mediate binding to the Galα 1–4 Gal saccharide in glycolipids of the globoseries. Type-1 fimbriae bind specifically to mannose residues. *Escherichia coli* strains harboring S-fimbriae are primarily responsible for UTI and newborn meningitis (NBM). The bacterial ligands and their corresponding eukaryotic receptor structures have only been identified and characterized for two (SfaI and SfaII) of the four members of the S-fimbrial family. The adhesin proteins and their cognate receptors of two other members of the S super family, F1C- and Sfr-fimbriae, which are also involved in UTI, are not yet identified. Despite the significant sequence similarities among the major and minor subunits of S-, F1C- and Sfr-fimbrial complexes, F1C- and Sfr-fimbriated bacteria do not bind to the receptor (2-3 sialyl lactose residues) of the S-fimbrial adhesin nor do they show a hemagglutinating property[5,6].

In the present study we investigated the binding ability of F1C fimbriated recombinant *E. coli* strain (HB101-110-54) to several different cell lines.

*Genes and Proteins Underlying Microbial Urinary Tract Virulence*
Edited by L. Emödy *et al.*, Kluwer Academic/Plenum Publishers, 2000

Additionally, a glycolipid receptor for F1C fimbriated bacteria was also identified.

## 2.      ELISA BASED ADHERENCE STUDIES

In order to identify the binding specificity of F1C fimbriated recombinant bacteria, binding assays were carried out with different cell lines as shown in Table 1. F1C fimbriated bacteria bound to the monolayers grown in microtiter plates in a dose dependent manner (Table 1). The bacteria of the nonfimbriated phenotype failed to bind. Interestingly, F1C fimbriated *E. coli* do not show binding to all of the cell lines to which the two other members of this family (SfaI and SfaII) bind (Table 1). These results suggest that the difference in binding of F1C- and SfaI-or SfaII-fimbriated bacteria could be due to the presence or absence of certain binding epitopes on the surface of those cell lines (Table 1). These finding also confirmed the previous

*Table 1.* Binding efficiencies of serially diluted nonfimbriated recombinant *E. coli* HB101 (control), F1C-, SfaI- and SfaII-fimbriated recombinant strains to the monolayers of several different cell lines grown on microtiter plates. Bacterial binding was determined by an ELISA based assay.

| Cell Lines | Origin | Control | Fimbrial Type | | |
|---|---|---|---|---|---|
| | | | F1C | SfaI | SfaII |
| | **Epithelium** | | | | |
| HKEPC | Human Kidney | - | ++ | ++ | ++ |
| LLCPK1 | Pig Kidney | - | - | ++ | ++ |
| MDCK | Canine Kidney | - | - | ++ | ++ |
| VERO | Monkey Kidney | - | - | - | - |
| A6-112 | Pigeon Kidney | - | - | - | + |
| T24 | Human Urinary Bladder | - | - | + | + |
| RT112 | Human Urinary Bladder | - | ++ | ++ | ++ |
| CaCo2 | Human Intestine | - | + | ND | ND |
| | **Endothelium** | | | | |
| HUVEC* | Human Umbilical. Cord | - | - | ++ | ++ |
| EA-hy926 | Human Umbilical Cord | - | - | + | + |
| HGMEC | Human Glomerulus | - | ++ | ++ | ++ |
| RGMEC | Rat Glomerulus | - | ++ | ++ | ++ |
| HBMEC | Human Brain | - | - | ++ | ++ |

(*) Primary cells, (-) No binding, (+) Weak binding, (++) Strong binding, (ND) Not determined

observation that F1C fimbriae do not interact with the receptor of SfaI- and SfaII-fimbrial adhesins [5,6].

# 3.     ADHERENCE STUDIES

In order to identify the binding specificity of F1C fimbriated recombinant bacteria, binding assays were carried out with human bladder carcinoma cell line RT112 as shown in figure1. Light microscopic studies demonstrated a distinct adherence of F1C fimbriated bacteria to the monolayers grown in chamber slides (Fig 1, panel A). The bacteria of the nonfimbriated phenotype failed to bind (Fig 1, panel B).

A       B

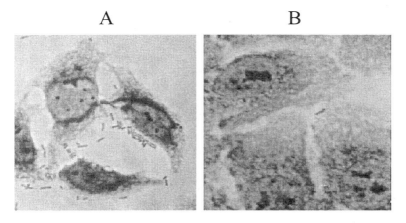

*Figure 1.* Adherence of F1C fimbriated recombinant *E. coli* HB101-110-54 (A) and non fimbriated control strain HB101-pBR (B) to RT112 cells. Cells were cultured in tissue culture chambered slides and after incubation with bacteria and fixing with methanol, the slides were Giemsa stained (X 1000).

# 4.     IDENTIFICATION OF F1C GLYCOLIPID RECEPTORS

To identify the F1C receptor(s), glycolipids were extracted from human intestinal epithelial cell line (CaCo2) and separated on high performance thin layer chromatographic plates (HPTLC). Glycolipids were detected by carbohydrate staining (Fig. 2 Panel A). Thin layer chromatography overlay assay with biotinylated and streptavidin-peroxidase conjugated F1C fimbriated bacteria highlighted essentially two closely migrating bands in the

CaCo2 glycolipid extract (Fig 2 Panel B). Nonfimbriated bacteria failed to show any binding (Fig 2 Panel C).

A    B    C

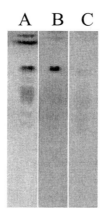

*Figure 2.* HPTLC separation and overlay analysis. Chromatograms of glycolipids extractracted from CaCo2 cell lines. Glycolipids (20µg/lane) separated on HPTLC silica gel 60, stained with orcinol (panel A) overlaid with biotinylated streptavidin-peroxidase conjugated F1C fimbriated (panel B) and nonfimbriated (control, panel C) recombinant bacteria ($10^9$ bacteria/ml) are shown. Bacterial binding is determined by diaminobenzidine and $H_2O_2$.

## 5.    CONCLUSIONS

The ability of F1C fimbriated bacteria to bind to the human urinary tract could be demonstrated by performing binding studies using several different cell lines as shown in table 1, and by performing direct binding assay using human bladder epithelial cell line RT112 as shown in Fig 1.

These results further suggest that similar to the the P-, S-, and 987P-fimbriae of uropathogenic and enterotoxigenic *E. coli*[4,5], F1C fimbriae of uropathogenic *E. coli* strains also mediate the binding of those strains to the glycolipid receptors on cell surfaces.

## ACKNOWLEDGEMENTS

This work was supported by grants from the Deutsche Forschungsgemeinschaft (KH23/2-1), the SFB 479, as well as by the Fonds der Chemischen Industrie.

# REFERENCES

1. Mühldorfer, I., and Hacker, J., 1994, Genetic aspects of Escherichia coli virulence. *Microbial Pathogenesis* **16:** 171-181.
2. Khan, A. S., Mühldorfer, I., Demuth, V., Wallner, U., Korhonen, T., and Hacker, J., Functional analysis of the minor subunits of S fimbrial adhesins (Sfa I) in pathogenic *Escherichia coli. Mol. Gen. Genet.* in press.
3. Khan, A. S., and Schifferli, D. M., 1994, A minor 987P protein different from the structural fimbrial subunit is the adhesin. *Infect. Immun.* **62:** 4223-4243.
4. Khan, A. S., Johnston, N. C., Goldfine, H., and Schifferli, D. M., 1996, Porcine 987P glycolipid receptors on intestinal brush borders and their cognate bacterial ligands. *Infect Immun.* **64:** 3688-3693.
5. Hacker, J., and Morschhäuser, J., 1994, *S and F1C fimbriae.* In Fimbriae, Adhesion, Genetics, Biogenesis, and Vaccines, (P. Klemm, ed.), CRC press, Boca Raton, pp. 27-36.
6. Marre, R., Kreft, B., and Hacker, J., 1990, Genetically engineered S and F1C fimbriae differ in their contribution to adherence of *Escherichia coli* to cultured renal tubulus cells. *Infect. Immun.* **58:** 3434-3437.

# THIN AGGREGATIVE FIMBRIAE ON URINARY
# *ESCHERICHIA COLI* ISOLATES

Eszter Pátri, Edina Szabó, Tibor Pál and Levente Emődy
*Department of Medical Microbiology and Immunology, University Medical School, Pécs, Hungary*

## 1.    INTRODUCTION

Thin aggregative fimbriae, also called curli, have been detected on *Escherichia coli* and *Salmonella enteritidis* isolates of both human and animal sources[1,2,3]. These morphologically and biochemically unique surface appendages are also called *GVVPQ* fimbriae referring to the N-terminal amino acid sequence of their fimbrin subunit. The whole fimbria is a homopolymer of subunits sizing 17 and 18 kDa in *S. enteritidis* and *E. coli*, respectively. Expression of this fimbria species requires special culture conditions, and it does not appear on the bacterial surface when grown on culture media conventionally used for processing clinical specimens. Optimal expression occures on a simple agar medium containing 1 % Tryptone as the sole nutrient. Grown on this medium bacteria are surrounded by copious vegetation of thin curled filamentous appendages. Bacterial cells expressing curli stick strongly to the surface of culture plates, bind intensively the hydrophobic dye congo red, and show a tendency to autoaggregate. Thin aggregative fimbriae also confer the capability for bacteria to interact with extracellular matrix components like fibronectin, laminin and various types of collagen [1,7].

Unlike other fimbria species curli is best expressed at ambient temperature. Its synthesis, assembly and regulation are governed by a collection of genes including the *csg* line and the *crl* regulatory cistron. The expression is also under the influence of the RpoS "starvation" sigma factor.

Earlier studies have revealed that representation of curli is quite common on *S. enteritidis* and on some groups of *E. coli* causing enteric infections [2,3,6]. Far less is, however, known about the frequency of curli producing strains among extraintestinal isolates, including uropathogenic *E. coli*.

## 2. AIM OF THE STUDY

As no data is available on the production of thin aggregative fimbriae by uropathogenic *E. coli* strains we decided to investigate the occurence of these surface appendages on urinary *E. coli* isolates.

We also studied if curli on urinary *E. coli* strains show an antigenic relationship with the prototype *GVVPQ* fimbria of *S. enteritidis*.

The wide distribution of *csg*A and *crl* genes among *E. coli* strains prompted us to investigate the presence of these gene sequences in both curli positive and negative strains involved in this study.

## 3. MATERIALS AND METHODS

### 3.1 Bacterial Strains

50 randomly selected positive urine cultures yielding $>10^5$ *E. coli* cells per mL as the single pathogen were included in the study. The *GVVPQ* fimbria producing *S. enteritidis* 27655-3b, its curli negative derivative and the PCR control *E. coli* ETEC CG-98-K51-2 and *S. aureus* strains were from our strain collection.

### 3.2 ELISA

Parallel wells of ELISA plates (Linbro) containing 200 µL colonisation factor (CF) broth[8] were inoculated with the test strains and incubated at 30 °C or 37 °C for 48 h. The curli positive *S. enteritidis* strain and its curli negative derivative were included in all plates as positive and negative controls. The ELISA reaction was carried out as described[9] using a polyclonal antibody raised against the curli (SEF17) of *S. enteritidis* 27655-3b[2]. The reaction was considered positive (i.e. the strain to carry curli) if the OD reached at least the 50 % value of the positive control. In case of a positive reaction the expression of curli was taken as temperature-regulated if the $OD_{30^{\circ}C}/OD_{37^{\circ}C}$ ratio exceeded 2 or, alternatively, it was below 0.5.

## 3.3 **Electronmicroscopy**

For electronmicroscopy bacteria were grown on T medium[2] containing 0.01 % congo red at the appropriate temperature for 48 h. Red colonies were suspended into distilled water and a drop was placed onto formvar coated grids. After staining with 0.1 % phosphotungstic acid the grids were examined on a JEOL-JEM-1200 electronmicroscope.

## 3.4 PCR

A loopful of cells grown as described above was suspended in distilled water and boiled at 97 °C for 15 min. One µL of this extract served as template in the reaction with 500 pMol forward and reverse PCR primers in the PCRMix (Gibco BRL) as described by the manufacturer. Two sets of primers were used, one for the *csg*A structural gene (theoretically providing a fragment of 200 bp) and one for the *crl* regulator gene (providing a fragment of 250 bp)[4]. Extract of a *S. aureus* strain and that of the curli positive ETEC CG-98-K-51-2 strain were included in every assay as negative and positive controls. The amplification products were analysed by agarose gel electrophoresis in 1 % gels with a 100 bp Gene Ruler DNA ladder molecular weight standard (MBI Fermentas).

## 4. RESULTS

Altogether 50 urinary *E. coli* isolates were investigated for the presence of thin aggregative fimbriae. Electronmicroscopy revealed the presence of this structure on the surface of 29 strains (58 %). The appendages showed the typical morphology described for curli. The degree of expression was variable from abundant vegetation surrounding the bacterial cells (Fig 1.) to much less fimbriation of other strains showing only patchy bundles on sections of the bacterial surface.

All the above strains were evaluated for ELISA reactivity with an immune serum specific for *GVVPQ* fimbriae of *S. enteritidis* (Table 1.) Twenty six isolates (52 %) exhibited a positive reaction, and the majority of them presented with a positive result only at ambient temperature. There were three strains positive under the electronmicroscope, while negative by ELISA at both temperatures.

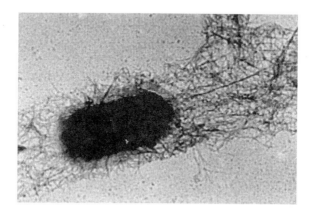

*Figure 1.* Electronmicrograph (x 10,000) of negatively stained *E. coli* with curli.

*Table 1.* Detection of curli by ELISA

|  | Positive at 30 °C | Positive at 37 °C | Positive at 30 and 37 °C | Negative |
|---|---|---|---|---|
| Number of strains | 25 (50 %)* | 1 (2 %)* | 0 | 24 (48 %) |
| Heat regulated | 22 (88 %)** | 1 (4 %)** | - | - |

  \* % of total

  \*\* % of the positive strains

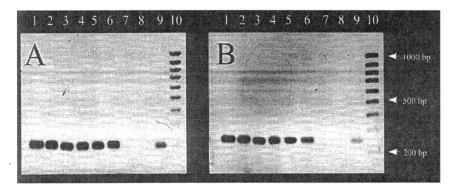

*Figure 2.* PCR reaction of representative urinary *E. coli* isolates with *csg*A and *crl* specific primers. Lanes. 1-4: selected curli negative isolates; 5-6: selected curli positive strains; 7: no DNA; 8: *S. aureus extract* (negative control); 9: *E. coli* ETEC CG-98-K51-2 (positive control); 10: molecular weight standard

Four curli expressing strains and all the negative ones were investigated for the presence of the *csg*A and *crl* genes by PCR reaction. All the strains examined harboured DNA sequences specific for these two genes. PCR reaction with representative strains is shown on Fig 2.

## 5. CONCLUSION

In the present work we investigated the occurrence of curli (thin aggregative fimbriae) on *E. coli* strains isolated from urinary tract infections with significant bacteriurea. In our collection of fresh isolates more than 50 % of the strains expressed surface structures morphologically indistinguishable from curli. ELISA reaction with anti-serum to the analogous thin aggregative fimbriae of *S. enteritidis* revealed a strong antigenic relationship between curli fimbriae of representatives of these two different bacterial genera. While 29 *E. coli* strains were positive ba electronmicroscopy, only 26 of them presented with positive result in the ELISA reaction. It needs further analysis if some of the *E. coli* strains may express thin aggregative fimbriae antigenically entirely distinct from that of *S. enteritidis*. Another possibility is that our criteria for ELISA positivitiy were too strict.

Expression of thin aggregative fimbriae of urinary *E. coli* isolates is in most cases under thermoregulatory control with an expression preference at ambient temperature.

Considering the fact that curli is rarely present at body temperature it is not clear if any pathogenetic role could be attributable to it. One can speculate that aggregative bacterial surface structures with an expression preference at 30-32 °C might be involved in primary colonisation of external surfaces like the perineal region and the orificium of the urinary tract.

## ACKNOWLEDGEMENTS

The work from our laboratory was supported by grants OTKA 016193 to L.E., OTKA 030201 to T.P., and ETT 16/96 to L.E.

## REFERENCES

1. Olsén, A., 1989, Fibronectin binding mediated by a novel class of surface organelles on *Escherichia coli. Nature.* **338**: 652-655.
2. Collinson, S.K., Emödy, L., Müller, K.H., Trust, T.J., and Kay W.W., 1991, Purification and characterization of thin aggregative fimbriae from *Salmonella enteritidis.* J. Bacteriol. **171**: 4773-4781.
3. Collinson, S.K., Emödy, L., Trust, T.J., and Kay, W.W., 1992, Thin, aggregative fimbriae from diarrheagenic *Escherichia coli. J. Bacteriol.* **173**: 4490-4495.
4. Maurer, J.J., Brown, T.P., Steffens, W.L., and Thayer, S.G., 1998, The occurence of ambient temperature-regulated adhesins, curli, and the temperature-sensitive hemagglutinin Tsh among avian *Escherichia coli. Avian. Dis.* **42**: 106-118.
5. Sjöbring, U., Pohl, G., and Olsén, A., 1994, Plasminogen, absorbed by *Escherichia coli* or by *Salmonella enteritidis* expressing thin aggregative fimbriae, can be activated by simultaneously captured tissue-type plasminogen activator (t-PA). *Mol. Microbiol.* **14**: 443-452.
6. Doran, J.L., Collinson, S.K., Burian, J., Sarlós, G., Todd, E.C.D., Munro, C.K., Kay, C.M., Banser, P.A., Peterkin, P.I., and Kay, W,W., 1993, DNA-based diagnostic tests for *Salmonella* species targeting *agf*A, the structural gene for thin, aggregative fimbriae. *J. Clin. Microbiol.* **31**: 2263-22672.
7. Emödy, L., Ljungh, A., Pál, T., Sarlós, G., and Wadström, T., 1991, Expression and possible biological functions of curli on infantile diarrhoea *Escherichia coli* isolates. In *Molecular Pathogenesis of Gastrointestinal Diseases* (T. Wadström, P.H. Mäkelä, A.-M. Svennerholm and H. Wolf-Watz, eds.), Plenum Press, London, pp. 303-306.
8. Evans, D.G., Evans, D.J., and Tjoa, W., 1977, Hemagglutination of human group A erythrocytes by enterotoxigenic *Escherichia coli* isolated from adults with diarrhea: correlation with colonization factor. *Infect. Immun.* **18**: 330-337.
9. Floderus, F., Pál, T., Karllson, K., and Lindberg, A.A.,1995, Identification of *Shigella* and enteroinvasive *Escherichia coli* strains by a virulence-specific, monoclonal antibody-based enzyme immunoassay. *Eur. J. Clin. Microbiol. Infect. . Dis.* **14**: 111-117.

# TYPE 1 PILI OF *CITROBACTER FREUNDII* MEDIATE INVASION INTO HOST CELLS

Petra Hess, Neda Daryab, Kai Michaelis, Anita Reisenauer, and Tobias A. Oelschlaeger

*Institut für Molekulare Infektionsbiologie, Universität Würzburg, Germany*

## 1.     INTRODUCTION

*Citrobacter freundii*, originally designated *Salmonella ballerup*, are Gram-negative, motile rod-shaped bacteria of the family *Enterobacteriaceae*. They are wide spread in nature and can be found in the environment in soil and water as well as in foodstuffs. *Citrobacter freundii* was also isolated from a wide variety of animals like household pets, birds, cattle and fish. Although *C. freundii* is often considered a commensal of the human intestinal flora, this organism may cause urinary tract infections, diarrhea and severe cases of gastritis, wound infections and nosocomial infections like pneumonia and rarely meningitis in newborns. Several probable virulence factors have been identified in *C. freundii*. Citrobacter isolates are often multidrug resistant. In addition, some of the corresponding antibiotic resistance genes (e.g. tetracycline, chloramphenicol, streptomycin) are located on transferable plasmids. The production of toxins has also been reported for *C. freundii* strains. Isolates from humans and beef samples were positive for the production of shiga(-like) toxin II. This toxin is much likely involved in enteropathogenicity caused by *C. freundii*. Futhermore, strains from patients with diarrhea produced a heat-stable enterotoxin identical to the 18-amino-acid *Escherichia coli* heat-stable enterotoxin STIa. Another probable virulence factor is a capsule, which is closely related to the Vi capsule of *Salmonella typhi*. Finally, invasion ability for several cell lines has been observed. Invasiveness *in vivo* would provide *C. freundii* with several advantages. Intracellular localization would result in protection from the host's (humoral) immune system, from the action of many antibiotics and could therefore prolong the infection time. Invasion ability could also

*Genes and Proteins Underlying Microbial Urinary Tract Virulence*
Edited by L. Emödy *et al.*, Kluwer Academic/Plenum Publishers, 2000

be used for penetrating through host barriers. Here, we report important properties of the *Citrobacter freundii* invasion pathway and evidence for a type 1 pili like determinant to constitute an invasion system in *Citrobacter freundii* strain 3009.

## 2.       INVESTIGATION OF THE *IN VITRO* INVASION ABILITY OF *CITROBACTER FREUNDII*

### 2.1      Invasion Efficiencies and Intracellular Localization

The two isolates investigated, 3009 and 3056, came from patients with urinary tract infections. Therefore, the gentamicin protection assay was performed with cultivated human urinary bladder epithelial cells (T24)[1]. However, because the gut might serve as a reservoir for *C. freundii* human cell lines originating from the digestive tract were included in these assays (INT407; HCT-8). The *C. freundii* strains 3056 and 3009 were invasive for all cell lines tested, however with varying efficiencies. Invasion efficiencies of both Citrobacter strains were comparable or higher than the invasion efficiency of *Salmonella typhi* Ty2 into T24 cells. In contrast, uptake into the gut epithelial cell lines INT407 and HCT-8 was less efficient for the Citrobacter strains than for the *S. typhi* strain Ty2 (Table 1).

*Table 1.* Invasion efficiencies of *Citrobacter freundii* human urinary tract isolates into human epithelial cell lines compared to those of *Salmonella typhi* and *Escherichia coli* K-12

| Cell line | % Invasion | | | |
| --- | --- | --- | --- | --- |
| | *Citrobacter freundii* | | *S. typhi* | *E. coli* |
| | 3009 | 3056 | Ty2 | HB101 |
| T24 | 12.8 | 9.3 | 6.3 | 0.02 |
| INT407 | 0.7 | 1.0 | 10.2 | 0.02 |
| HCT-8 | 10.0 | 8.4 | 8.4 | 0.07 |

Invasion efficiencies are given as the percentage of the inoculum surviving the gentamicin treatment.

Still, the invasion rates of *C. freundii* strains 3056 and 3009 into INT407 and HCT-8 cells were much higher than those observed for the negative control strain HB101 (Table 1). That the bacteria surviving the gentamicin treatment are really located intracellulary was demonstrated by transmission electronmicroscopic examination (TEM) of infected cells. *C. freundii* bacteria are enclosed in vacuoles inside the cytoplasm of T24 bladder epithelial cells as was observed for *S. typhi* Ty2. However, *E. coli* strain HB101, which was recovered after gentamicin treatment of infected epithelial cells at very low numbers, was never observed intracellularly by TEM.

## 2.2    Characterization of the Internalization Pathway

The internalization of bacteria into eukaryotic cells is either mediated by the zipper or the trigger mechanism. If uptake occurs via the zipper mechanism, a surface protein of the bacterium acts as a ligand connecting the bacterium with the host cell via binding to a specific eukaryotic receptor. This interaction leads to internalization. Well characterized examples of this mode of internalization are the uptake of *Yersinia* spp. via the outer membrane protein invasin (Inv) and *Listeria monocytogenes* via the surface protein internalin A (InlA)[2,3]. The corresponding eukaryotic receptor for Inv are β1-subunits of integrins and E-cadherin for InlA[4,5]. This uptake pathway is also characterized by a close approximation of the bacterial surface to the host cell surface, which can be observed by electronmicroscopic examination and it resembles very much internalization of particles by professional phagocytes, termed phagocytosis. In contrast, uptake via the trigger mechanism does not rely on a very close contact between bacterium and host cell because of bacterial ligand - eukaryotic receptor interaction. Rather, bacterial effector molecules are translocated by the invading bacterium into the host cell, which induce internalization. This can be achieved via type three secretion systems (TTSS) encoded by many pathogenic bacteria[6]. *Salmonella* and *Shigella* spp. are the prototypes of bacteria internalized via the trigger mechanism resembling macropinocytosis[7,8].

However, no matter what kind of uptake pathway is induced by bacteria, rearrangement of the cytoskeleton is essential either to form the pseudopode-like protrusion zipping around Yersinia or Listeria or the ruffles, which finally collapse over the bacteria and fuse with the cytoplasmic host cell membrane, thereby enclosing Salmonella or Shigella.

## 2.3    The Role of the Cytoskeleton

Most well established invasive bacteria are internalized in a microfilament (MF)-dependent way. This was demonstrated in gentamicin protection assays with host cells pretreated with the microfilament depolymerizing drug cytochalasin D (CD). Uptake into eukaryotic cells treated with CD was dramatically reduced. A prototype of a microorganism internalized in a MF-dependent way is Salmonella. Surprisingly, internalization of *C. freundii* into T24 bladder epithelial cells was not inhibited, if the T24 cells had been pretreated with CD (Figure 1). Obviously, the uptake of *C. freundii* into this cell line is not dependent on intact MFs. However, if the microtubules (MTs) were disrupted in the epithelial cells by colchicine or nocodazole prior to infection with Citrobacter, then a pronounced reduction of internalization was observed (Figure 1).

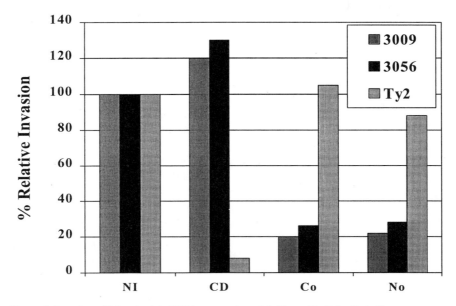

*Figure 1.* Invasion efficiencies into T24 human urinary bladder epithelial cells in the presence of no inhibitor (NI), 1μg/ml cytochalasin D, 10μM colchicine, or 20μM nocodazole. The effects of the inhibitors employed were determined for *C. freundii* strains 3009 and 3056 as well as for *S. typhi* strain Ty2.

In contrast, *C. freundii* invasion of other cell lines (e.g. INT407, HCT-8) was inhibited by CD and colchicine or nocodazole. However, Salmonella internalization in any of the cell lines tested was strongly dependent on intact MFs but independent of intact MTs (Figure 1). In summary, *C. freundii* internalization into T24 cells relys solely on intact MTs and in other cells additionally on intact MFs. Solely or in addition to MFs MTs are also involved in the uptake pathways of *Campylobacter jejuni*[9], *Chlamydia trachomatis*[10], enterohemorrhagic *E. coli* (EHEC)[11], enteropathogenic *E. coli* (EPEC)[12], newborn meningitis-causing *E. coli* (MENEC)[13], certain uropathogenic *E. coli* (UPEC)[14], *Listeria monocytogenes*[15,16], *Klebsiella pneumoniae*[17], *Mycobacterium bovis* BCG[18], *Mycobacterium tuberculosis*[19], *Mycoplasma penetrans*[20], *Neisseria gonorrhoeae*[21], and *Porphyromonas gingivalis*[22].

## 2.4 The Internalization Receptor

Futhermore, engulfment of Citrobacter could be reduced by interfering with receptor-mediated internalization. This was demonstrated by treatment of the epithelial cells with monodansylcadaverine, a substance that interferes with the recycling of receptors, thereby inhibiting receptor mediated endocytosis[23].

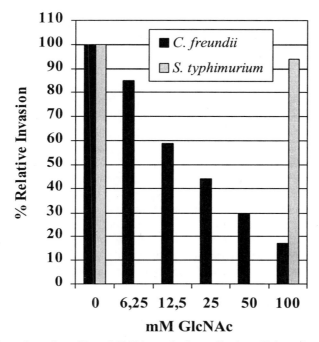

*Figure 2.* Dose dependent effect of GlcNAc on the internalization efficiency into T24 human urinary bladder epithelial cells of *Citrobacter freundii* 3009 and *Salmonella typhimurium* C17.

Again, this was specific for Citrobacter uptake, because Salmonella invasion was not affected by MD. Epithelial cells are covered by the glycocalyx. This is a composition of various sugar structures many of which are part of glycolipids or glycoproteins. We hypothesized, that invading bacteria might encounter first and interact with certain sugar components of the glycocalyx. If so, this interaction should be sensitive to lectins. Lectins are proteins specifically binding to defined sugar structures. Therefore, a variety of lectins was employed in the gentamicin protection assay. The pretreatment of the host cells with lectins prior to infection with *C. freundii* reduced internalization only if the lectin employed was able to bind GlcNAc residues.

The receptor structure used by *C. freundii* strain 3009 seems to be GlcNAc residues of N-glycosylated proteins. Strong evidence for this notion are (i) the dose dependent inhibitory effect of GlcNAc on internalization of *C. freundii* into T24 cells (Fig 2); (ii) inhibition of N-glycosylation of eukaryotic proteins by tunicamycin also resulted in a strong reduction of *C. freundii* internalization; (iii) the specific removal of glycan chains from only N-glycosylated proteins decreased the internalization efficiency of *C. freundii* into T24 cells to a similar degree as the treatment with tunicamycin. Other glycosidases tested had no adverse effect on *C. freundii* uptake. Again, the observed effects were specific for Citrobacter, because *S. typhimurium* engulfment was never affected by any of the treatments of the cell lines. Work is now in progress to identify the protein part of the N-glycosylated protein(s) acting as an internalization receptor for *C. freundii*.

## 3.    THE INVASION DETERMINANT FROM *CITROBACTER FREUNDII*

Bacterial invasion determinants might consist of only one gene as the *inv* invasion system of Yersinia. Other invasion systems like those from Salmonella or Shigella consist of more than thirty genes. Some of these genes encode a TTSS, whereas others encode regulators or the effector proteins translocated via the TTSS into the host's cell cytosol. At the beginning of the research work on *Citrobacter freundii* invasiveness, it was unclear if *C. freundii* encodes a rather simple or more complex invasion system.

### 3.1    Cloning an Invasion Determinant from *Citrobacter freundii*

Cosmid cloning was chosen in order to molecularly clone longer chromosomal DNA fragments, in case *C. freundii* might encode an invasion system consisting of several genes. The noninvasive *E. coli* K-12 strain HB101 was chosen to be transformed with the recombinant cosmids. Selection for recombinant HB101 clones which have received a cosmid conferring invasiveness was achieved by employing the clones in a gentamicin protection assay. Noninvasive clones were killed by gentamicin due to their extracellular location. An invasive HB101 cosmid clone was identified in this way and the about 50 kb cosmid was isolated and digested in parallel with several restriction endonucleases. After religation and transformation of *E. coli* HB101, the gentamicin protection assay was again used to select invasive clones with down sized cosmids. The smallest plasmid obtained was pTO3 with 13.5 kb in size, resulting from *Pvu*II digestion. Restriction analysis revealed, that this was not a cosmid anymore, because the *cos*-site had also been deleted by PvuII restriction. To ensure that invasion ability was mediated directly by pTO3 and not by a regulatory effect of pTO3 on a gene cluster otherwise silent in HB101, other K-12 strains were also transformed with pTO3. All the resulting recombinant *E. coli* K-12 strains were indeed invasive after transformation with pTO3.

## 3.2 Sequence and Analysis of the Cloned Citrobacter Invasion Determinant

The insert of pTO3 was sequenced and analysis of the sequence obtained revealed the highest identity rate with sequences of type 1 pili genes from Salmonella. As in Salmonella the type 1 like determinant from Citrobacter (*fim*<sub>Cf</sub>) consists of 10 open reading frames (ORFs) termed *fimA, I, C, D, H, F, Z, Y, W*, and *U*. However,

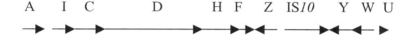

*Figure 3.* The cloned type 1 pili like determinant from *C. freundii* 3009. It consists of 10 *fim* genes as the *fim* gene cluster of *Salmonella typhimurium*. However, an IS*10* element is inserted between *fimZ* und *fimY* in the *C. freundii* determinant.

in contrast to the determinant in Salmonella, the gene cluster of Citrobacter contains an IS*10* element between *fimZ* and *fimY* (Fig 3). Futhermore, the arrangement of the *fim*<sub>Cf</sub> genes is identical with the *fim* genes of Salmonella (Fig 3). The inactivation or deletion of the most likely regulatory genes *fimZ, Y, W*, and *U* did not result in loss of the ability of the resulting plasmids to confer invasiveness on noninvasive *E. coli* K-12 clones. Invasiveness was however lost, if *fimA*, the gene for the major subunit in Salmonella type 1 pili was interrupted by insertion of an IS*1* element. Therefore, the conclusion was drawn, that the genes coding for regulators (*fimZ, fimY, fimW, fimU*) are not essential for mediating invasion ability in contrast to those Citrobacter genes, with high identity rates to type 1 Salmonella genes coding for the major subunit (*fimA*), minor subunits (*fimH, fimF*), a chaperon (*fimC*) or the usher (*fimD*).

To demonstrate the invasion ability mediated by pTO3 is not a general feature of all fimbrial determinants in our experimental setting, a variety of recombinant *E. coli* strains expressing different pili, were tested in the gentamicin protection assay. Non of the tested pili determinants and not even the *fim* determinant from *S. typhimurium* (*fim*$_{St}$), to which the Citrobacter invasion determinant showed such a high degree of homology were able to confer invasiveness on the noninvasive *E. coli* K-12 strain HB101. However, all of the pili determinants made the recombinant strains adhere to the same cell lines also employed in the gentamicin protection assay. Obviously, the type 1 like pili determinant from Citrobacter is different from other (type 1) pili determinants in being able to mediate invasion into host cells.

## 3.3    Functional Characterization of the Citrobacter Type 1 Pili Like Determinant

As expected, HB101 carrying pTO3 (HB101pTO3) was also able to agglutinate yeast. This agglutination was inhibitable by mannose. These are the typical features of type 1 pili, again strengthening the close relatedness of *fim*$_{Cf}$ with *fim*$_{St}$. Because invasion by Citrobacter was not inhibited by mannose but by GlcNAc, the effect of GlcNAc on yeast agglutination by HB101pTO3 was determined. Suprisingly, GlcNAc had no adverse effect on yeast agglutination by HB101pTO3. Another surprise was the finding, that *C. freundii* strain 3009 was not able to agglutinate yeast. This was not due to loss of the type 1 pili like determinant in the WT strain, because the presence of the *fim*$_{Cf}$ determinant in strain 3009 was again demonstrated in Southern blot experiments. However, *Citrobacter freundii* is known to express a Vi capsule, which might interfere with yeast agglutination[24]. In contrast, the recombiant *E. coli* HB101pTO3 strain does not express any capsule. Therefore, the capsule expression by *C. freundii* strain 3009 might interfere with yeast agglutination.

The mannose binding activity, which is responsible for yeast agglutination, is mediated by the FimH subunit in type 1 pili. However, it is still unclear which subunit protein encoded by *fim*$_{Cf}$ is responsible for binding to GlcNAc residues on the host cells thereby inducing the internalization process. Mutagenesis of the different subunit protein genes and complementation studies should help to answer this important question.

## 4.    CONCLUSION

*Citrobacter freundii* strains 3056 and 3009 are invasive for human epithelial cell lines. This invasion ability is heavily dependent on intact microtubules and in certain cell lines additionally on intact microfilaments. The host cell receptor structure used by *C. freundii* for invasion are GlcNAc residues of N-glycosylated proteins. GlcNAc residues on the host cell surface are also internalization receptor structures for newborn meningitis causing *E. coli* and *Klebsiella pneumoniae*[25,26]. It is unclear if the GlcNAc residues used by these microorganisms are part of the same protein(s) or if different N-gylcosylated proteins are the internalization receptors for these three species. The newborn meningitis causing *E. coli* interact via the outer membrane protein OmpA with GlcNAc residues[25]. The invasion protein of *K. pneumoniae* interacting with GlcNAc residues is unknown.

C. *freundii* 3009 encodes a type 1 pili like determinant, which is necessary for efficient internalization into human epithelial cell lines. If this determinant is transformed in noninvasive *E. coli* K-12 strains, it confers invasiveness on these strains. Suprisingly however, mannose does not interfere with internalization of *C. freundii* but GlcNAc, whereas mannose inhibits yeast agglutination of the recombinant invasive *E. coli* K-12 strains but not GlcNAc. This and other studies elucidate another important property of certain adhesins, the ability to mediate not only adhesion but also invasion. This was reported for type 1 pili of uropathogenic *E. coli*, opening an uptake pathway which results in intracellular survival inside macrophages[27]. Also Dr-pili of uropathogenic *E. coli* are able to mediate internalization into epithelial cells by binding to the SCR-3 domain of the decay-accelerating-factor protein on host cells[14]. Similarly, pili of the mouth pathogen *Porphyromonas gingivalis* allow this species to invade normal human gingival epithelial cells[28]. Obviously, adhesins are multi purpose tools for certain bacteria, as could be demonstrated for a type 1 pili like determinant from *Citrobacter freundii* clinical isolates, which functions also as an invasin.

# REFERENCES

1. Elsinghorst, E.A., 1994, Measurement of invasion by gentamicin resistance. *Methods Enzymol.* **236:** 405-420.
2. Young, V.B., Miller, V.L., Falkow, S., and Schoolnik, G.K., 1990, Sequence, localization and function of the invasion protein of *Yersinia enterocolitica. Mol. Microbiol.* **4:** 1119-1128.
3. Gaillard, J.L., Berche, P., Frehel, C., Gouin, E., and Cossart, P., 1991, Entry *of L. monocytogenes* into cells is mediated by internalin, a repeat protein reminiscent of surface antigens from gram-positive cocci. *Cell* **65:** 1127-1141.
4. Isber, R.R. and Leong, J.M., 1990, Multiple β1-chain integrins are receptors for invasin, a protein that promotes bacterial penetration into mammalian cells. *Cell* **60:** 861-871.
5. Mengaud, J., Ohayon, H., Gounon, P., Mege, R.-M., and Cossart, P., 1996, E-cadherin is the receptor for internalin, a surface protein required for entry of *L. monocytogenes* into epithelial cells. *Cell* **84:** 923-932.
6. Hueck, C.J., 1998, Type III protein secretion systems in bacterial pathogens of animals and plants. *Microbiol. Mol. Biol. Rev.* **62:** 379-433.
7. Brumell, J.H., Steele-Mortimer, O., and Finaly, B.B., 1999, Bacterial invasion: force feeding by *Salmonella. Curr. Biol.* **9:** R277-280.

8. Sansonetti, P.J. and Egile, C.,  1998, Molecular basis of epithelial cell invasion by Shigella flexneri. *Antonie Van Leeuwenhoek* **74:** 191-197.

9. Oelschlaeger, T.A., Guerry, P., and Kopecko, D.J., 1993, Unusual microtubule-dependent endocytosis mechanisms triggered by *Campylobacter jejuni* and *Citrobacter freundii. Proc. Natl. Acad. Sci. USA* **90:** 6884-6888.

10. Clausen, J.D., Christiansen, G., Holst, H.U., and Birkelund, S., 1997, *Chlamydia trachomatis* utilizes the host cell microtubule network during early events of infection. *Mol. Microbiol.* **25:** 441-449.

11. Oelschlaeger, T.A., Barrett, T.J., and Kopecko, D.J., 1994, Some structures and processes of human epithelial cells involved in uptake of enterohemorrhagic *Escherichia coli* O157:H7 strains. *Infect. Immun..* **62:** 5142-5150.

12. Donnenberg, M.S., Donohue-Rolfe, A., and Keusch, G.T., 1990, A comparison of Hep-2 cell invasion by enteropathogenic and enteroinvasive *Escherichia coli. FEMS Microbiol. Lett.* **69:** 83-86.

13. Meier, C., Oelschlaeger, T.A., Merkert, H., Korhonen, T.K., and Hacker, J., 1996, Ability of the newborn meningitis isolate *Escherichia coli* IHE3034 (O18:K1:H7) to invade epithelial and endothelial cells. *Infect. Immun.* **64:** 2391-2399.

14. Goluszko, P., Popov, V., Selvarangan, R., Novicki, S., Pham, T., and Nowicki, B.J., 1997, *Dr* fimbriae operon of uropathogenic *Escherichia* coli mediate microtubule-dependent invasion to the HeLa epithelial cell line. *J. Infect. Dis.* **176:** 158-167.

15. Guzman, C.A., Rohde, M., Chakraborty, T., Domann, E., Hudel, M., Wehland, J., and Timmis, K.N., 1995, Interaction of *Listeria monocytogenes* with mouse dendritic cells. *Infect. Immun.* **63:** 3665-3673.

16. Kuhn, M., 1998, The microtubule depolymerizing drugs nocodazole and colchicine inhibit the uptake of *Listeria monocytogenes* by P388D1 macrophages. *FEMS Microbiol. Lett.* **160:** 87-90.

17. Oelschlaeger, T.A. and Tall., B.D., 1997, Invasion of cultured human epithelial cells by *Klebsiella pneumoniae. Infect. Immun.* **65:** 2950-2958.

18. Buchwalow, I.B., Brich, M., and Kaufmann, S.H., 1997, Signal transduction and phagosome biogenesis in human macrophages during phagocytosis of *Mycobacterium bovis* BCG. *Acta. Histochem.* **99:** 63-70.

19. Bermudez , L.E. and Goodman, J., 1996, *Mycobacterium* tuberculosis invades and replicates within type II alveolar cells. *Infect. Immun.* **64:** 1400-1406.

20. Borovsky, Z., Tarshis, M., Zhang, P., and Rottem, S., 1998, Protein kinase C activation and vacuolation in HeLa cells invaded by *Mycoplasma penetrans. J. Med. Microbiol.* **47:** 915-922.

21. Grassme, H.U., Ireland, R.M., and van Putten, J.P., 1996, Gonococcal opacity protein promotes bacterial entry-associated rearrangement of the epithelial cell actin cytoskeleton. *Infect. Immun.* **64:** 1621-1630.

22. Lamont, R.J., Chan, A., Belton, C.M., Izutzu, K.T., Vasel., D., and Weinberg, A., 1995, *Porphyromonas gingivalis* invasion of gingival epithelial cells. *Infect. Immun.* **63:** 3878-3885.

23. VanLeuven, F., Cassiman, J.J., and Van Den Berge, H., 1980,  Primary amines inhibit recycling of $\alpha_2 M$ receptors in fibroblasts. *Cell* **20:** 37-43.

24. Ou, J.T., Baron, L.S., Rubin, F.A., and Kopecko, D.J., 1988,  Specific insertion and deletion of insertion sequence 1-like DNA element causes the reversible expression of the virulence capsular antigen Vi of *Citrobacter freundii* in *Escherichia coli. Proc. Natl. Acad. Sci. USA* **85:** 4402-4405.

25. Prasadarao, N.V., Wass, C.A., and Kim, K.S., 1996, Endothelial cell $GlcNAc\beta 1$-4GlcNAc epitopes for outer membrane protein A enhances traversal of *Escherichia* coli across the blood brain barrier. Infect. Immun. **64:** 154-160.

26. Fumagalli, O., Tall., B.D., Schipper, C., and Oelschlaeger, T.A., 1997, N-glycosylated

proteins are involved in efficient internalization of *Klebsiella pneumoniae. Infect. Immun.* **65**: 4445-4451.

27. Baorto, D.M., Gao, Z., Malaviya,R., Dustin, M.L., van der Merwe, A., Lublin, D.M., and Abraham, S.N., 1997, Survival of fimH-expressing enterobacteria in macrophages relies on glycolipid traffic. *Nature* **389**: 636-639.

28. Weinberg, A., Belton, C.M., Park, Y., and Lamont, R.J., 1997, Role of fimbriae in *Porphyromonas gingivalis* invasion of gingival epithelial cells. *Infect. Immun.* **65**: 313-316.

# SEROTYPES, SIDEROPHORE SYNTHESIS, AND SERUM RESISTANCE OF UROPATHOGENIC *KLEBSIELLA* ISOLATES

[1]Mine Anğ-Küçüker, [2]Ömer Küçükbasmacı, [2]Mehmet Tekin, [1]Didem Akbulut, [1]Özden Büyükbaba-Boral and [1]Özdem Anğ

[1]*University of Istanbul, Istanbul Faculty of Medicine, Department of Microbiology; [2]University of Istanbul, Experimental Medical Research Institute, Capa, Istanbul, Turkey*

## 1.     INTRODUCTION

*Klebsiella* species are frequently associated with human urinary tract infections. These bacteria are important gram-negative pathogens in nosocomial infections. They cause several endemic and epidemic outbreaks in urologic wards[1,2].

*Klebsiella* are typically enveloped by a polysaccharide capsule which is considered a major factor in the pathogenicity of these bacteria. Up to date 82 different capsular antigens have been reported[3]. Particular capsular types are associated with the site of isolation and some serotypes may in fact be more virulent than others[4]. *Klebsiella* strains have shown to produce siderophores[2]. Serum resistance in *K .pneumoniae* is found more commonly among isolates from clinical specimens than among fecal and environmental isolates[5].

In this study, we present epidemiologic data on virulence characteristics among *Klebsiella* strains isolated from patients with urinary tract infection. We investigated the capsular types, siderophore, enterobactin, aerobactin and serum resistance properties.

*Genes and Proteins Underlying Microbial Urinary Tract Virulence*
Edited by L. Emödy *et al.*, Kluwer Academic/Plenum Publishers, 2000

## 2.      MATERIALS AND METHODS

Bacteria: 20 *Klebsiella pneumonia*, and 6 *Klebsiella oxytoca* strains were isolated from urine samples. The isolates were identified using conventional methods.

Capsule typing: The isolates were serotyped by the capsular swelling method as described by Ullmann[6] in the Department of Medical Microbiology and Virology, University of Kiel, Germany.

Determination of siderophore production: For detection of siderophore production the chrome azurol S (CAS) agar was used as described by Schwyn and Neilands[7]. The cross-feeding bioassay of Hantke[8] was done for detecting enterobactin and aerobactin production.

Serum bactericidal assay: The susceptibility of bacteria to human serum was determined by the method of Podschun et al[5].

## 3.      RESULTS

Serotypes: Of the 26 isolates, 25 could be serotyped and 11 different capsule types were observed. Serotype K69 was the most common (34%). Serotypes K33 and K62 were found as second and third most frequent ones (15% each). K62 capsular type was especially predominant in *K. oxytoca* strains (50%).

Siderophores: All the strains expressed siderophore. 54% and 8% of the isolates expressed enterobactin and aerobactin, respectively. All aerobactin-producing isolates were *K. pneumoniae* (Table 1).

*Table 1.* Distribution of siderophore production among *Klebsiella* strains

|                        | Enterobactin | | Aerobactin | |
| --- | --- | --- | --- | --- |
|                        | n  | %  | N | % |
| *K.pneumoniae* (20)    | 11 | 55 | 2 | 10 |
| *K.oxytoca* (6)        | 3  | 50 | - | - |
| Total (26)             | 14 | 54 | 2 | 8 |

Serum resistance: The responses of the examined isolates to the bactericidal activity of normal human serum were recorded over 3 h and arranged into six grades, highly sensitive (grade 1 or 2), intermediately sensitive (3 or 4), or resistant (5 or 6). The majority of the strains (53%) were highly serum resistant, half of the *K .oxytoca* strains were serum sensitive (Table 2).

*Table 2.* Distribution of serum resistance among *Klebsiella* strains

| | Resistance categories and No.of strains represented | | | | | |
|---|---|---|---|---|---|---|
| | 1 | 2 | 3 | 4 | 5 | 6 |
| *K.pneumoniae* (20) | - | 3 | 5 | - | 3 | 9 |
| *K.oxytoca* (6) | 1 | 2 | 1 | - | - | 2 |
| Total (26) | 1 | 5 | 6 | - | 3 | 11 |

## 4.    DISCUSSION

Serotyping of *Klebsiella* isolates from hospital infections shows that a large number of capsular types are involved[2,9]. Epidemiologic studies on the incidence of particular serotypes produced different results, from total heterogenity to predominance of certain capsule types. Serotype K2 has been reported to be the most common in clinical strains[2,9,10]. Other studies found K2, K8, K9, K10 and K21 most commonly among urinary isolates. However, in our study we found K69, K33, K62 as the predominant capsular types. K69 which is the most frequent one (34%) in our study gives a strong cross-reaction with K2[11].

The ability of bacteria to avoid killing by normal serum is considered as a property which co-determines their virulence. Commensal or non-invasive gram negative bacteria are found to be usually sensitive to serum, whereas invasive pathogens are frequently serum resistant[2,5]. Serum resistance of urinary pathogens is related to the site of infection and the severity of symptoms[5,12]. In this study, we found the majority of the strains highly resistant (53%), and only 23% of them was serum sensitive. However, half of the *K. oxytoca* strains proved to be serum sensitive. That is clinical *K. pneumoniae* strains were more frequently serum resistant than *K.oxytoca*. This may – at least partly - explain the reduced virulence of *K. oxytoca* in comparison with *K. pneumoniae*.

The urinary tract represents an iron restricted environment to which bacterial pathogens may respond by producing iron-chelating compounds known as siderophores. Enterobactin seems to be the main siderophore of enterobacteria, but its effect is unclear[2]. The contribution of aerobactin to virulence has been shown clearly[13]. In the present study all the strains produced siderophore. 54% and 8% of the isolates express enterobactin and aerobactin, respectively. 50% of *K. pneumoniae* and 66% of *K.oxytoca* produce enterobactin. These percentages are rather low when compared with the findings of Williams et al[14]. Aerobactin synthesis has been correlated with the virulence of *K.pneumoniae*, but its production is less common in enteric bacteria than that of enterobactin [2,15]. Similarly to these observations we have found a low frequency of aerobactin expression in our strains.

In the present study 26 *Klebsiella* strains were examined. This work was planned as a preliminary study for a detailed epidemiologic assay of *Klebsiella* isolates in our University Hospital. Arbitrarily primed PCR (AP-PCR) typing technique, a relatively inexpensive and technically feasible method will also be applied in order to have a further possibility of distinction between the isolates.

## ACKNOWLEDGEMENT

We would like to thank to Prof. Dr. R. Podschun for capsular serotyping.

## REFERENCES

1. Montgomerie, J.Z., 1979, Epidemiology of Klebsiella and hospital associated infections. *Rev. Infect. Dis.* **1**: 736-53.
2. Podschun, R., Sievers, D., Fischer, A., and Ullmann, U., 1993, Serotypes, hemagglutinins, siderophore synthesis, and serum resistance of *Klebsiella* isolates causing human urinary tract infections. *J. Infect. Dis.* **168**: 1415-21.
3. Podschun, R., and Ulmann, U., 1998, *Klebsiella spp.* as nosocomial pathogens: Epidemiology, taxonomy, typing methods, and pathogenicity factors. *Clin. Microbiol. Rev.* **11**: 589-603.
4. Riser, E., and Noone, P., 1981, *Klebsiella* capsular types versus site of isolation. *J. Clin. Pathol.* **34**: 552-5.
5. Podschun, R., Teske, E., and Ullmann, U., 1991, Serum resistance properties of Klebsiella pneumoniae and K.oxytoca isolated from different sources. *Zentralbl. Hyg. Umweltmed.* **192**: 279-85.
6. Ullmann, U., 1983, The distrubition of *Klebsiella pneumoniae* serotypes from different sources and their sensitivity to cephalosporins. *Infection* **11(Suppl . 1)**: 28-31.
7. Schwyn, B., Neilands, J.B., 1987, Universal chemical assay for the detection and determination of siderophores. *Analyt. Biochem.* **160**: 47-56.
8. Hantke, K., 1990, Dihydrobenzoylserine- a siderophore for *E.coli. FEMS Microbiol. Lett.* **67**: 5-8.
9. Simoons-Smit, A.M., Verweij-van Vught, A.M.J.J., Kanis, I.Y.R., and MacLaren, D.M., 1985, Biochemical and serological investigations on clinical isolates of *Klebsiella. J. Hyg.* **95**: 265-76.
10. Smith, S.M., Digori, J.T., and Eng, R.H.K., 1982, Epidemiology of *Klebsiella* antibiotic resistance and serotypes. *J. Clin. Microbiol.* **16**: 868-73.
11. Ørskov, I., and Ørskov, F., 1984, Serotyping of *Klebsiella*. Methods in Microbiol **14**: 150-51.
12. Gower, P.E., Taylor, P.W., Koutsaimanis, K.G., and Roberts, A.P., 1972, Serum bactericidal activity in patients with upper and lower urinary tract infections. *Clin. Sci.* **43**: 13-22.
13. De Lorenzo, V., and Martinez, J.L., 1988, Aerobactin production as a virulence factor: a re-evaluation. *Eur. J. Clin. Microbiol. Infect. Dis.* **7**: 621-9.

14. Williams, P.H., Chart, H., Griffiths, E., and Stevenson, P., 1987, Expression of high affinity iron uptake systems by clinical isolates of Klebsiella. *FEMS Microbiol. Lett.* **44:** 407-12.
15. Martinez, J.L., Cercenada, J.L., Baquero, F., and Perez Diaz, J.C., 1987, Incidence of aerobactin production in gram-negative hospital isolates. *FEMS Microbiol. Lett.* **43:** 351-53.

# EPITOPE SPECIFICITY OF POLYCLONAL RABBIT ANTISERA AGAINST *PROTEUS VULGARIS* O-ANTIGENS

[1]Beata Bartodziejska, [1]Agnieszka Torzewska, [1]Dorota Babicka, [1]Marianna Wykrota, [1]Antoni Różalski, [2]Andrei V. Perepelov, [2]Filip V. Toukach and [2]Yuriy A. Knirel

[1]*Department of Immunobiology of Bacteria, Institute of Microbiology and Immunology, University of Łódź, 90-237 Łódź, Banacha 12/16, Poland: [2]N.D. Zelinsky Institute of Organic Chemistry, Russian Academy of Sciences, Leninsky Prospect 47, Moscow 117913, Russian Federation.*

## 1. INTRODUCTION

Bacteria of the genus *Proteus* cause mainly urinary tract infections, sometimes leading to acute or chronic pyelonephritis and formation of stones. Outer membrane lipopolysaccharide (LPS, endotoxin) is considered to be a virulence factor of *Proteus* sp. Based on the O-specific polysaccharide chains of LPS (O-antigens), two species, *P. mirabilis* and *P. vulgaris* were classified into 60 O-serogroups[1]. Chemical and immunochemical studies of *Proteus* LPS are important for the understanding of the molecular basis of the immunospecificity of *Proteus* strains and for their classification based on structural and serological data. In most *Proteus* O-serogroups, the O-specific polysaccharides (OPS) of LPS were found to be acidic due to the presence of uronic acids and various non-carbohydrate acid components[2]. OPSs of *P. vulgaris* are the last studied among *Proteus* species. Recently, we have determined the structure of acidic OPSs of *P. vulgaris* O8, O22, O25, O32 and O45.

*Genes and Proteins Underlying Microbial Urinary Tract Virulence*
Edited by L. Emődy *et al.*, Kluwer Academic/Plenum Publishers, 2000

## 2.      MATERIAL AND METHODS

All bacterial strains used in this study came from the Czech National Collection of Type Cultures (Institute of Epidemiology and Microbiology, Prague). LPSs were isolated from dried bacterial cells by phenol/water extraction. Alkali treated LPS (LPSOH) was prepared by saponification of LPS with 0.25 NaOH. The structures of O-specific polysaccharides were established by $^1$H and $^{13}$C-NMR spectroscopy, including two dimensional NOESY and H-detected $^1$H, $^{13}$C heteronuclear multiplequantum coherence (HMQC) experiments. Serological studies were performed by use of enzyme immunosorbent assay (EIA), passive immunohemolysis (PIH) and their inhibition tests, as well as DOC/PAGE and Western blot analysis. In these studies polyclonal rabbit anti - O-specific antisera, as well as homologous and heterologous LPSs, released O-specific polysaccharides (OPS), Smith degraded polysaccharides and synthetic antigens were used. All methods were described[3,4].

## 3.      RESULTS

### 3.1     Structural Analysis

On the basis of the chemical data the following structures of *P. vulgaris* O-antigens were established (Fig 1).

**P. vulgaris O8**

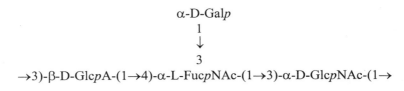

*P. vulgaris* **O22**

**P. vulgaris O32**

→2)-α-L-Rha*p*-(1→2)-α-L-Rha*p*-(1→4)-β-D-Gal*p*A-(1→3)-β-D-Glc*p*NAc-
(1→4)-α-D-Gal*p*A-(1→

**P. vulgaris O45**

$$\begin{array}{c} \text{β-D-Glc}p\text{A} \\ 1 \\ \downarrow \\ 4 \end{array}$$

→4)-α-D-Gal*p*NAc3Ac-(1→3)-β-D-Gal*p*NAc-(1→3)-β-D-Gal*p*NAc-(1→

*Figure 1.* The structures of O-specific polysaccharides of *P. vulgaris* strains[3,4,5,6].

## 3.2    Serological studies

By use of polyclonal rabbit O-specific antisera and a number of *Proteus* LPSs, OPSs and synthetic antigens with known structures, we were able to reveal the molecular basis for the antigenic specificity of four *P. vulgaris* O-antigens.

*P. vulgaris O8.* It was found that anti-(*P. vulgaris* O8) serum reacted with homologous LPS (titer 1:51,200 in EIA and PIH) and with LPS of *P. mirabilis* O6 (1:3,200 and 1: 6,400 in PIH and EIA, respectively). Both LPSs contain α-L-Fuc*p*NAc-(1→3)-β-D-Glc*p*NAc disaccharide in the O-specific part of LPS, thus it was concluded that this epitope is important for the specificity of *P. vulgaris* O8 O-antigen[5].

*P. vulgaris O22 and O32.* Results of immunochemical and serological studies of O-specific polysaccharides from *P. vulgaris* O22 and O32 (Table 1. and 2.) suggested that these O-antigens had a common antigenic determinant containing α-L-Rha*p*-(1→4)-β-D-UA-(1→3)-β-D-GlcNAc where UA is GalA and GlcA in O32 and O22 O–antigens, respectively[3,6]. β configuration of GalA is of little immunological importance in *P. vulgaris* O32 O-antigen (Table 2).

*Table 1.* Reactivity of LPS with anti – (*P. vulgaris* O22 and O32) sera

| LPS of P. vulgaris | Reactivity in: | | | |
|---|---|---|---|---|
| | PIH | | EIA | |
| | Reciprocal titer | | | |
| | O22-antiserum | O32- antiserum | O22- antiserum | O32-antiserum |
| O22 | 12,800 | 800 | 512,000 | <200 |
| O32 | 3,200 | 12,800 | 250 | 64,000 |

*Table 2.* Inhibition of PIH in the system of *P. vulgaris* O32 LPSOH/anti-(*P.vulgaris* O32) serum

| Inhibitor | Inhibitory dose [ng] |
|---|---|
| *P. vulgaris* O32 LPS-OH | 9,8 |
| *P. vulgaris* O22 LPS-OH | 78,1 |
| α-D-GalA-polyacrylamide | 15,6 |
| β-D-GalA-polyacrylamide | >2000 |

P. vulgaris O45. We have found that anti-(P. vulgaris O45) serum contains at least two types of antibodies having different specificities. The major antibodies recognise an O45-serogroup-specific epitope with the lateral β-D-GlcA residue as the immunodominat sugar (Table 3). Results of DOC/PAGE-Western blot (data not presented) showed, that the minor fraction are core-specific antibodies, which react with common epitope presents in the LPS core regions of P. vulgaris O45 and O25[4].

*Table 3.*Reactivity of *Proteus* LPSs with anti – (*P. vulgaris* O45) serum

| Antigen | PIH (reciprocal titer) | Inhibition of PIH [ng] |
|---|---|---|
| *P. vulgaris* O45 LPS-OH | 25,600 | 2,44 |
| *P. vulgaris* O45 OPS | ND* | 2,44 |
| *P. vulgaris* O45 OPS Smith degraded | ND | >5000 |
| *P.vulgaris* O25 LPS-OH | 1,600 | >5000 |
| *P. vulgaris* O22 LPS-OH | 400 | ND* |

*not determined

## 4.    CONCLUSIONS

Acidic components, which are characteristic for many *Proteus* O-specific polysaccharides play an important role in manifesting immunospecificity of three out of four *P. vulgaris* O-antigens investigated in this paper. It was found that the immunological role of acidic components was determined also by other factors, such as the configuration of the glycosidic iinkage and the type of neighbouring sugars.

The acidic nature of polysaccharides, which are present on the surface of *Proteus* strains, is believed to contribute to the formation of stones in urinary tract[7] and to facilitate the migration of swarm cells from these bacteria[8].

## ACKNOWLEDGMENTS

This work was supported by grant 4 P05A 140 14 of the Sciences Research Committee (KBN) Poland, and grants 96-04-50460 and 96-15-97380 of the Russian Foundation for Basic Research.

## REFERENCES

1.  Różalski, A., Sidorczyk, Z., Kotełko, K., 1997, Potential virulence factors of *Proteus* bacilli. *Microbiol. Molec. Biol. Rev.* **61:** 65-89.
2.  Knirel, Y. A., Kaca, W., Różalski, A., Sidorczyk, Z., 1999, Structure of the O-antigenic polysaccharides of *Proteus* bacteria. *Pol. J. Chem.* **73:** 895-907.
3.  Bartodziejska, B., Shashkov, A. S., Babicka, D., Grachev, A. A., Torzewska, A., Paramonov, N. A., Chernyak, A. Y., Różalski, A., Knirel, Y. A., 1999, Structural and serological studies on a new acidic O-specific polysaccharide of *Proteus vulgaris* O32. *Eur. J. Biochem.* **259:** 212-217.
4.  Bartodziejska, B., Shashkov, A. S., Torzewska, A., Grachev, A. A., Ziółkowski, A., Paramonov, N. A., Różalski, A., Knirel, Y. A., 1999, Structure and serological specificity of a new acidic O-specific polysaccharide of *Proteus vulgaris* O45. *Eur. J. Biochem.* **256:** 488-493.
5.  Perepelov, A. V., Babicka, D., Shashkov, A. S., Arbatsky, N. P., Senchenkova, S. N., Różalski, A., Knirel, Y. A., 1999, Structure and cross-reactivity of the O-antigen of *Proteus vulgaris* O8. *Carbohydr. Res.* **318:** 186-192.
6.  Toukach, F. V., Bartodziejska, B., Senchenkova, S. N., Wykrota, M., Shashkov, A. S., Różalski, A., Knirel, Y. A., 1999, Structure and cross-reactivity of a new acidic O-antigen of *Proteus vulgaris* O22 containing *O*-acetylated 3-acetamido-3,6-dideoxy-D-glucose. *Carbohydr. Res.* **318:** 146-153
7.  Dumanski, A. J., Hedelin, H., Edin-Liljegren, A., Beauchemin, D., McLean, R. J., 1994, Unique ability of the *Proteus mirabilis* capsule to enhance mineral growth in infectious urinary calculi. *Infect Immun.* **62:** 2998-3003.
8.  Gygi, D., Rahman, M. M., Lai, H. C., Carlson, R., Guarr-Petter, J., Hughes, C., 1995, A cell-surface polysaccharide that facilitates rapid population migration by differentiated swarm cell of *Proteus mirabilis*. *Mol. Microbiol.* **17:** 1167-1175.

# VIRULENCE FACTORS OF *ESCHERICHIA COLI* ISOLATED FROM URINE OF DIABETIC WOMEN WITH ASYMPTOMATIC BACTERIURIA

[1]Suzanne E. Geerlings, [2]Ellen C.Brouwer, [3]Wim Gaastra, and [1,2]Andy M. Hoepelman

[1]*Dept. Med.,Div. Infect Dis. & AIDS:* [2]*Eijkman-Winkler Lab. Med. Microbiol. Univ. Hospital Utrecht:* [3]*Dept. Bact., Vet. Faculty, Utrecht University, The Netherlands*

## 1. INTRODUCTION

A higher prevalence of <u>asymptomatic</u> and <u>symptomatic</u> bacteriuria has been found in women with diabetes mellitus (DM) than in those without DM.[1] *Escherichia coli* is the most common causative microorganism of urinary tract infections (UTIs) in patients with and without DM[1,2]. Different virulence factors and O:K:H serotypes of uropathogenic *E. coli* have been described[3-12]. It is known that *E. coli* isolated from patients with a <u>symptomatic</u> urinary tract infection (UTI) express fewer virulence factors when the patient has an abnormal urinary tract or is immunocompromised (including diabetic patients) compared with *E. coli* isolated from healthy controls[13]. This suggests that in compromised patients the infecting *E. coli* strain can be less "virulent" than in healthy controls. We hypothesized that *E. coli* isolated from compromised (for example DM) patients with <u>asymptomatic</u> bacteriuria (ASB) also express fewer virulence factors than *E. coli* isolated from non-compromised patients with ASB. Therefore, we decided to study the virulence factors of causative *E. coli* isolated from urine of diabetic women with ASB.

*Genes and Proteins Underlying Microbial Urinary Tract Virulence*
Edited by L. Emödy *et al.*, Kluwer Academic/Plenum Publishers, 2000

## 2.    MATERIALS AND METHODS

### 2.1    Patients

Women, aged 18-75 years, with either DM type 1 or DM type 2 were recruited in the diabetes outpatient clinics of one university tertiary care and three nonuniversity hospitals. Exclusion criteria were: Pregnancy, recent hospitalisation or surgery (< 4 months), known urinary tract abnormalities, symptoms of a UTI or the use of antimicrobial drugs in the previous 14 days.

### 2.2    Urine

One or two midstream urine specimens were collected for evaluation of bacteriuria with an interval of 2-4 months. Urine culture was performed according to standard procedures. When three or more different microorganisms were isolated, the urine was called contaminated and another specimen was collected.

#### 2.2.1    Hemagglutination

The phenotypic expression of type 1 fimbriae was measured by the occurrence of mannose sensitive hemagglutination (MSHA), of P, S fimbriae and AFA by mannose resistant hemagglutination (MRHA) according to standard procedures with guinea pig an human erythrocytes respectively[3,14].

### 2.4    Hemolysin Production

*E. coli* isolates were tested for hemolysis by inoculating them onto 5% sheep blood agar plates. Hemolysis was defined as a distinct zone of clearing around isolated bacterial colonies after an incubation of 24 and 48 hours at 37 $^\circ$C.

### 2.5    Polymerase Chain Reaction (PCR)-Assays

*E. coli* genomic DNA was purified as described previously and performed according to standard procedures[15] with primers for the following groups: the major subunit A (papA) of P fimbriae; G-adhesin (class I, II, and III G-adhesin) of P fimbriae; type 1 fimbriae (type1); S fimbriae (SFA);

afimbrial adhesin (AFA); cytotoxic necrotizing factor (CNF1, CNF2), and aerobactin (Table 1). All assays with negative results were repeated.

## 2.6    O:K:H Serotyping

Isolates were O:K:H serotyped according to the standard method of the National Institute of Public Health and Environmental Protection (RIVM, Bilthoven, The Netherlands (S.O.P. nr LIS/BBT/M521)).

## 2.7    Definitions

Following the 1985 WHO criteria we defined DM as a fasting glucose concentration of at least 7.8 mmol/l or a 2 h glucose concentration of at least 11.1 mmol/l or higher[16].

ASB was defined as the presence of at least $10^5$ cfu/ml of one or two microorganisms in a culture from a clean-voided midstream urine of a patient without symptoms of a UTI or fever $(>38.3^0C)$[17]. Cleared strains were defined as strains, which were isolated from the first urine of a patient with a sterile urine culture 2-4 months later. Persistent strains were defined as strains, which were cultured from the first urine of a patient with a positive urine culture with the same *E. coli* strain (considering the virulence factors) 2-4 months later. Known uropathogenic O-serotypes are O1, O2, O4, O6, O7, O8, O16, O18, O25 and O75[18].

## 2.8    Statistics

Number (and percentages) of different virulence factors were counted for all strains and for cleared and persistent strains separately. The Mann Whitney U-test was used to compare the different virulence factors in one strain. The Chi-square test was used to compare the differences in virulence factors between the cleared and persistent strains.

## 3.    RESULTS

## 3.1    Study Population

In total 111 *E. coli* strains were isolated (48 from the university hospital and 63 from the non-university hospitals) from urine of diabetic women with ASB. A total of 43 of these women collected a second urine culture 2-4 months later. Of these patients 19 had a sterile second urine culture (strain from first culture was called cleared strain) and 15 had a positive second culture with the same (considering the virulence factors) *E. coli* strain (strain from first culture was called persistent strain.)

## 3.2    Prevalence of Virulence Factors

The number (and percentages) of the various virulence factors are shown in Table 1.

*Table 1.* Characteristics of 111 isolated *Escherichia coli*. P-values of differences in numbers of virulence factors between cleared and persistent strains are given. Primers for type 1 fimbriae (type1), P fimbriae (papA), three alleles of the G-adhesin of type P fimbriae (papG-I, papG-II, papG-III), S fimbriae (SFA), afimbrial adhesin (AFA), cytotoxic necrotizing factor (CNF), and aerobactin were used. O-UTI= known uropathogenic O-serotypes (O1, O2, O4, O6, O7, O8, O16, O18, O25, O75). Phenotypes were also determined: MSHA = mannose-sensitive hemagglutination; MRHA = mannose-resistant hemagglutination; and hemolysin.

| Virulence Factors | Numbers in all strains (n=111) | Numbers in persistent strains (n=15) | Numbers in cleared strains (n=19) | p-value |
|---|---|---|---|---|
| Type1 | 96 (86%) | 13 (87%) | 19 (100%) | 0.6 |
| MSHA | 65 (59%) | 8 (53%) | 15 (79%) | 0.6 |
| PapA | 22 (20%) | 1 (7%) | 3 (16%) | 0.1 |
| PapG-I | - | - | - | - |
| PapG-II | 5 (5%) | - | 1 (5%) | 0.4 |
| PapG-III | 16 (14%) | 1 (7%) | 3 (16%) | 0.3 |
| SFA | 33 (30%) | 2 (13%) | 5 (26%) | 0.09 |
| AFA | 6 (5%) | 2 (13%) | - | 0.2 |
| MRHA | 21 (19%) | 1 (7%) | 2 (11%) | 0.2 |
| Aerobactin | 35 (32%) | 3 (20%) | 7 (37%) | 0.4 |
| CNF | 21 (19%) | 1 (7%) | 2 (11%) | 0.2 |
| Hemolysis | 36 (32%) | 6 (40%) | 7 (37%) | 0.6 |
| O-UTI | 21 (19%) | - | 2 (11%) | 0.05 |

The most prevalent virulence factor was type 1 fimbriae (86% by genotyping and 59% by phenotyping respectively). Genes coding for P or S fimbriae and known uropathogenic O-serotypes were more common in cleared than in persistent strains.

## 3.3    Virulence Factors In One Strain

Associations were found between the presence of the genes coding for papA and CNF, papA and papG-III, CNF and papG-III, the gene coding for papA and MRHA or hemolysis, the gene coding for CNF and hemolysis or

MRHA, the gene coding for papG-III and MRHA, the gene coding for SFA and haemolysis or MRHA, and haemolysis and MRHA (all p<0.001.)

## 4.   CONCLUSIONS

1. Type 1 fimbriae is the most prevalent virulence factor in *E. coli,* isolated from urine of diabetic women with ASB.
2. *E. coli,* isolated from urine of diabetic women with ASB, express comparable numbers of virulence factors as *E. coli* isolated from urine of noncompromised patients with ASB.

## ACKNOWLEDGEMENTS

This work was supported by the Dutch Diabetes Fund (number 95.123) and "Stichting de Drie Lichten".

## REFERENCES

1.   Patterson, J.E., and Andriole, V.T., 1997, Bacterial urinary tract infections in diabetes. *Infect. Dis. Clin. North Am.* **11**: 735-750.
2.   Svanborg, C., and Godaly, G., 1997, Bacterial virulence in urinary tract infection. *Infect. Dis. Clin. North Am.* **11**: 513-529.
3.   Johnson, J.R., 1991, Virulence factors in *Escherichia coli* urinary tract infection. *Clin. Microbiol. Rev.* **4**: 80-128.
4.   Johnson, J.R., 1998, PapG alleles among *Escherichia coli* strains causing urosepsis: Associations with other bacterial characteristics and host compromise. *Infect. Immun.* **66**: 4568-4571.
5.   Mitsumori, K, Terai, A., Yamamoto, S., and Yoshida, O., 1998, Identification of S, F1C and three PapG fimbrial adhesins in uropathogenic *Escherichia coli* by polymerase chain reaction. *FEMS Immunol.. Med. Microbiol.* **21**: 261-268.
6.   Orskov, I., Svanborg Eden, C., Orskov, F., 1988, Aerobactin production of serotyped *Escherichia coli* from urinary tract infections. *Med. Microbiol. Immunol.* **177**: 9-14.
7.   Ulleryd, P., Lincoln. K., Scheutz. F., and Sandberg, T., 1994, Virulence characteristics of *Escherichia coli* in relation to host response in men with symptomatic urinary tract infection. *Clin. Infect. Dis.* **18**: 579-584.
8.   Hagberg, L., Jodal, U., Korhonen, T,K,, Lidin Janson, G., Lindberg, U. and, Svanborg Eden, C., 1981, Adhesion, hemagglutination, and virulence of *Escherichia coli* causing urinary tract infections. *Infect. Immun.* **31**: 564-570.
9.   Opal, S.M., Cross, A.S., Gemski, P., and Lyhte, L.W., 1990, Aerobactin and alpha-hemolysin as virulence determinants in *Escherichia coli* isolated from human blood, urine, and stool. *J Infect Dis* **161**: 794-796.
10.  Marild, S., Wettergren, B., Hellström, M., Jodal, U., Lincoln, K., Orskov, I., Orskov, F., and Svanborg Eden, C., 1988, Bacterial virulence and inflammatory response in infants with febrile urinary tract infection or screening bacteriuria. *J. Pediatr.* **112**: 348-354.
11.  Blanco, J., Alonso, M.P., Gonzalez, E.A., Blanco, M., and Garabal, J.I., 1990, Virulence

factors of bacteraemic *Escherichia coli* with particular reference to production of cytotoxic necrotising factor (CNF) by P-fimbriated strains. *J. Med. Microbiol.* **31**: 175-183.

12.  Lindberg, U., Hanson, L.A., Jodal, U., Lidin-Janson, G., Lincoln, K., and Olling, S., 1975, Asymptomatic bacteriuria in schoolgirls. *Acta Paediatr.Scand.* **64**: 432-436.

13.  Johnson, J.R., Roberts, P.L., and Stamm, W.E., 1987, P fimbriae and other virulence factors in *Escherichia coli* urosepsis: association with patients' characteristics. *J. Infect. Dis.* **156**: 225-229.

14.  Schlager, T.A., Whittam, T.S., Hendley, J.O., Hollis, R.J., Pfaller, M.A., Wilson, R.A., Stapleton, A., 1995, Comparison of expression of virulence factors by *Escherichia coli* causing cystitis and *E. coli* colonizing the periurethra of healthy girls. *J. Infect. Dis.* **172**: 772-777.

15.  Kärkkäinen, U.M., Kauppinen, J., Ikäheimo, R., Katila, M.L., and Siitonen, A., 1998, Rapid and specific detection of three different G adhesin classes of P-fimbriae in uropathogenic *Escherichia coli* by polymerase chain reaction. *J. Microbiol. Methods* **34**: 23-29.

16.  Wahl, P.W., Savage, P.J., Psaty, B.M., Orchard, T.J., Robbins, J.A., and Tracy, R.P., 1998, Diabetes in older adults: comparison of 1997 American Diabetes Association classification of diabetes mellitus with 1985 WHO classification. *Lancet* **352**: 1012-1015, 1998

17.  Members of the Medical Research Council Bacteriuria Committee, 1979, Recommended terminology of urinary tract infection. *Br. Med. J* **.2**: 717- 719.

18.  Johnson, J.R., Brown, J.J., and Maslow, J.N., 1998, Clonal distribution of the three alleles of the Gal(alpha1-4)Gal- specific adhesin gene *papG* among *Escherichia coli* strains from patients with bacteremia. *J. Infect. Dis.* **177**: 651-661.

# CYTOKINE SECRETION IS IMPAIRED IN WOMEN WITH DIABETES MELLITUS

[1]Suzanne E. Geerlings, [2]Ellen C.Brouwer, [2]Kok P.M. van Kessel, [3]Wim Gaastra, and [1,2]Andy M. Hoepelman
[1]Dept. Med.,Div. Infect Dis. & AIDS: [2]Eijkman-Winkler Lab. Med. Microbiol. Univ. Hospital Utrecht: [3]Dept. Bact., Vet. Faculty, Utrecht University, The Netherlands

## 1.      INTRODUCTION

Cytokines are small proteins that play an important role in the regulation of host defences against systemic and local bacterial infecions.[1-3]They are also involved in endothelial cell functioning and atherogenesis.[4]Tumor necrosis factor-alpha (TNF-$\alpha$) is a pro-inflammatory cytokine[2] that induces a cascade of inflammatory reactions involving the production of other cytokines.[3] Monocytes and macrophages are the main producers of TNF-$\alpha$ and lipopolysaccharide (LPS) is one of its strongest inducers.[3] Interleukin-6 (IL-6) is another pro-inflammatory cytokine,[2] an endogenous pyrogen, that stimulates hepatocytes to produce acute-phase reactants like C-reactive protein and fibrinogen. It can be synthesized by a variety of cells, including endothelial and renal tubular epithelial cells.[5] Interleukin-8 (IL-8) is a chemokine (chemotactic cytokine), that is induced in monocyte/ macrophages and neutrophils by bacteria, LPS, TNF-$\alpha$, interleukin-1 (IL-1), or interleukin-2 (IL-2).[1,6,7] Human renal mesangial cells and tubular epithelial cells also synthesize and release this chemokine.[5,8,9] An elevation of the urinary cytokines IL-8 and IL-6, has been observed in non-diabetic patients with either symptomatic UTI or ASB compared with non-bacteriuric controls.[10-12]

*Genes and Proteins Underlying Microbial Urinary Tract Virulence*
Edited by L. Emödy *et al.*, Kluwer Academic/Plenum Publishers, 2000

Women with diabetes mellitus (DM) have an increased prevalence of ASB compared to women without DM.[13] We measured, IL-8 and IL-6 levels in the urine of diabetic women with ASB to achieve insight into inflammation in these women. The aims of the present study were: 1. to study the IL-8 and IL-6 concentrations in the urine of diabetic females with ASB and compare them with those of non-diabetic bcteriuric controls; 2. to study the ability of women with diabetes mellitus (DM) to secrete cytokines after stimulation of whole blood or isolated monocytes and compare it with that of women without DM.

## 2.        MATERIALS AND METHODS

### 2.1      Patients

Midstream urine was collected from four groups of patients: Group 1, diabetic females with ASB; Group 2, diabetic females without ASB; Group 3, non-diabetic females with ASB; and Group 4, non-diabetic females without ASB. Moreover, blood was collected from three groups of patients: Group A, females with DM type 1; Group B, females with DM type 2; and Group C, non-diabetic females. Age of all patients ranged between 18 and 75 years. Haemoglobin A1c (HbA1c), as a measurement of diabetes regulation, was measured in all patients. ASB was defined as the presence of at least $10^5$ cfu/ml of one and the same micro-organism in two consecutive cultures from a patient without symptoms of a UTI or fever.[14] DM was defined according to the 1985 WHO criteria: a fasting glucose concentration of greater than or equal to 7.8 mmol/l or a 2 hour glucose concentration of 11.1 mmol/l or higher.[15] DM type 1 was defined as an absolute deficiency of insulin secretion and, according to the data of the treating physician, measured as the absence of C-peptide. DM type 2 was defined as a combination of resistance to insulin action and an inadequate compensatory Exclusion criteria for Groups 1 and 2 were symptoms of a UTI (at that moment and/or in the previous 14 days), pregnancy, known urinary tract abnormalities (also diabetic cystopathy), recent hospitalization or surgery, and the use of antibiotics or immunosuppressive medication (at that moment and/or in the previous 14 days). Exclusion criteria for Groups A and B were: recent onset of DM (<2 years), the presence of symptoms of an infection, and/or the use of antimicrobial or anti-inflammatory drugs (at that moment and/or during the previous 14 days). In the same months, all women in the eye and surgery outpatient clinic (for example, before an elective eye operation or with a bone fracture) were asked to provide two midstream urine specimens. Women with positive urine culture results were placed in Group 3. Exclusion criteria were, besides the presence of DM, the same as for Groups 1 and 2. Urine and blood from healthy ambulant non-diabetic women (working in the hospital), with a negative urine culture, were used for the Groups 4 and C. All urines were stored at -20 $^0$C before use. All blood samples were used directly. All women gave informed consent and the study was approved by the Medical Ethical Committee of our hospital.

## 2.2    Quantitation of TNF-α, IL-8 and IL-6

Concentrations of TNF-α, IL-8, and IL-6 were determined by enzyme-linked immunosorbent assay (ELISA) kits (Central Blood Transfusion Laboratory, Amsterdam, The Netherlands), according to the manufacturer's instructions. The lowest detection limits for the TNF-α, IL-8 and IL-6 assays were respectively 10, 1.5 and 7 pg/ml.

## 2.3    Leukocyturia and Glucosuria

The urinary leukocyte cell counts were divided into the following groups: 0, 5-10, 10-25, and >25 leukocytes/high-power field. The following levels of glucosuria were differentiated: 0 mg/dl, 50 mg/dl, 100 mg/dl, 300 mg/dl, and 1,000 mg/dl (Combur-Test$^R$, Boehringer-Mannheim, Almere, The Netherlands).

## 2.4    Whole Blood Cytokine Induction

Blood was collected aseptically from the three patient groups. Whole blood (100 µl heparinized blood) was mixed with 100 µl  ReLPS (*Salmonella* Minnesota Re595, Sigma-Aldrich Chemie BV, Zwijndrecht, The Netherlands) in different concentrations (30, 100, 300, and 1,000 pg/ml) in a sterile 96-well tissue culture plate (Costar, Badhoevedorp, The Netherlands). EDTA-blood was used as a non-stimulated control. After mixing gently, the plate was stimulated for 4 hours, at 37 $^0$C in a humidified 5% $CO_2$ atmosphere. All samples were tested in duplicate. After 4 hours, the samples were centrifuged (first for 10 min at 420 x g and then for 5 min at 1000 x g) and the supernatants were stored in duplicate at –20 $^0$C.

## 2.5    Isolated Monocyte Stimulation

Peripheral blood mononuclear cells (PBMC) were isolated from Phosphate Buffered Solution (PBS), diluted whole blood (1:1 v/v) by density centrifugation over *Ficoll-Hisopaque* (Pharmacia Biotech, Uppsala, Sweden).  Cells (5 x 10$^6$ PBMC/ml) were enriched for monocytes by incubating 100 μl/well for 90 minutes in a 96-well tissue culture plate (Costar) suspended in RPMI supplemented with 5% fetal calf serum (FCS) at 37 $^0$C in a humidified 5% $CO_2$ atmosphere. Non-adherent cells were removed by gently washing the wells twice with warm RPMI/FCS. The remaining cells (>80% monocytes) were then stimulated (in duplicate) with 100 μl of different LPS concentrations (30, 100, and 300 pg/ml) in the presence of 1% normal pooled human serum (NHS) (of non-diabetic controls) for 18 hours at 37 $^0$C in a humidified 5% $CO_2$ atmosphere. After stimulation, the microplate was centrifuged (10 min at 1000 x g) and the supernatant was stored at -20 $^0$C in duplicate.

## 2.6     Statistics

The Wilcoxon rank sum W test and the logistic regression analysis were used for statistical analyses.

## 3.     RESULTS

## 3.1     Clinical Characteristics

IL-8 and IL-6 were measured in the urine of diabetic females with (n=26, Group 1) and without (n=36, Group 2) ASB and in the urine of non-diabetic females with (n=10, Group 3) and without (n=16, Group 4) ASB. Except for the higher age of the women in both bacteriuric groups, there were no differences in clinical characteristics between the four groups. Whole blood stimulation was conducted on different days with blood samples of 5 different women with DM type 1, 3 women with DM type 2 and 10 women without DM (mean age DM type 1: 46 years, DM type 2: 49 years, controls: 39 years, mean HbA1c for DM type 1: 8,1%, for DM type 2: 7,5%). Blood samples of 8 other women with DM type 1, 7 women with DM type 2, and 8 women without DM were selected for isolated monocyte stimulation on different days (mean age DM type 1: 35 years, DM type 2: 61 years, controls: 36 years, mean HbA1c for DM type 1: 6,5%, for DM type 2: 8,0%).

## 3.2     Urinary IL-6 and IL-8 Concentrations

IL-6 was measurable in 2 of the 23 patients in Group 1, in none of the patients in Group 2, in 9 of the 10 patients in Group 3 (median concentration 23 pg/ml), and in 5 of the 10 patients in Group 4 (median concentration 8 pg/ml) (see Figure 1). The difference in IL-6 concentrations between Group 1 (diabetic females with ASB) and Group 2 (diabetic females without ASB) was not statistically significant (p=0.46). Lower urinary IL-6 concentrations were found in Group 1 (diabetic females with ASB) than in Group 3 (nondiabetic females with ASB). This difference was highly significant (p<0.001).

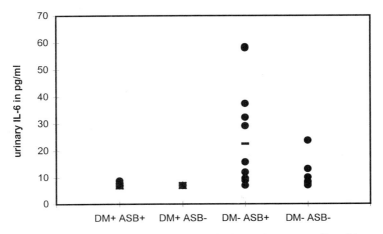

*Figure 1.* Urinary IL-6 concentration in pg/ml of the four patient groups. Dots (•) represent the median concentration in one patient, dashes ( - ) the median value of the whole patient group. Determinations were performed in duplicate.

The median urinary IL-8 concentration was 133 pg/ml (range 15-601) in Group 1, 11 pg/ml (range 3-84) in Group 2, 258 pg/ml (range 25-674) in Group 3 and 67 pg/ml (range 2-468) in Group 4. As expected, higher urinary IL-8 concentrations were found in Group 1 (diabetic females with ASB) than in Group 2 (diabetic females without ASB)(p=0.004). Like the IL-6 concentrations, urinary IL-8 concentrations were also lower in Group 1 (diabetic females with ASB) than in in Group 3 (non-diabetic females with ASB). This difference was, however, not significant (p=0.11).

## 3.3 Relationship Between Urinary IL-6 and IL-8 Concentrations and Patient Characteristics, Glucosuria, Leukocyturia

Higher urinary IL-6 and IL-8 concentrations were correlated with higher urinary leukocyte cell counts. These correlations were highly significant (p=0.008 and p=0.04 for IL-6 and IL-8, respectively). As expected, therefore, lower urinary leukocyte cell counts were found in diabetic than in non-diabetic females (p=0.01 and p=0.003 for IL-6 and IL-8, respectively). No correlations were found between the amount of glucosuria and the urinary IL-6 or IL-8 concentrations. No differences in urinary IL-6 and IL-8 concentrations were seen between *E. coli* and other causative micro-organisms.

## 3.4    Whole Blood and Isolated Monocytes: TNF-α-Concentrations

Since lower IL-6 and IL-8 concentrations were found in urine of diabetic women with ASB compared with that of non-diabetic women with ASB, we wanted to evaluate the cytokine secretion capacity of women with DM. To do this, whole blood of 5 women with DM type 1, 3 women with DM type 2, and 10 women without DM was stimulated *(ex-vivo)* with LPS. Lower TNF-α concentrations were found in women with DM type 1 after stimulation of whole blood (p<0.008 for all LPS concentrations). Since this impairment of cytokine production could be due to a cellular defect or a difference in plasma components, we collected blood from 8 other women with DM type 1, 7 with DM type 2, and 8 without DM to study cytokine excretion in isolated monocytes. Lower TNF-α concentrations were found in women with DM type 1 than women without DM after stimulation of isolated monocytes (p= 0.008 for 30 pg/ml LPS, p=0.03 for 100 pg/ml, and p=0.10 for 300 pg/ml, Figure 2). These differences were not found between women with DM type 2 and controls.

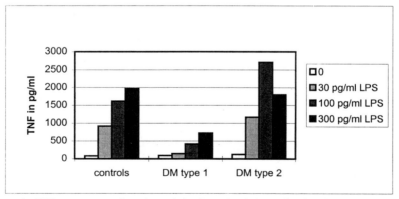

*Figure 2.* TNF-α concentrations in pg/ml after stimulation of isolated monocytes with different (0,30,100,300 pg/ml) LPS concentrations in women without DM (controls), women with DM type 1, and women with DM type 2. Values are means with standard deviations.

## 3.5     Relationship Between Blood TNF-$\alpha$ Concentrations and Patient Characteristics

No correlation's could be demonstrated between the age of the women or the HbA1c and the TNF-$\alpha$ and IL-6 concentrations.

## 4.     CONCLUSIONS

1.  Diabetic women with ASB have lower urinary IL-6 concentrations than non-diabetic bacteriuric controls.

2.  Monocytes of women with DM type 1 secrete lower TNF-$\alpha$ after *ex-vivo* stimulation with LPS than monocytes of women without DM.

## ACKNOWLEDGEMENTS

This study was supported by grants from the Dutch Diabetes Fund (number 95.123)

## REFERENCES

1. Luster, A.D:, 1998, Chemokines - Chemotactic cytokines that mediate inflammation. *New Engl. J. Med.* **338:** 436-445.
2. Poll, vd T., Speelman, P., and Deventer, van S.J.H., 1998, Immunologie in de medische praktijk. VIII. De rol van cytokinen in de pathogenese van bacteriele infecties. *Ned. Tijdschr. Geneeskd.* **142:** 14-17.
3. Bemelmans, M.H.A., Tits. L.J.H., and Buurman, W.A., 1996, Tumornecrosis factor: Function, release and clearance. *Crit. Rev. Imuunology* **16:** 1-11, 1996
4. Epstein, F.H., and Ross, R., 1999, Atherosclerosis - An inflammatory disease. *New Engl. J. Med.* **340:** 115-126, 1999
5. Agace, W., Hedges, S., Andersson, U., Andersson, J., Ceska, M., and Svanborg, C., 1993, Selective cytokine production by epithelial cells following exposure to *Escherichia coli*. *Infect. Immun.* **61:** 602-609.
6. Jacobson, S.H., Hylander, B., Wretlind, B., and Brauner, A, 1994, Interleukin-6 and interleukin-8 in serum and urine in patients with acute pyelonephritis in relation to bacterial virulence-associated traits and renal function. *Nephron* **67:** 172-179.
7. Arnold; R:, and König., W., 1998, Immune response to infection – Interleukin-8 release from human neutrophils after phagocytosis of *Listeria monocytogenes* and *Yersinia enterocolitica*. *J. Med. Microbiol.* **47:** 55-62.
8. Kusner, D.J., Luebbers, E.L., and Nowinski, R.J., Konieczkowski, M., King, C.H., and Sedor, J.R., 1991,Cytokine- and LPS-induced synthesis of interleukin-8 from human mesangial cells. *Kidney Int.* **39:** 1240-1248.

9. Gerritsma, J.S.J., Hiemstra, P.S., Gerritsen, A.F., Prodjosudjadi, W,. Verweij, C.L., Es, van L.A., and Daha, M.R., 1996, Regulation and production of IL-8 by human proximal tubular epithelial cells in vitro. *Clin. Exp. Immunol.* **103:** 289-294.
10. Svanborg, C., Agace, W., Hedges, S., Lindstedt, R., and Svensson, M.,L., 1994, Bacterial adherence and mucosal cytokine production. *Ann. N. Y. Acad. Sci.* **730:** 162-181.
11. Benson, M., Jodal, U., Agace, W., Hellström, M., Marild, S., Rosberg, S., Sjöström, M., Wettergren, B., Jonsson, S., and Svanborg, C., 1996, Interleukin (IL)-6 and IL-8 in children with febrile urinary tract infection and asymptomatic bacteriuria. *J. Infect. Dis.* **174:** 1080-1084.
12. Ko, Y., Mukaida, N., Ishiyama, S., Tokue, A., Kawai, T., Matsushima, K., and Kasahara, T., 1993, Elevated interleukin-8 levels in the urine of patients with urinary tract infections. *Infect. Immun.* **61:** 1307-1314.
13. Patterson, J.E., and Andriole, V.T., 1997, Bacterial urinary tract infections in diabetes. *Infect. Dis. Clin. North Am.* **11:** 735-750.
14. Members of the Medical Research Council Bacteriuria Committee, 1979, Recommended terminology of urinary tract infection. *Br. Med. J.* **2:** 717-719.
15. Wahl, P.W., Savage, P.J., Psaty, B.M., Orchard, T.J., Robbins, J.A., and Tracy, R.P., 1998, Diabetes in older adults: comparison of 1997, American Diabetes Association classification of diabetes mellitus with 1985 WHO classification. *Lancet* **352:** 1012-1015.

# CHARACTERISATION AND ADHERENCE MECHANISMS OF *ESCHERICHIA COLI* STRAINS CAUSING INFECTIONS IN PATIENTS WITH A RECONSTRUCTED BLADDER

[1]Sally J. Keegan, [1]Carlos E. Hormaeche, [2]Jeffery P. Pearson, and [3]David L. Gally

*Departments of Microbiology[1] and Physiology[2], Medical School, University of Newcastle upon Tyne, NE2 4HH. [3]Department of Veterinary Pathology, Royal (Dick) School of Veterinary Studies, University of Edinburgh, EH9 1QX.*

## 1. INTRODUCTION

Since the 1950s bladder reconstruction by enterocystoplasty has replaced the need to use urinary diversion as a means of treating a wide range of conditions. This form of corrective surgery has improved the quality of life for the patient and provided them with a urinary tract that resembles that of a normal lower urinary tract as closely as possible. In most cases, patients are able to void without the use of clean intermittent self-catheterisation (ISC). The type of bowel tissue used to create a 'new' bladder and the procedure undertaken, are dictated by the underlying cause of the bladder dysfunction. In brief three types of enterocystoplasty are currently implemented, 1) augmentation (enlargement by the addition of tissue, none of the existing bladder wall is removed), 2) substitution (partial bladder resection before reconstruction) and 3) orthotopic bladder replacement (entire bladder, and possibly the urethra and sphincter mechanisms are replaced by refashioned bowel segments)[1]. Segments of stomach, ileum, caecum, and colon have been used in all types of

*Genes and Proteins Underlying Microbial Urinary Tract Virulence*
Edited by L. Emödy *et al.*, Kluwer Academic/Plenum Publishers, 2000

reconstructive surgery[2]. In the long-term, studies have revealed that intermittent and/or chronic bacterial infections are almost invariably present among patients with a reconstructed bladder[3]. The frequency of urinary tract infections (UTIs) is believed to be due to the presence of the bowel tissue in the urinary tract. In patients that have a history of renal failure/damage these infections can be life threatening, and for the remainder they can seriously effect the quality of life. As persistent colonisation of the reconstructed bladder may cause pain and irreversible damage to the extent that the operation itself is declared a failure as the tissue is rejected. In an attempt to alleviate the problems imposed by UTIs, patients are often enrolled in a long term program of prophylactic antibiotic therapy. Certain infections still prove to be unmanageable, as studies[4] have shown that up to 60 % of patients receiving enterocystoplasty presented with chronic bacteriuria that is resistant to prophylactics. Other complications of enterocystoplasty are linked to the implementation of ISC and the physiology of the augmented tissue. Excessive mucus production, for example, may contribute to the development and persistence of UTIs in these patients.

Little is known about the bacterial isolates causing infections in patients with a reconstructed bladder and what role the augmented tissue may have in presenting a colonisation site to predispose for an infection and/or facilitate the persistence of an infection.

## 2. MATERIALS AND METHODS

### 2.1 Sample Collection and Bacterial Isolates

Twenty-nine patients with enterocystoplasty were enrolled into a study based at the Urology Clinic Freeman Hospital, Newcastle upon Tyne. None of the patients were shown to have any evidence of reflux, uretral obstruction or calcui. In this study the patients were required to attend on a monthly basis over a 5-9 month period. On each visit the patients were interviewed with regards to their health, and requested to provide a fresh mid-stream or catheter sample of urine. Additional visits were made when the patients believed themselves to be symptomatic. Urine samples collected from all of the clinic visits were sent to the Microbiology Department, Freeman Hospital to be screened for bacteriuria.

*E. coli* isolates causing a community acquired cystitis infection were collected by Dr. C. Graham at the Clinical Microbiology Department, University of Newcastle upon Tyne.

Isolates from both study groups were cultured at 37 °C on Luria-Bertani (LB) and MacConkey agar plates, and then stored at -70 °C in 20 % glycerol.

## 2.2    Genotypic Characterisation

### 2.2.1    Polymerase chain reaction (PCR) using specific primers

Crude extracts of deoxyribonucleic acid (DNA) were prepared from the isolates of both study groups in order to screen for virulence determinants by PCR using primers (Table 1) previously characterised and tested at the Institute for the Molecular Biology of Infectious Diseases (MBID), University of Wuerzburg.   PCR conditions were 94 °C (5 min) then 34

*Table 1.* Primer information

| Virulence determinant | Primer name | Oligonucleotide sequence (5' → 3') | Primer temp.(°C) | PCR product (bp) |
|---|---|---|---|---|
| S family | SFAM I | ATG TCT GTG CAG CGG GTT CT | 61 | 420 |
| | SFAM II | ATT ACC GGC CTT TAC CGG AA | | |
| P family | PFAMA | GTG CAG ATT AAC ATC AGG GG | 60 | 430 |
| | PFAMB | ATG CTC ATA CTG GCC GTG GT | | |
| Type 1 fimbriae | TYPE IA | GCC GGA TTA TGG GAA AGA A | 54 | 643 |
| | TYPE IB | AGT GAA CGG TCC CAC CAT | | |
| Aerobactin | AER I | TTC GGC GAT GAC CGC TAC TG | 62 | 800 |
| | AER II | TTC CAG CGT GAA GCC AGT G | | |
| Cytotoxic necrotising factor 1 | CNF IA | CCA TGA ACG CCT TAA ATC GC | 54 | 530 |
| | CNF IB | ATA CCT CCG GGA CTA CGA TA | | |
| α–haemolysin | HYL A1 | TAT GAA TTC ACT CAT ATC AAT GG. | 59 | 700 |
| | HYL A2 | TCT GAA TTC TGA TTA GAG ATA TCA CCT GAC TC. | | |

cycles of 94 °C (45 s), primer specific annealing temperature (45 s), 72 °C (60 s), plus a final extension at 72 °C (10 min).

### 2.2.2   Pulsed-field gel electrophoresis (PFGE)

PFGE analysis was carried out on the *E. coli* isolates obtained from patients with a reconstructed bladder.   In brief, chromosomal DNA was prepared in agarose plugs and then cleaved with the restriction enzyme *Xba*I. PFGE running conditions were 24 h with increasing pulse times from 5 to 50s.  Assistance with PFGE was provided by Dr G. Blum-Oehler at MBID, University of Wuerzburg[5].

## 3.     RESULTS

## 3.1    Study

26 patients took part in this study, 19 males and 7 females, with an average age of 53 years.    Fig 1 shows the distribution of surgical reconstruction procedure performed and which section of the bowel was used.  The majority of reconstruction procedures utilise a combination of the two bowel tissues, the ileum and caecum.

56 % of all the asymptomatic bacteriuria cases were shown to be due to *E. coli* ($2x10^4$ -$1x10^5$ cells/ml).  Fig. 2 shows the percentage of bacterial spp causing asymptomatic bacteriuria in the study group patients.  In 50 % of all symptomatic infections *E. coli* was identified as the causative spp.  In one of these cases the patient was hospitalised with septicaemia due to *E. coli*. Other bacterial spp implicated in causing a symptomatic infection were *Proteus* spp, *Klebsiella* spp and an unidentified coliform.  Only 1 out of 26 patients, who was not taking any prophylactic antibiotics had no evidence of bacteria present in their urine over the minimum sampling period of 5 months.

On entering into this study 11 out of the 26 patients complained of recurrent UTIs, although the remaining 15 agreed to take part due to problems with UTIs in the past.  In 5 of these 11 patients *E. coli* was previously documented to be the main or only causative bacterial spp.  In this study, 2 out of these 5 patients still had persistent bacteriuria with *E. coli*. Of the remaining 6 patients, 4 had previous chronic recurrent episodes of UTI and were taking prophylactic antibiotics, either Cephalexin, Trimethoprim or Nalidixic acid.  In this study, 3 of these 4 had persistent bacteriuria, one with only *E. coli*.

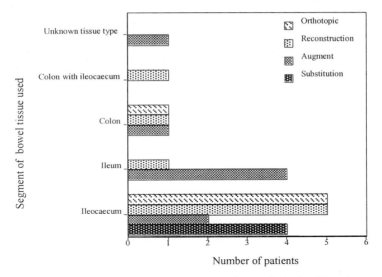

*Figure 1.* Reconstructive surgery procedure performed and bowel segment used in the twenty-six patients.

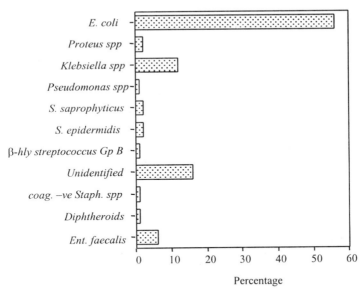

*Figure 2.* Percentage of bacterial spp causing asymptomatic bacteriuria in patients with a reconstructed bladder.

## 3.2     Virulence Determinant Characterisation

For the purpose of this analysis, the *E. coli* isolates obtained from each patient with enterocystoplasty on consecutive visits are treated separately. Table 1 shows the percentage distribution of virulence determinants among the two study groups.

Type 1 fimbriae occur at a higher frequency among the *E. coli* isolates from patients with a reconstructed bladder than those isolates causing a cystitis infection. The other virulence determinants occur at a significantly lower frequency in the isolates from a reconstructed bladder as shown by the paired student t-test ($P < 0.05$).

*Table 2.* Distribution of virulence determinants among isolates of *E. coli* from the two study groups.

| Virulence determinant | Isolates from patients with urinary reconstruction. | Cystitis community acquired isolates. |
| --- | --- | --- |
| Type 1 | 36/37 (97.3) | 42/46 (91.3) |
| P family adhesin | 22/30 (73.3) | 48/48 (100) |
| S family adhesin | 14/34 (41.2) | 28/44 (63.6) |
| α-haemolysin | 15/34 (44.1) | 17/35 (48.6) |
| CNF 1 | 19/37 (51.4) | 35/47 (74.5) |
| Aerobactin | 13/34 (38.2) | 31/46 (67.4) |

## 3.3     Pulsed-field Gel Electrophoresis (PFGE)

Genomic DNA was isolated from 10 of the 26 patients and digested with *Xba*I, then analysed by PFGE. PFGE patterns obtained with isolates cultured from two of the 26 patients, BR 16 and 17 are shown in Fig 1. The patterns for the *E. coli* isolate cultured on consecutive visits from each patient are almost identical. In addition, the isolates cultured from individual patients have a unique PFGE pattern. Band deletions are evident between the PFGE patterns obtained for the isolates cultured from BR 16 and 17. For instance, a band of 130 Kb is absent from the isolates BR 16 V2 and V3, as is a band of 340 Kb from the isolate BR 17 V3.

## 4.     CONCLUSION

This study has highlighted the problems patients with a reconstructed bladder have with UTIs.    The majority of both asymptomatic and symptomatic bacteriuria has been shown to be due to isolates of *E. coli*. It is has also given an indication that the prescription of prophylactic antibiotics is not effective.

The majority of isolates from a reconstructed bladder have the ability to encode an array of fimbrial adhesins (type 1 and P family) that facilitate bacterial attachment and subsequent colonisation. The significance of type 1 fimbriae for colonising a reconstructed urinary tract has been   indicated   by

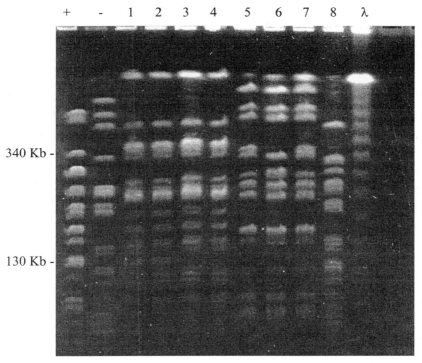

*Figure 3.* PFGE analysis of *E. coli* isolates cultured from two different patients, BR 16 and 17. Lane +: *E. coli* 536, lane -: *E. coli* HB101, Lane 1:BR16V1, Lane 2:BR16IVi, Lane 3:BR16V2, Lane 4:BR16V3, Lane 5:BR17V1, Lane 6:BR17V1, Lane 7:BR17V5, Lane 8:MG1655, Lane λ: molecular weight marker.

Nakano et al.,[6]   who suggested that bacterial isolates expressing type 1 are more commonly associated with asymptomatic bacteriuria in patients with enterocystoplasty.

Even though the frequency in the isolates from a reconstructed bladder for the toxins α-haemolysin and CNF 1 is lower than that of the cystitis study group, it is significantly higher from that reported for faecal isolates from healthy individuals in previous studies (Table 3).

Despite the isolates possessing established virulence determinants, the true pathogenicity of these isolates cannot be assessed until they have been compared in detail to a third study group, the faecal isolates from healthy individuals. This work is currently in progress.

*Table 3.* Distribution of virulence determinants among isolates of *E. coli* from healthy individuals and patients with a reconstructed bladder.

| Virulence determinant. | Faecal isolates from healthy individuals. | Isolates from patients with urinary reconstruction. |
|---|---|---|
| α-haemolysin | 13 % [a] | 44.1 % |
| CNF 1 | 3 % [b] | 51.4 % |

[a]Dudgeon *et al.*[7], [b]Caprioli *et al.*[8]

PFGE analysis of the *E. coli* isolates from the same patient on consecutive visits has shown that they have an almost identical banding profile, whether the patients were attending for a routine visit, or as a consequence of a symptomatic infection (interim visit). This would imply that the isolates of *E. coli* are persisting in patients with enterocystoplasty and in some instances in spite of antibiotic treatment. The small number of band deletions shown could be of significance as it may mean that the isolates have lost or gained a piece of DNA which harbours important virulence determinants.

Future work will determine whether the use of bowel tissue to reconstruct the bladder provides a natural colonisation site for *E. coli* and consequently predisposes for infection and/or facilitates the persistence of an infection. From a medical perspective, information will be gathered to help clinicians to decide which cases of asymptomatic bacteriuria need to be treated and the benefit of prophylactic antibiotic prescription.

## ACKNOWLEDGEMENT

This study was supported by the Dr. William Edmund Harker Foundation at the University of Newcastle upon Tyne. Thank you to Professor J. Hacker and Dr. G. Blum-Oehler at the MBID, Germany for the use of their PFGE equipment and continual support.

## REFERENCES

1. Webster, G.D., and Ramon, J., 1992, Bladder Augmentation and Reconstruction. In *Surgical Management of Urologic Disease, an Anatomic Approach* (M.J. Droller, ed.) Mosby-Year Book, Inc. pp. 601-617.

2. Rowland, R.G., 1991, Intestine for Bladder Augmentation and Substitution In *Bladder Reconstruction and Continent Urinary Diversion.* (L.R. King, A. R. Stone, and G. D. Webster, ed.) Mosby-Year book, Inc.pp-25-28.

3. Gonzalez, R., and Reinberg, Y., 1987, Localisation of bacteriuria in patients with enterocystoplasty and nonrefluxing conduits. *The Journal of Urology.* **138:** 1104-1105.

4. Gonzalez, R., Sidi, A.A., and Zhang, G., 1986, Urinary undiversion: indications, technique and results in 50 cases. *The Journal of Urology.* **136:** 13-16.

5. Blum, G., Muhldorfer, I., Kuhnert, P., Frey, J., and Hacker J., 1996, Comparative methodology to investigate the presence of *Escherichia coli* K-12 strains in environmental and human stool samples. *FEMS Microbiology Letters.* **143:** 77-82.

6. Nakano, Y., Fujisawa, M., Matsui, T., Arakawa, S., and Kamidono, S., 1999, The significance of the difference in bacterial adherence between bladder and ileum using rat ileal augmented bladder. *The Journal of Urology.* **162:** 243-247.

7. Dudgeon, L.S., Wordley, E., and Bawtree, F, 1921, On *Bacillus coli* infections of the urinary tract, especially in relation to haemolytic organisms. *The Journal of Hygiene.* **20:** 137-164.

8. Caprioli, A., V. Falbo, F. M. Ruggeri, L. Baldassarri, R. Bisicchia, G. Ippolito, E. Romoli and G. Donelli. 1987. Cytotoxic necrotising factor production by haemolytic strains of *Escherichia coli* causing extraintestinal infections. *Journal of Clinical Microbiology.* **27:** 758-761.

# IMMUNODOMINANT PROTEINS IN HUMAN SEPSIS CAUSED BY METHICILLIN RESISTANT *STAPHYLOCOCCUS AUREUS*

[1]Udo Lorenz, [2]Knut Ohlsen, [3]Helge Karch, [1]Arnulf Thiede and [2]Jörg Hacker
[1]*Department of Surgery, The University of Würzburg,, Germany: *[2]*Institute for Molecular Biology of Infectious Diseases, The University of Würzburg,, Germany: *[3]*Institute for Hygiene and Microbiology, The University of Würzburg, 97080 Würzburg, Germany*

## 1.    INTRODUCTION

*Staphylococcus aureus* is the most common cause of nosocomial infections with a significant morbidity and mortality. In addition, the percentage of methicillin resistant *Staphylococcus aureus* (MRSA) as causative agent for nosocomial infections has become increasingly prevalent since the 1980s [1,2]. Infections due to MRSA are seen more often in intensive care units due to the immunocompromised state of many patients. Taking this into account, there are only few published data about immune response during human infections caused by *Staphylococcus aureus* and even more by MRSA.

## 1.1    Aim

The objective of this study was to analyze the humoral immune response in human sepsis against MRSA, to assess differences in antibody profiles between healthy individuals and patients with sepsis caused by MRSA, and finally, to determine significant immunodominant cell components.

*Genes and Proteins Underlying Microbial Urinary Tract Virulence*
Edited by L. Emödy *et al.*, Kluwer Academic/Plenum Publishers, 2000

## 2.       METHODS

### 2.1       Patients and Serum Samples

Antibody response was investigated in sera of 10 individuals. Five patients developed nosocomial sepsis caused by MRSA. Serum samples were obtained several times during the course of sepsis. As control, sera of five healthy individuals were used.

### 2.2       Strains

All MRSA strains were isolated from the septic patients investigated in this study.

### 2.3       Sodium       Dodecyl       Sulphate       Polyacrylamide       Gel Electrophoresis (SDS-PAGE)

A modified version of SDS-PAGE technique by Laemmli was carried out.

### 2.4       Immunoblot (Western Blot)

For immunoblot experiments, separated proteins were transferred to nitrocellulose sheets by semidry electro-blotting. The nitrocellulose sheets were incubated with human sera. Bound antibodies were detected with horseradish peroxidase conjugated anti-human IgM, IgG, IgA secondary antibody (Dako, Hamburg, Germany).

### 2.5       N-Terminal Amino Acid Sequence Analysis

For N-terminal amino acid sequencing, staphylococcal whole cell extract with soluble proteins was concentrated and Tricine-SDS-PAGE was performed.

### 2.6       DNA Sequence Analysis of Immunodominant Proteins

The detected N-terminal amino acid sequence of immunodominant proteins were compared with known amino acid sequences of various protein data banks and with data of unfinished *Staphylococcus aureus* genome sequencing. Large contigs, which include sequences that matched to 100 % with the predicted N-terminal amino acid sequence of immunodominant proteins were analyzed for open reading frames (ORFs). ORFs, where the presumed molecular weight of the protein product was similar to the molecular weight of immunodominant protein determined by immunoblotting, were cloned in *Escherichia coli* and subsequently sequenced.

## 2.7 Enzyme-Linked Immunosorbent Assay (ELISA)

In order to confirm the specificity of the antibody reactions, the recombinant staphylococcal proteins were used in ELISA assays with different sera.

## 3. RESULTS AND DISCUSSION

### 3.1 Immune Response of Healthy Adults Against MRSA

A representative immunoblot of serum gained from a healthy donor against MRSA is shown in Fig 1. A complex pattern of antibody response to a wide range of protein antigens was detected. Up to 25 immunodominant proteins were detectable depending on the investigated MRSA isolate. Similiar immunoblots were also obtained with sera of other healthy individuals (data not shown).

### 3.2 Immune Response of Septic Patients Against MRSA

Representative immunoblotting experiments with sera of a septic patient is shown in Fig 2.

In contrast to that determined for healthy individuals, the profile of immunodominant proteins after sepsis shows significant differences. One characteristic feature is a clear enhancement of immunodominant proteins. In particular, a 29 kDa protein, was identified as an abundant antigen. The enhancement of antibody response to protein of 29 kDa was recognized with all sera of septic patients (data not shown). A second remarkable feature is the detection of antibodies against other abundant protein antigens with apparent molecular weights of 17 and 10 kDa, respectively. Antibodies to the protein antigen of 10 kDa were prominent in three of five sera from patients with sepsis and antibodies to the protein antigen of 17 kDa could be observed in immunoblots of all septic patients.

### 3.3    Immune Response Against Extracellular Proteins

Immunoblots of culture supernatant of MRSA strains were obtained to investigate the nature of the immunodominant proteins. As an example, immunoblot of culture supernatant from MRSA probed with serum of a septic patient is shown in Fig 3. Among other immunodominant antigens, the prominent protein of 29 kDa was detected in all preparations of MRSA strains.

### 3.4    Molecular Analysis of Immunodominant Proteins

Analysis of protein of 29 kDa revealed an entire gene and amino acid sequence which was assigned to GenBank/EMBL (Accession no. AF144681). The protein exhibited 29 % identity with secreted protein SceA precursor of *Staphylococcus carnosus*. The gene and amino acid sequence of protein of 17 kDa was assigned to GenBank/EMBL (Accession no. AF144682). No homology to any currently known protein could be found. The two novel proteins were named IsaA (29 kDa) and IsaB (17 kDa), respectively Interestingly, the preparation of immunodominant proteins of 10 kDa harbored two different proteins. One protein exhibited 100 % identity to phosphocarrier protein Hpr in *Staphylococcus aureus* and the other protein exhibited 88 % identity to cold shock protein CspB and CspC, respectively in *Staphylococcus aureus*.

### 3.5    ELISA Test with Immunodominant Proteins

As indicated in Fig 4, serum from septic patient strongly reacted with the antigens IsaA, IsaB, Hpr and CspB. No signal was detected against CspC. These data confirm our finding, that the staphylococcal proteins IsaA, IsaB, Hrp and an epitope of CspB act as strong antigens in episodes of human sepsis.
The presence of native circulating antibodies throughout individuals in a normal population does not provide necessarily a strong protection from infection, since patients at the onset of sepsis also showed an immune response (data not shown) which is comparable to healthy individuals. It was found that patients who developed sepsis had a different antibody response compared to healthy individuals to at least four proteins. IsaA specific antibodies were detected in all healthy adults as well as in patients suffering from sepsis. In general, antibody response in healthy adults was clearly weaker than in septic patients. This might be indicate that seroconversion against IsaA as an essential step in host immune defense. Most important, the IsaA protein was also detected in culture supernatant. Similarity of IsaA

to secreted protein SceA precursor of *Staphylococcus carnosus* is in agreement with this finding. IsaB, the protein of 17 kDa was only detected in small amounts in immunoblots using sera from three healthy adults.

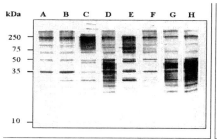

FIG. 1    Immunoblot probed with serum of healthy individual against whole cell lysate proteins of different MRSA strains. Molecular weight of proteins were determined with Rainbow RPN 800 recombinant protein marker (Amersham, Buckinghamshire, England).

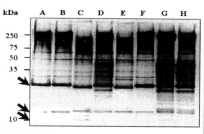

FIG. 2    Immunoblot probed with serum from septic patient against whole cell lysate proteins of different MRSA strains. Serum sample was drawn 14 d after detection of MRSA in blood culture. Immunodominant proteins of 29, 17 and 10 kDa are marked by an arrow. Molecular weight marker is arranged as in Fig. 1.

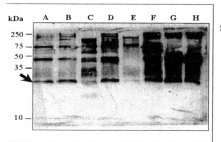

FIG. 3    Immunoblot of culture supernatant of different MRSA strains probed with serum from septic patient. Serum sample was drawn 14 d after detection of MRSA in blood culture. Immunodominant protein of 29 kDa is marked by an arrow. Molecular weight marker is arranged as in Fig. 1.

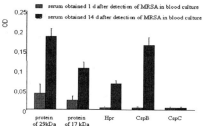

FIG. 4    Antibody reaction of sera from septic patient against overexpressed and purified immunodominant proteins as determined with ELISA tests

Otherwise, all septic patient showed an increase in antibody response against IsaB. However, the native function of IsaA and IsaB, respectively and their possible role in pathogenesis of infections due to MRSA is unknown. The other two detected immunodominant proteins are known proteins. The amino acid sequence and structural analysis of phosphocarrier protein Hpr of the phosphoenolpyruvate sugar phosphotransferase system in *Staphylococcus aureus* have been characterized extensively [3]. In case of the other protein of 10 kDa, the presumed cold shock protein, analysis of the entire gene and corresponding amino acid sequence needs to be performed. So far, it is known that CspB but not CspC of *Staphylococcus aureus* carries the immonogenic epitope, according to the results obtained by the ELISA tests This study demonstrates that human sepsis caused by methicillin resitant *Staphylococcus aureus* results in the development of a specific antibody response. Identification of at least four immunogenic proteins, where seroconversion occurs, is likely to be of direct clinical value.

## ACKNOWLEDGMENTS

This work was supported by a grant from the BMBF no. 01KI9608 and the 'Fond der Chemischen Industrie'. We thank J. Hoppe, Department of Physiological Chemistry II, University of Würzburg, for protein sequencing. Sequencing of *Staphylococcus aureus* was accomplished with support from the National Institute of Allergy and Infectious Diseases and the Merck Genome Research Institute.

## REFERENCES

1. Centers for Disease Control and Prevention, 1996, National Nosocomial Infection Surveillance System report: data summary from October 1986-April 1996, Atlanta (GA): U.S. Department of Health and Human Services.
2. Panlilio, A.L., Culver, D.H., Gaynes, R.P., Banerjee, S., Henderson, T.S., Tolson, J.S., and Martone, W.J., 1992, Methicillinresistant *Staphylococcus aureus* in U.S. hospitals, 1975-1991. *Infect. Control. Hosp. Epidemiol.* **13**: 582-586.
3. Beyreuther, K., Raufuss, H., Schrecker, O., and Hengstenberg, W., 1977, The phosphoenolpyruvate-dependent phosphotransferase system of *Staphylococcus aureus*. 1. Amino-acid sequence of the phosphocarrier protein HPr. *Eur. J. Biochem.* **75**: 275-286.

# MODERN CONCEPT OF ANTIBIOTIC THERAPY OF URINARY TRACT INFECTIONS

Raymond Auckenthaler
*Division of Infectious Diseases, University Hospital Geneva, 24, Micheli du Crest, CH-1211 Geneva, Switzerland*

## 1.    INTRODUCTION

Urinary tract infections (UTI) are among the most commonly seen bacterial infections in adults. In the USA there are about 8,000,000 visits to physicians per year, mostly for cystitis and >100,000 admissions to hospitals for acute pyelonephritis.[1,2] Women suffer more frequently from UTI than men. Each year about 5% of women present with dysuria and frequency. About half of them have a urinary tract infection with a significant number of bacteria in the urine. The others have symptoms in the absence of bacterial infection, a condition referred to as urethral syndrome. This article reviews the approach to diagnosis and treatment of the most frequent manifestations of UTI.

## 2.    EPIDEMIOLOGY

The prevalence UTI varies according sex and age[3]. The female gender is more prone to infection for anatomical reasons: short and straight urethra and short distance between the ostium of the urethra and the anus contribute to the easy colonization of the periurethral region with enteric bacteria equipped with appropriate pili, fimbriae, etc attaching to the mucosal surface. In female the prevalence is 1% in newborns (congenital defects with functional or anatomic reflux), 4-5% in toddlers for the same reasons, 4-5%

*Genes and Proteins Underlying Microbial Urinary Tract Virulence*
Edited by L. Emődy *et al.*, Kluwer Academic/Plenum Publishers, 2000

in schoolgirls (reflux), 20% in young sexually active women (more frequent when using spermicides), 35% in middle age women (lack of oestrogen, surgery, prolapsus, incontinence, residual urine) and 40% for women >65 year for the same reasons and /or indwelling catheters and incontinence. In males the prevalence of UTI is 1% (functional or anatomic reasons), 0.5% in preschool boys (no circumcision, sexual abuse) <0.5% from 5-35 years, 20-40% and increasing with age due to prostata hyperplasia, surgery, indwelling catheters or incontinence.

The most frequent organisms causing UTI are *Escherichia coli*, less common are *Klebsiella* spp. *Enterobacter* spp, *Proteus* spp, *Staphylococcus syprophyticus* (women only), *Pseudomonas* spp, *Acinetobacter* spp, streptococci group B and enterococci, whereas *Haemophilus influenzae*, salmonella, shigella, anaerobes, yeasts or mycobacteria are rare. A clear link to UTI has not been established for *Gardnerella vaginalis*, *Ureaplasma urealyticum* and *Mycoplasma hominis*.

For therapeutic reasons it is useful to distinguish between uncomplicated and complicated infections. Uncomplicated infections are due to the most common microorganisms (*E. coli*, klebsiellae, *P. mirabilis*, *S. saprophyticus*) in the absence of functional or anatomical abnormalities. They are often linked to a positive personal or family history with UTI, the use of diaphragm or spermicides. This type of infection can be treated with a short course of antibiotics.

In contrast, complicated UTI, more frequently due to *S. aureus* or *P. aeruginosa*, are linked to functional or anatomical dysfunctions, to instrumentation, catheterization or to recent use of antibiotics. Risk factors for complicated UTI include males, elderly persons, previous or actual hospitalization, pregnancy, duration of symptoms > 7 days, presence of stones, indwelling catheter, recent instrumentation, anatomical abnormalities, history of UTI in childhood, immunosuppression or recent use of antibiotics. These infections need a prolonged antibiotic treatment to be cured.

## 3.        UNCOMPLICATED BACTERIAL CYSTITIS

Uncomplicated bacterial cystitis is characterized by dysuria, frequency, urgency, suprapubic pain and pyuria, in the absence of fever. Elevated temperature points to pyelonephritis or complicated infection. If there are no risk factors for a complicated infection (see above), it is sufficient for the diagnosis, to establish the presence of nitrate and/or leukocyte esterase with a rapid dipstick method as summarized in Fig 1. If positive, a culture is not necessary and the patient should be treated with a 3-days course of antibiotics. Key to the successful treatment is the impregnation of the urinary tract with antibiotics during > 72 hours. Many treatments have been evaluated. It has been clearly demonstrated, that cotrimoxazole or fluoroquinolones are more efficient than betalactam antibiotics[4,5]. The following 3-days regimens are frequently used: trimethoprim 300 mg q24h, cotrimoxazol 960 mg q12h, norfloxacin 400 mg q12h, ciprofloxacin 250 mg q12h, or fosfomycine 3g (as a single dose). General measures include drinking to increase the urinary output. Once the treatment is completed, the urine sediment should be normal and the urine culture negative after 10-14 days.

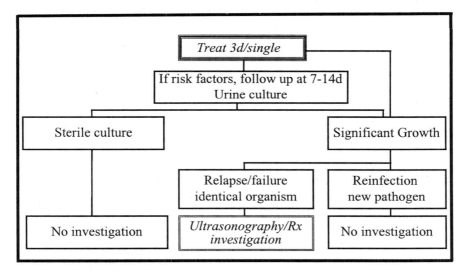

*Figure 1*  Approach of uncomplicated bacterial cystitis.

## 4.     URINE CULTURES

Urine cultures should be performed only if essential for the management of the patient: to control the efficacy of treatment, in complicated UTI including paraplegic patients, neurogenic bladder, chronic bacterial prostatitis, after renal transplantation, in the setting of gynecological or urological surgery or in any other particular clinical situation. Asymptomatic bacteriuria must be searched in pregnancy, in immunocompromised patients, in presence of lithiasis and diabetes mellitus.

Urine cultures are often performed on midstream urine. Correct collection and transportation to the laboratory are essential. In young women it has been shown that cleaning of the genitalia with soap, disinfectants or water does not improve the quality of the results[6]. More important, female patient should be seated on the toilet in order to move the legs apart and to separate the labia with one hand. Male patients should retract the prepuce. The patient should start urinating and then catch a portion of the midstream (!) with a clean cup or sterile tube without interrupting the miction. Urine must be cultured within 2 hours if maintained at room temperature, within 48 h if refrigerated or introduced in a special tube containing boric acid. The dipslide method is useful if used appropriately: slides should not be dried out because of inadequate storing, slides should be inoculated evenly once they have reached room temperature (if previously stored at 4°C), there should be no residual moisture in the transportation tube, incubation at 35-37°C during 24 h, inspection for growth should be done under good illumination and interpretation according to manufacturer instructions.

## 5.        RECURRENT CYSTITIS

Positive cultures after adequate treatment occur in 20% of patients, mainly in women and should be categorized as persistence, recidive or reinfection. Persistence can be due to lack of compliance, insufficient absorption of the antibiotic, stones, resistant organisms or, rarely, structural or functional abnormalities which need further investigations with ultrasonography, radiologic imaging and eventually an urologist advice. Relapse occurs in general within one week after stopping therapy and is due to incomplete killing of organisms in relation with persistence and/or chronic bacterial prostatitis or other deep seated infections. Reinfection is the most frequent form of recurrent cystitis (90%). It occurs more than two weeks after the initial treatment and is due to a new microorganism introduced by ascending way from the vaginal or digestive flora. Factors favoring recurrent infections include use of diaphragm, incomplete voiding, sexual intercourse, instrumentation, genetic particularities, diabetes etc.

The treatment of recurrent cystitis is difficult and a confident relation between the patient and the physician is mandatory[7]. A precise history is essential to decide how to prevent further episodes. The therapeutic attitude in the absence of structural abnormalities varies according the clinical situtation. If new episodes can not be linked to particular circumstances, the patient should be instructed for a self-start therapy for each new episode[8]: in the presence of characteristic symptoms and after collection of a midstream urine for culture, a 3-days course of antibiotics (see above) can be started. If recurrent cystitis is linked to sexual intercourse, a postcoital prophylaxis with a single dose of either cotrimoxazol (80/400mg) or nitrofurantoin (50mg) is recommended. In case of many recurrent episodes within 6 months, a long-term low-dose prophylaxis during 3-6 months might be useful (cotrimoxazol 80/400mg or nitrofurantoin 100 mg each night)[9]. Prophylaxis for recurrent UTI should also be considered in children with abnormal urinary tract or recurrent UTI, in paraplegic patients without catheters or in presence of neurogenic bladder. In all circumstances discussed, repeated cultures with identification and susceptibilities are essential to detect development of resistance and for the correct choice of antibiotics[10]. In chronic bacterial prostatitis a prolonged treatment (6 weeks to 3 months) is necessary in therapeutic dosis with antibiotics penetrating and biologically active in this particular tissue namely with: cotrimoxazol, fluoroquinolones or doxycycline are the drugs of choice.

Besides antibiotic use, hygienic measures should be instructed : daily washing of the external genitalia with water and mild soap (no disinfectants), no vaginal shower, use of clean cotton underwear, wiping after micturition without contaminating the vulva with perineal flora, no use of spermicides or diaphragm, voiding after sexual intercourse, increased daily fluid intake, etc. It is not clearly proven that cranberry juice, vitamin C and others prevent recurrent cystitis. Elderly women suffering from recurrent cystitis and atrophic vagina should be treated with local applications of oestriol cream (0.5 mg twice a week) in order to reconstitute the normal vaginal flora[11].

# 6.    URETHRAL SYNDROME

The urethral syndrome, also known as dysuria-pyuria syndrome, is an acute UTI with low number of microorganisms, $10^2$-$10^5$cfu/ml observed in women only. The cause can be an infection with *Ureaplasma urealyticum*, *Chlamydia trachomatis* or other sexually transmitted diseases confined to the proximal urethra or an infection of the para-urethral glands with lactobacilli. Some cases are due to chemical irritation with deodorants, bubble bath etc., to mechanical or psychological trauma. The therapeutic measures are the same as those mentioned for recurrent cystitis. Specific treatment with doxycycline (200 mg daily for 10 days, azithromycine (1 g in a single dose) or fluoroquinolones (10 days) is indicated for *Ureaplasma urealyticum*, or *Chlamydia trachomatis*.

## 7.    ACUTE PYELONEPHRITIS

Acute pyelonephritis is characterized by fever, lumbar pain, nausea and vomiting. Lower UTI symptoms may be absent. The severity of clinical symptoms is variable and can go from sepsis to multi-organ failure. There is no adequate laboratory test for localization: antibody-coated bacteria are neither sensitive, nor specific and have been abandoned. Leucocyturia and significant bacteriuria (in 20% $< 10^5$cfu/ml) are always present, blood cultures are positive in 15-20%. Fifty percent of acute pyelonephritis are uncomplicated and observed mainly in young women. The other 50% concern mainly elderly men with prostata hyperplasia with recent or indwelling catheters. Patients with acute pyelonephritis should be hospitalized if complicated or severely ill, unstable, immunocompromised, pregnant, or if they are children or men. Persistent vomiting, unsuitable home situation and any suspicion of abscess, obstruction or kidney stones are also indications for hospitalization[12].

The diagnostic workup includes urine sediment and culture, blood cultures, ultrasonography and additional imaging as requested, blood count, surveillance of electrolytes, renal function and hemostasis. General measures include adequate fluid/electrolyte control, hemodynamic surveillance and analgesics. In mild to moderate cases, after 1-2 doses of iv third generation cephalosporin or fluoroquinolones a 10-14 days course of oral treatment with one of the following antibiotics is adequate: cotrimoxazole, fluoroquinolones, amoxicillin/clavulanic acid or second (third) generation cephalosporins[12,13]. Severe cases should be hospitalized and started on iv medication with these antibiotics. Adjunction of few doses of aminoglycoside might be useful. Once the patient is stable, a switch from iv to oral treatment should be considered. Prerequisite is that the patient is afebrile and able to take fluid by mouth, is not vomiting, has an adequate gut function and the chosen peroral drug should be adapted to the susceptibility results, have a good bioavailability, generates high urine concentrations and be well tolerated. If the compliance is reliable the iv-oral switch allows the patient to leave the hospital earlier, contributing to important cost-savings. Patients should be treated for 14-21 days in the absence of major complications.

## 8.    CATHETER-RELATED UTI

Most indwelling catheters are colonized with bacteria within 2 weeks. Bacteriuria is therefore not an indicator for catheter related infection. Favorable factors include prolonged duration of catheterization, female gender, elderly patients, and renal insufficiency. Attempts to prevent colonization with daily disinfection of the meatus, disinfectant of the drainage bag, irrigation of the bladder with antibiotics or disinfectants or use of silver-coated catheters have not proven effective. More useful is to consider the indication of the catheter, to limit the duration of catheterization, to observe strict aseptic insertion, to use a closed antireflux drainage system and to maintain a urine volume of > 1.5 liters/day[14]. Suprapubic catheters are less prone to colonization, probably because the fixation to the skin is easier and more efficient. It has the advantage that if colonization occurs it is mainly with coagulase negative staphylococci and not with enterobacteriaceae. Also, the patient is still able to urinate normally, which is important for the reeducation after removal of the catheter.

The diagnosis of catheter related UTI is based on clinical signs such as turbid urine, abnormal odor, pain, secretions along the external part of the catheter and or the meatus and low urine production. General signs are atypical, mainly in elderly patients, and include one or several symptoms such as mental confusion, anorexia, depression, increased tendency to fall, nausea, vomiting and any manifestation from no fever to sepsis syndrome. Treatment should be iv or po according the severity and should be of short duration: 5-7 days are sufficient and should not be prolonged because of the risk that bacteria develop resistance mechanisms. Initial treatment should start with a broad spectrum betalactam, eventually combined with aminoglycosides. Urine cultures are mandatory and treatment should be adapted as early as possible to the organism identified and to susceptibility results[15]. The indwelling catheter should be changed after the first 24 hours of therapy.

## 9.     ASYMPTOMATIC BACTERIURIA

Asymptomatic bacteriuria usually does not need any treatment and therefore should not be looked for. Bacteriuria varies according age and gender. In females it is observed in schoolgirls (1-2%), sexually active women (2-4%), women >60y (6-8%), women > 80y (20%), in old institutionalized patients (30-50%). In men asymptomatic bacteriuria is observed in childhood to middle age (<1%), men 60-65y (1-3%), men >80y (>10%), elderly institutionalized (20-40%). Asymptomatic bacteriuria should not be treated with antibiotics for several reasons: antibiotic treatment has only a transient effect, favors development of resistance and has not shown a beneficial effect on morbidity and mortality[16]. Exception to this rule is the asymptomatic bacteriuria in pregnancy which favors acute pyelonephritis, and small for date neonates. Pregnant women should be monthly controlled with urine cultures and treated with antibiotics, in general betalactam, if necessary. Regular urine surveillance cultures are performed in renal transplant patients, in immunocompromised patients and in the presence of lithiasis and difficult to control diabetes mellitus.

## 10.    CONCLUSIONS

UTI remain among the most frequent infections in community and in hospitals. The treatment depends on age, sex, likely site of infection, predisposing factors, recurrence and pregnancy. Nitrite and leucocyte esterase tests are sufficient for the diagnosis and a 3 day treatment of uncomplicated UTI. Urine cultures are necessary for the correct management of complicated UTI which need a 10-14 days course of antibiotics. In this case an initial iv treatment can be switched to peroral treatment as soon as the patient is stable. Catheter-related infections are treated only if symptomatic and for a short period of time to avoid the development of resistance.

## REFERENCES

1. Patton, J.P., Nah, D.B., and Abrutyn, E.,1991, Urinary tract infection : economic considerations. *Med. Clin. North Am.* **75:** 495-513.
2. Harding, G.K.M., and Ronald, A.R., 1994, The management of urinary infections: what have we learned in the past decade ? *Int J Antimicrob Agent*, **4:** 83-88.
3. Kunin C.M., 1997, Detection, prevention and management of urinary tract infections. 5$^{th}$ ed. Baltimore : Williams and Wilkins, pp. 28-164.
4. Norby, S.R., 1990, Short term treatment of uncomplicated lower UTI in women. *Rev. Infect. Dis.* **12:** 458-467.
5. Hooton, T.M., and Stamm, W.E., 1997, Diagnosis and treatment of uncomplicated urinary tract infection. *Infect. Dis. Clin. North. Am.* **11:** 551-581.
6. Baerheim, A., Digranes, A., and Hunskaar, S., 1990, Evaluation of urine sampling technique :  bacterial contamination of samples from women students. *Br. J. Gen. Pract.* **42:** 241-343.
7. Stapleton, A., and Stamm,W.E., 1997, Prevention of urinary tract infection. *Infect. Dis. Clin. North. Am.* **11:** 719-733.
8. Engel, D., and Schaeffer, A.J., 1998, Evaluation of and antimicrobial therapy for recurrent urinary tract infections in women. *Urol. Clin. North. Am.* **25:** 685-701.
9. Brumfitt, W., and Hamilton-Miller, J.M.T., 1990, Prophylactic antibiotics for recurrent urinary tract infections. *J. Antimicrob. Chemother.* **25:** 505-512.
10. Gupta K., Scholes, and D. Stamm, W.E., 1999, Increasing prevalence of antimicrobial resistance among uropathogens causing acute uncomplicated cystitis in women. *JAMA* **281:** 736-738.
11. Raz, R., and  Stamm, W.E., 1993, A controlled trial of intravaginal estriol in postmenopausal women with recurrent urinary tract infections. *N. Engl. J Med.* **329:**

753-566.

12. Richard, G.A., Kjlimberg, I.N., Fowler, C.L., Callery-D'Amico, S., and Klim, S.S., 1998, Levofloxacin versus ciprofloxacin versus lomefloxacin in acute pyelonephritis. *Urology,* **52:** 51-55.

13. Stamm, W.E., Hooton, T.M., 1993, Management of urinary tract infections in adults *N. Engl. J. Med.* **329:** 1328-1334.

14. Saint, S., and Lipsky, B.A., 1999, Preventing catheter-related bacteriuria, should we, can we, how ? *Arch. Intern. Med.* **159:** 800-808.

15. Warren, J.W., 1997, Catheter-associated urinary tract infections *Infect. Dis. Clin. North Am.* **11:** 609-622.

16. Baldassarre, J.S., and Kaye, D., 1991, Special problems of urinary tract infection in the elderly *Med. Clin. North Am.* **75:** 375-390.

# THE ROLE OF ANAEROBIC BACTERIA IN PROSTATITIS

[1]Elisabeth Nagy, [1]Ildikó Szöke, [2]László Török and [2]László Pajor
[1]*Department of Clinical Microbiology:* [2]*Department of Urology, Albert Szent-Györgyi Medical University, Szeged, Hungary*

## 1.    INTRODUCTION

Prostatitis is an enigmatic condition which affects up to 50% of men at some point according to different estimations. Unlike benign prostatic hyperplasia (BHP) and prostate cancer, which are diseases of older men, prostatitis affects men of all ages. Although prostatitis has been reffered to as the third most important disease of the prostate gland[1], data from the National Center of Health Statistics showed that there were actually more physician visits for prostatitis than for BPH or prostate cancer in the USA in 1985[2]. Certainly, for many patients, chronic prostatitis is the most important disease of the prostate gland.  A recent study[3], utilizing data from the National Ambulatory Medical Care Surveys between 1990-1994 revealed that there were almost 2 million US physician visits annually with prostatitis listed as a diagnosis, only 4% of which were listed as acute prostatitis, suggesting that chronic prostatitis is indeed common.

The US National Institute of Health have recently committed themselves to the development and validation of a new classification system which has become the reference standard for research studies on these diseases and disorders[4]. The category I, the **acute bacterial prostatitis**, means the acute infection of the prostate gland with positive culture results mostly with common uropathogens. The category II, the **chronic bacterial prostatitis** is a recurrent infection of the prostate with the same aerobic pathogens. The

*Genes and Proteins Underlying Microbial Urinary Tract Virulence*
Edited by L. Emődy *et al.*, Kluwer Academic/Plenum Publishers, 2000

289

category III, the **chronic abacterial prostatitis/chronic pelvic pain syndrome** with no demonstrable infection was split in two subcategories. IIIA is **the inflammatory chronic pelvic pain syndrome**, where white cells are present in the semen, in the expressed prostatic secretions or post-prostatic massage urine. IIIB is the **non-inflammatory chronic pelvic pain syndrome**, where no white cells can be detected in the different materials. The category IV is the **asymptomatic inflammatory prostatitis**. In this case no subjective symptoms are present, but the inflammation can be detected either by prostate biopsy or by the presence of white cells in expressed prostatic secretion or semen during evaluation for other disorders like infertility.

To assess prostatitis patients, a widely accepted classification system can be used on the basis of the standardized sequential bacteriological localization technique introduced by Meares and Stamey in 1968[5], including analysis of expressed prostatic secretions (EPS) for presence of increased numbers of leukocytes[6].

Between 5% and 10% of patients with chronic bacterial prostatitis are infected by *E. coli*. Other *Enterobacteriaceae*, such as *Proteus mirabilis* and various *Klebsiella* and *Pseudomonas* spp., may also be implicated. More than one species can often be demonstrated simultaneously in the prostatic secretion. The etiologic role of Gram-positive cocci in acute or chronic bacterial prostatitis is unclear[7]. Non-bacterial prostatitis is also very common, however it is difficult to know whether the condition is caused by organisms such as *Chlamydia*, which are hard to isolate, or by unknown organisms, or whether the symptoms are simply a result of commensal organisms colonizing damaged tissue. In both acute and chronic cases, often no definite infecting organism can be identified. Patients have symptoms and signs of prostatitis, but the causative organism cannot be conclusively demonstrated. Anatomical changes may also contribute to the chronicity of prostatitis; once the normal architecture of the prostate is altered by cystic changes or stone formation, it becomes difficult to eliminate microorganisms[8]. Stones or cysts may become coated by a bacterial biofilm, and this may explain the relapse after an apparently adequate course of antibiotic treatment. There is evidence that the bacteria in a biofilm may survive concentrations of antibacterial agents which would be bactericidal in the absence of the biofilm[9, 10].

The role of anaerobic bacteria in chronic bacterial prostatitis has not been investigated widely especially in those cases, which do not respond empiric antibiotic therapy and are culture negative after using conventional methods. To elucidate the role of anaerobic bacteria as causative organisms in chronic bacterial prostatitis, we have investigated their incidence in the prostatic fluid obtained after prostatic massage of chronic prostatitis patients where infecting organisms could previously not be identified. The urethral samples and seminal fluid of urethritis patients and of healthy men were also investigated.

## 2.    MATERIALS AND METHODS

### 2.1    Clinical Methods

109 male patients (age 25-56 years), with clinical symptoms of chronic prostatitis but *resistant* to empirical quinolon therapy, were involved in this study. In each of the 109 patients, physical examination demonstrated typical symptoms of prostatitis: perianal discomfort, an aching sensation on the inner aspects of the thighs, suprapubic or deep perineal discomfort, and characteristical changes by rectal examination. They were asked to assess their symptoms as mild, moderate or severe to be able to asses differences in the symptomes after therapy. A similar assessment was made after treatment. Increased numbers of leukocytes ( $\geq 10$ per high power field) were found in the EPS after prostatic massage in 89 of the cases. The methods applied to establish the clinical diagnosis of chronic prostatitis included ultrasonographic examinations. These transabdominal, scrotal and transrectal prostate ultrasonographic examinations were carried out with Acuson 128 and Hitachi EUB-450 equipment. The ultrasonographic examinations revealed that 98 of the 109 chronic prostatitis patients exhibited signs of prostatovesiculitis. All patients had previously undergone several routine bacteriological investigations, involving quantitative aerobic cultures of specimens from the urethra, the bladder and of the EPS by the method of Meares and Stamey[5], without positive culture result. Patients sufferenig of chronic prostatitis and having positive culture results for the common aerobic uropathogens were excluded from this study.

### 2.2    Microbiological Methods

During this study, after an antibiotic-free period of at least 2 weeks, urethral sample and prostatic fluid was collected with swabs after prostatic massage and immediately placed in an anaerobic transport medium (Stuart medium). A direct smear of the EPS was also examined after Gram staining and leukocytes were counted per high-power field (5 high-power field/sample). The prostatic fluid was defined as purulent if an average of >10 white blood cells were seen per high-power field at a magnification of x400. They were cultured on Columbia agar (Pasteur Sanofi) supplemented with 5% cow blood for 48 hours at 37 °C in 5% $CO_2$ for aerobic and facultative anaerobic bacteria, and on Columbia agar supplemented with 5% cow blood, 100 µg/ml vitamin $K_1$ and 300 µg/ml cysteine for 6 days at 37 °C in an anaerobic chamber (Sheldon, USA). For the detection of *Gardnerella vaginalis,* the same agar supplemented with 5% human blood was used and incubated anaerobically. The presence of *Chlamydia trachomatis, Mycoplasma/Ureaplasma, Trichomonas vaginalis* and *Candida* species was also recorded.   As controls, the urethral sample of 30 male patients with clinical symptoms of urethritis and the seminal fluid of 30 healthy subjects were cultured in a similar way. The isolated aerobic and anaerobic bacteria were identified by conventional methods[11,12].


## 3.        RESULTS

Of the 109 patients investigated, in the samples of 48 patients, only anaerobic bacteria were found in $>10^6$ CFU/ml, while in 8 patients 1 aerobic and 3 or more anaerobic bacteria could be cultured (Table 1). *Mycoplasma hominis, Ureaplasma urealyticum* were isolated from 8 and 5 samples, respectively, while *Chlamydia trachomatis* was detected in the samples of 2 patients. The specimens of 33 patients were negative for all pathogens (Table 1). Of these 33 patients 10 were also negative ultrasonographically and < 10 leukocytes were seen per high-power field. The distribution of aerobic and anaerobic bacteria isolated from the EPS of the patients yielding positive culture results is to be seen in Table 2. Gram-positive aerobic bacteria (*S. epidermidis, Streptococcus α-haemolyticus* and *Corynebacterium* spp.) were isolated in low numbers ($<10^4$ CFU/ml) from 7 patients and *Citrobacter freundii* and *Providencia stuartii* from 1 and 2 patients, respectively. The most frequently isolated anaerobic Gram-positive bacteria were *Peptostreptococcus* spp. and *Propionibacterium* spp., and the most frequent Gram-negative bacteria were *Bacteroides ureolyticus, Bacteroides spp, Prevotella* spp. and *Porphyromonas* spp. Altogether 299 anaerobic bacteria were isolated from  71 patients alone or together with other pathogens, which means an average of  4.2 anaerobic bacteria/positive patient; in contrast, 11 aerobic bacteria were isolated from 8 patients, an average of 1.4 aerobic bacteria/positive in this group of patients  (Table 3.). All patients who gave positive EPS culture results for anaerobic bacteria or for mixed aerobic/anaerobic bacteria underwent 3 to 6 weeks of antibiotic therapy against the anaerobic bacteria found in the specimens. Amoxicillin/clavulanic acid was applied in a dose of 3x375 mg/day or clindamycin in a dose of 3x150 mg/day. During the treatment the patients were followed up, they were seen again in 3 weeks and 6 weeks. After the completion of therapy, ultrasonographic examinations and culture procedures after prostatic massage were repeated.  The cultures were then negative for anaerobic bacteria or only Gram-positive anaerobic species of normal moucosal flora (*Peptostreptococcus* spp. and *Propionibacterium* spp.) were growing in low number ($<10^2$ CFU/ml). Out of the 56 patients where anaerobes dominated the flora of the EPS, after finishing therapy in parallel with the negative culture results a decrease (10 patients) or total elimination (46 patients) of the symptoms was detected, but in some cases the transrectal ultrasonographic examination revealed residual abnormalities in the prostatic glands for weeks after the treatment.  Those patients who had positive cultures for *Mycoplasma hominis, Ureaplasma urealyticum* or *Chlamydia trachomatis*  received  specific therapy against these pathogens.

The 33 patients who were negative for all pathogens examined were treated according the treatment protocol of prostatodynia.

*Table 1.* Culture results on EPS of 109 chronic prostatitis patients

| Culture results | No. of patients |
|---|---|
| Only aerobic bacteria | 0 |
| Only anaerobic bacteria | 48 |
| Aerobic and anaerobic bacteria | 8 |
| *Mycoplasma hominis* | 8* |
| *Ureaplasma ureolyticum* | 5* |
| *Chlamydia trachomatis* | 2* |
| *Candida* spp. | 5 |
| Negative | 26 |

* isolated in the presence of anaerobic bacteria

*Table 2.* Distribution of aerobic and anaerobic species isolated from EPS of chronic prostatitis patients

| Species | No. of isolates |
|---|---|
| Gram-positive aerobes | |
| *Staphylococcus epidermidis* | 2 |
| *Streptococcus α-haemolyticus* | 3 |
| *Corynebacterium* spp. | 2 |
| *Enterococcus faecalis* | 1 |
| | |
| Gram-negative aerobes | |
| *Citrobacter freundii* | 1 |
| *Providencia* spp | 2 |
| | |
| Total aerobes | 11 |
| | |
| Gram-positive anaerobes | |
| *Peptostreptococcus* spp. | 51 |
| *Propionibacterium* spp. | 31 |
| *Bifidobacterium* spp. | 11 |
| *Eubacterium* spp. | 9 |
| *Actinomyces* spp. | 8 |
| *Clostridium* spp | 5 |
| | |
| Gram-negative anaerobes | |
| *Bacteroides ureolyticus* | 28 |
| *Prevotella* spp. | 36 |
| *Porphyromonas* spp. | 35 |
| *Veillonella* spp. | 23 |
| *Bacteroides* spp. | 32 |
| *Fusobacterium* spp. | 28 |
| *Tissierella* spp. | 1 |
| *Mobiluncus* spp. | 1 |
| | |
| Total anaerobes | 299 |

*Table 3.* Average number of bacteria/positive patient

| No.of patients /positive patient | Positive for | | Average no. of bacteria | |
|---|---|---|---|---|
| | aerobic bacteria | anaerobic bacteria | aerobic | anaerobic |
| Chronic prostatitis (50) | 8 | 48 | 1.4 | 4.2 |
| Urethritis (30) | 25 | 9 | 1.2 | 2.2 |
| Healthy donors (30) | 3 | 0 | 1.0 | 0 |

*Table 4.* Culture results on urethral discharges from 30 urethritis patients and the seminal fluid from 30 healthy donors

| Culture results | No. of Urethritis patients | No. of healthy donors |
|---|---|---|
| Only aerobic bacteria | 18 | 3 |
| Only anaerobic bacteria | 2 | 0 |
| Aerobic and anaerobic bacteria | 7 | 0 |
| *Mycoplasma hominis* | 0 | 0 |
| *Ureaplasma ureolyticum* | 3 | 0 |
| *Chlamydia trachomatis* | 3 | 0 |
| *Candida* spp. | 0 | 0 |
| Negative | 1 | 24 |

As concerns the two control groups, the urethral sample of 30 men with typical symptoms of urethritis were cultured similarly. 25 of these patients were infected by aerobic bacteria, either alone (18 cases) or together anaerobes (7 cases). Only 2 patients displayed anaerobic bacteria alone. Three patients exhibited *U. urealyticum,* and 3 *Chlamydia trachomatis* (Table 4). The distribution of the aerobic and anaerobic isolates obtained from the urethritis patients is shown in Table 5. Typical aerobic uropathogens could be isolated from 10 patients. Peptostreptococci were the most frequently isolated anaerobic bacteria. Thirty aerobic bacteria were isolated from 25 patients (1.2 bacteria/positive patient), and 20 anaerobic bacteria from 9 patients (2.2 bacteria/positive patient) (Table 3).

The aerobic and anaerobic culture results on the seminal fluid of healthy donors revealed no anaerobic bacteria, and aerobic bacteria were present in only few cases, with a low CFU/ml ($<10^2$) (Table 3 and 4).

*Table 5.* Distribution of species isolated from urethral discharge of 30 urethritis patients

| Species | No. of isolates |
|---|---|
| Gram-positive aerobes | |
| *Streptococcus α-haemolyticus* | 5 |
| *Streptococcus agalactiae* | 2 |
| *Enterococcus faecalis* | 7 |
| *Staphylococcus* spp. | 2 |
| *Corynebacterium* spp. | 1 |
| | |
| Gram-negative aerobes | |
| *Esherichia coli* | 7 |
| *Klebsiella* spp. | 2 |
| *Enterobacter* spp. | 1 |
| *Proteus* spp. | 1 |
| *Haemophylus influenzae* | 1 |
| | |
| Fungi | |
| *Candida glabrata* | 1 |
| | |
| Total aerobes | 30 |
| | |
| Gram-positive anaerobes | |
| *Peptostreptococcus* spp | 8 |
| *Propionibacterium* spp. | 3 |
| *Eubacterium* spp | 2 |
| *Bifidobacterium* spp. | 2 |
| | |
| Gram-negative anaerobes | |
| *Prevotella* spp. | 1 |
| *Porphyromonas* spp. | 1 |
| *Veillonella* spp. | 3 |
| | |
| Total anaerobes | 20 |
| | |
| Others | |
| *Chlamydia trachomatis* | 3 |
| *Ureaplasma urealyticum* | 3 |

# 4. DISCUSSION

Prostatitis is a difficult and puzzling syndrome, which rarely affects younger male adults, but is relatively frequent among men aged 30 years or more [13, 14]. It is recognized that there are several distinct forms of the syndrome and successful treatment depends on a specific diagnostic procedure. Chronic bacterial prostatitis requires special bacteriological investigation by the Stamey test and microscopic evaluation of the presence of leukocytes in the specimen[6]. It is well documented that streptococci and usual urinary pathogens such as *E. coli* and other members of the *Enterobacteriaceae* may be responsible for the chronic infection. However, in some cases, where ultrasonographic investigation of the prostate and the presence of leukocytes in the urine sample or in the EPS after prostatic massage suggest prolonged bacterial infection, the customary routine culture techniques may not reveal the pathogens. In some prostatitis cases, considered to be non-bacterial because of the negative culture results, it is difficult to know whether only improper laboratory methods are responsible for the diagnostic failures. In the present study, a careful culture technique was used to isolate aerobic, facultative anaerobic and strict anaerobic bacteria from the EPS of 109 patients with prolonged symptoms of chronic prostatitis, despite empiric quinolone therapy. The primary plates for anaerobic bacteria were incubated for a longer period (6 days) than usually applied in the routine procedures. From 71 patients, an average of 4.2 anaerobic bacteria were isolated. In 8 patients, the mixed anaerobic bacteria were accompanied by few aerobic species. The low numbers of *S. epidermidis*, *S. α-haemolyticus* and *Corynebacterium* spp., but not *C. freundii* and *P. stuartii* can be considered contaminants derived from the skin flora in these cases. The lowest number of different anaerobic species was 3, whereas 35 patients had ≥5 different anaerobic species in their EPS after prostatic massage. All patients who exhibited mixed anaerobic bacteria in their EPS had previously undergone several routine culture tests using the Stamey criteria, without any positive culture results because in most laboratories anaerobic culture methods are not routinly used for these patients.

The role of anaerobic bacteria in chronic prostatitis has not yet been studied in detail. Only a few reports have been published on attempts to isolate anaerobic bacteria from the prostatic fluid of patients with chronic bacterial or non-bacterial prostatitis [15, 16].

The normal flora of the male urethra and prostatic fluid of 46 healthy subjects was evaluated by Ambrose et al.[17]. No anaerobes were recovered from the urethra and only 2 *Bacteroides* spp. were found in the prostatic fluid. On the other hand, Finegold et al.[18] studied "urethral" urine (the first 10 to 20 ml of voided urine) in 17 subjects, and recovered anaerobes (together with aerobes) from 8 of these specimens. The colony counts of anaerobes were ≤$10^4$/ml. The organisms recovered included anaerobic Gram-positive cocci and bacilli, as well as *Bacteroides* spp. In our study, only 9 of 30 urethritis patients displayed anaerobic bacteria in the urethral sample (mostly *Peptostreptococci*, *Propionibacterium* and Gram-positive non-spore-forming bacilli). The average number of anaerobic species/positive patient was 2.2. Anaerobic bacteria were not isolated from the seminal fluid of 30 healthy donors.

Treatment of chronic prostatitis patients with positive culture results for anaerobes was carried out for 3 to 6 weeks with amoxicillin/clavulanic acid or clindamycin. This decreased or totally eliminated the complaints of the patients and the typical clinical symptoms of prostatitis, and the post-treatment cultures of the EPS obtained after prostatic massage were negative for anaerobes or only Gram-positive anaerobic bacteria such as peptostreptococci or *Propionibacteria* were grown in low number.

In general, for chronic bacterial prostatitis patients a prolonged course of treatment, an increased dose of antibiotic, or both is suggested [7, 15]. The most widely-used antibiotics are the fluoroquinolones because of their broad spectrum of action against Gram-positive and Gram-negative aerobic bacteria and their good penetration into the prostatic tissues [9, 19, 20]. In our cases amoxicillin/clavulanic acid or clindamycin was used for the prolonged treatment because of their good activity against anaerobic bacteria and their good penetration into the inflamed prostatic tissue[20].

In this study, *B. ureolyticus* was isolated from mixed cultures, of more than 39% of the positive patients (28 of 71 patients) with chronic prostatitis. *B. ureolyticus* is considered to be part of the normal flora in both the male and female genital tract, but it has also been isolated from mixed cultures of infections of virtually every organ system in men [22]. It has previously been found to be associated with male non-gonococcal urethritis, where it was suggested that this organism may have a pathogenic role [23, 24]. Eley et al.[25] studied the pathogenicity of *B. ureolyticus* in animals and established that a pure culture of *B. ureolyticus* is capable of producing infection when it is injected subcutaneously in mice. The frequent isolation of *B. ureolyticus* together with other Gram-positive and Gram-negative anaerobes from mixed cultures among our patients indicated its possible pathogenic role in chronic bacterial prostatitis.

Our results suggests that anaerobic bacteria may be etiological agents in some cases of therapy-resistant, chronic bacterial prostatitis, and anaerobic culture methods involving prolonged incubation may be required for the laboratory diagnosis of chronic prostatitis.

## ACKNOWLEDGEMENTS

This study was partly supported by the National Research Grant OTKA T 016222.

## REFERENCES

1. Roberts, R.O., Lieber, M.M., Bostwick, D.G.and Jacobsen, S.J., 1997, A review of clinical and pathological prostatitis syndromes. *Urology* **49:** 809-821
2. National Kidney and Urological Advisory Board. Long-Range Plan Window on the 21st Century. Bethesda: United States Department of Health and Human Services, 1990, (NIH Publication No.90-583), p 20.

3. McNaughton Collins, M., and Barry, M.J., 1998, Epidemiology of chronic prostatitis. *Current Opinion in Urology* **8**: 33-37.

4. Nickel, J.C. 1998, Prostatitis: considerations for the next millenium. *Current Opinion in Urology* **8**: 31-32.

5. Meares, E. M. Jr., and Stamey, T. A, 1968, Bacteriologic localization patterns in bacterial prostatitis and urethritis. *Investigative Urology* **5**: 492- 518.

6. Drach, G.W., Meares, E. M. Jr., Fair, W.R., and Stamey, T. A., 1978, Classification of benigndisease associated with prostatic pain: prostatitis or prostatodynia ? *Journal of Urology* **120**: 266.

7. Aagard, J., and Madsen, P.O., 1992, Diagnostic and therapeutic problems in prostatitis. Therapeutic position of ofloxacin. *Drugs-Aging.* **2**: 196-207.

8. De la Rosette, J.J.M.C.H., Karthaus, H.F.M., and Debruyne, F.M.J., 1992, Ultrasonographicfindings in patients with bacterial prostatitis. *Urologia Internationalis.* **48**: 323-326.

9. Nickel, J.C., 1991, New concepts in the pathogenesis and treatment of prostatitis. *Current Opinion in Urology* **2**: 37-43.

10. Anwar, H., Strap, J.L., and Costerton, J.W., 1992, Establishment of ageing biofilms: possiblemechanism of bacterial resistance to antimicrobial therapy. *Antimicrobial Agents and Chemotherapy* **36**: 1347-1351.

11. Summanen, P., Baron, E. J., Citron, D.M., Strong, C., Wexler, H. M., Finegold, S. M., 1993, *Wadsworth Anaerobic Bacteriology Manual*, 4th ed. Star Publishing Company, Belmont, California.

12. Murray, P.R., 1995, *Manual of Clinical Microbiology*, 6th ed. ASM, Wasington.

13. Weidner, W., 1984, Prostatitis diagnosis. Studies on objectivation and differential diagnosis of various forms of prostatitis. *Fortschritte der Medizin*, **102**: 1113-1116.

14. De la Rosette, J.J.M.C.H, Hubregtse, M.R., Meulemann, E.J.H., Stolk-Engelaar, M.V.M., and Debruyne F.M.J., 1993, Diagnosis and treatment of 409 patients with prostatitis syndromes. *Urology* **41**: 301-307.

15. Leigh, D.A., 1993, Prostatitis - an increasing clinical problem for diagnosis and management. *The Journal of Antimicrobial Chemotherapy* **32**: Suppl. A, 1-9.

16. Mardh, P-A., and Colleen, S., 1975, Search for urogenital tract infections in patients with symptoms of prostatitis: Studies on aerobic and strictly anaerobic bacteria, mycoplasmas, fungi, trichomonad and viruses. *Scandinavian Journal of Urology and Nephrology* **9**: 8-12.

17. Ambrose, S.S., Taylor, W.W., and Josefiak, E.J., 1961, Flora of the male lower genitourinarytract. *Journal of Urology* **85**: 365-.369.

18. Finegold, S.M., Miller, S.G., Merril, S.L, and Posnick, D.J., 1965, Significance of anaerobicand capnophilic bacteria isolated from the urinary tract. In: *Progress in pyelonephritis.* (E.H. Kass and E.H. Davis, eds.,) Philadelphia, Pennsylvania pp. 159178.

19. Naber, K.G., Kinzig, M., Sorgel, F., Weigel, D., 1993, Penetration of ofloxacin into prostatic fluid, ejaculate and seminal fluid . *Infection* **21**: 98-100.

20. Nielsen, O.S. Frimodt-Moeller, N., Maigaard, S., Hoyme, U., Baumueller, A., and Madsen, P.O., 1980, Penicillanic acid derivates in the canine prostate. *Prostate* **1**: 79-85.

21. Dalhoff, A., and Weidner, W., 1984, Diffusion of ciprofloxacin into prostatic fluid. *European Journal Clinical Microbiology* **3**: 360-362.

22. Duerden, B.I., Benne, K.W.,and Faulkner, J., 1982, Isolation of *B. ureolyticus* from clinical infections. *Journal of Clinical Pathology* **35**: 309-312.

23. Hawkins, D.A., Fountaine, E.A.R., Thomas, B.J., Boustouller, Y.K., and Taylor-Robinson, D., 1988, The enigma of non-gonococcal urethritis: role of *B. ureolyticus.* *Genitourinary Medicine* **64**: 10-13.

24. Balmelli T., Stamm J., Dolina-Giudici M., Peduzzi, M., Piffaretti-Yanez A., and Balerna, M., 1994, *Bacteroides ureolyticus* in men consulting for infertility. *Andrologia* **26:** 35-38.

25. Eley, A., Start, R.D., and Potter, C.W., 1995, Animal model of pathogenicity for *Bacteroides urealyticus*. In: *Medical and Dental Aspects of Anaerobes* (B.I. Duerden, W.G. Wade, J.S.Brazier, A. Eley, B, Wren and M.J. Hudson, eds.), Science Reviews, Northwood, UK, pp. 325-328.

# URINARY TRACT INFECTION IN DOGS
*Analysis of 419 urocultures carried out in Portugal*

[1]Constança P. Féria, [1]José D. Correia, [2]Jorge Machado, [3]Rui Vidal, and [1]José Gonçalves

[1]CIISA, Faculdade de Medicina Veterinária, Universidade Técnica de Lisboa, Portugal;[2]Centro de Bacteriologia, Instituto Nacional de Saúde, Portugal; [3]Faculdade de Farmácia de Lisboa, Portugal

## 1. INTRODUCTION

Bacterial infections of the urinary system are among the most frequent infections in small animal practice. During their lifetime 14% of dogs may experience urinary tract infection[1]. Gram negative fecal flora constitutes the majority of uropathogenic strains isolated. However isolation frequencies differ between studies being 36 to 59 % for *Escherichia coli*, 9 to 32% for *Proteus mirabilis*, 5 to 8% for *Klebsiella pneumoniae*, 0 to 5% for *Pseudomonas spp*, 9 to 22% for *Streptococcus spp* and 11 to 19% for *Staphylococcus spp* [2,3,4,5,6].

Microbiological analysis of urine allows the detection of significant bacteriuria and sensitivity testing of isolated uropathogens, and hence provides a definitive diagnosis and a rational therapeutical approach.

This is the first antimicrobial sensitivity study performed with pathogenic bacteria isolated from dogs with urinary infection that we are aware of, in Portugal.

## 2. SIGNIFICANT BACTERIURIA

Four hundred and nineteen urocultures were performed at request due to clinical suspicion. Urine specimens were collected via cystocentesis,

*Genes and Proteins Underlying Microbial Urinary Tract Virulence*
Edited by L. Emödy *et al.*, Kluwer Academic/Plenum Publishers, 2000

301

catheterization or voided midstream catch. Significant bacteriuria criteria used in this study were as follows: for cystocentesis samples- $>10^2$ UFC/ml; for catheter samples- $>10^3$ or $10^4$ UFC/ml; for midstream urine- $>10^5$ UFC/ml. The presence of leucocyturia was a valuable parameter taken into consideration in the above criteria.

Significant bacteriuria was found in 165 specimens (39%), from 81 males and 70 females, 14 unknown, of all ages (18 less than a 1 year old, 62 between 1 and 7 years old, 51 more than 7 years old and 34 unknown age).

## 3.        UROPATHOGENIC BACTERIA

Uropathogenic bacteria isolated were identified to genera or species level, the majority being Gram negative rods (76,4%). Frequencies are as follows: *Proteus mirabilis* (35,2%), *Escherichia coli* (32,7%), *Staphylococcus spp* (16,4%), *Streptococcus spp* (7,3%), *Pseudomonas spp* (1,8%) and other enterobacteriaceae (6,6%).

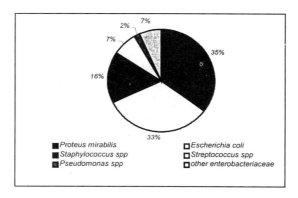

*Figure 1.* Uropathogenic bacteria frequencies isolated from canine urine specimens.

## 4.        ANTIMICROBIAL SENSITIVITY TESTING

Twelve strains (7,3%) were susceptible to all antibiotics tested by the Kirby-Bauer method (ampicillin - amp, amoxicillin/clavulanic acid - amc, cephalothin - Kf, chloramphenicol - C, tetracycline - T, gentamicin - Gm, nalidixic acid - Na, enrofloxacin - Enr, trimethoprim/ sulfamethoxazole - Stx, nitrofurantoin - F) and 92,7% were resistant at least to one compound.

In the *Proteus mirabilis* group all strains were found to be resistant to tetracycline and nitrofurantoin (natural resistance) and thus 18/58 (31,0%)

were wild type phenotypes. Major resistance found in *Proteus mirabilis* was towards chloramphenicol (33,9%), trimethoprim /sulfamethoxazole (29,3%) and ampicillin (28,1%).

In *Escherichia coli*, important resistance was found to ampicillin (47,2%), tetracycline (34,9%), trimethoprim/sulfamethoxazole (28,3%) and nalidixic acid (30,4%).

In *Staphylococcus spp*, resistance was high towards nalidixic acid (71,4%), followed by tetracycline (57,7%) and in *Streptococcus spp* to tetracycline (55,6%).

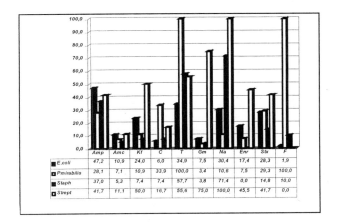

|  | Amp | Amc | Kf | C | T | Gm | Na | Enr | Stx | F |
|---|---|---|---|---|---|---|---|---|---|---|
| E.coli | 47,2 | 10,9 | 24,0 | 6,0 | 34,9 | 7,5 | 30,4 | 17,4 | 28,3 | 1,9 |
| P.mirabilis | 28,1 | 7,1 | 10,9 | 33,9 | 100,0 | 3,4 | 10,6 | 7,5 | 29,3 | 100,0 |
| Staph | 37,0 | 5,3 | 7,4 | 7,4 | 57,7 | 3,8 | 71,4 | 0,0 | 14,8 | 10,0 |
| Strept | 41,7 | 11,1 | 50,0 | 16,7 | 55,6 | 75,0 | 100,0 | 45,5 | 41,7 | 0,0 |

*Figure 2.* Uropathogenic bacteria antimicrobial resistance.

## 5. CONCLUSION

In our study, negative cultures were 60,6%, perhaps because of concurrent antimicrobial therapy or poor clinical evaluation. In this work, *Proteus mirabilis* is the major pathogen, followed by *E. coli*, probably because *Proteus mirabilis* is commonly associated with recurrent urinary tract infections in dogs thus providing easily detectable clinical signs (haematuria).

Susceptibility testing revealed diversity in resistance patterns and phenotypes in the different genera of uropathogens, which corroborates the importance of urine culture and bacterial identification in the diagnosis and treatment of urinary tract infection in dogs.

## ACKNOWLEDGMENTS

This work was financially supported by Centro de Investigação Interdisciplinar em Sanidade Animal (CIISA).

Our special thanks to Lurdes Anciães and Maria Helena Brito for all their dedication and technical assistance.

## REFERENCES

1. Polzin, D.J., 1997, Management of recurrent bacterial urinary tract infections. *Supl. Compend. Contin. Educ. Pract. Vet.* **19:** 47.
2. Ihrke, P.J., Norton, A.L., Ling, G.V., and Stannard, A.A., 1985, Urinary infection associated with long-term corticosteroid administration in dogs with chronic skin diseases. *JAVMA* **186:** 43-46.
3. Finco, D.R., Shotts, E.B., Cromwell, W.A., 1979, Evaluation of methods for localization of urinary tract infection in the female dog. *Am. J. Vet. Res.* **40:** 707-712.
4. Garvey, M.S., and Aucoin, D.P., 1984, Therapeutic strategies involving antimicrobial treament of disseminated bacterial infection in small animals. *JAVMA* **185:** 1185-1189.
5. Ling, G.V., Biberstein, E.L., and Hirsch, D.C., 1979, Bacterial pathogens associated with urinary tract infection. *Vet. Clin. North. Am.*, **9:** 617-630.
6. Rohrich, P.J, Ling, G.V., Ruby, A.L., Jang, S.S., and Johnsson, D.L., 1983, *In vitro* susceptibilities of canine urinary tract bacteria to selected antimicrobial agents. *JAVMA* **183:** 863-867.

# DETECTION OF VIRULENCE FACTORS IN UROPATHOGENIC ESCHERICHIA COLI ISOLATED FROM HUMANS, DOGS AND CATS IN PORTUGAL

[1]Constança P. Féria, [1]José D. Correia, [1]José Gonçalves, [2]Jorge Machado
[1]CIISA, Faculdade de Medicina Veterinária, Universidade Técnica de Lisboa, Portugal; [2]Centro de Bacteriologia, Instituto Nacional de Saúde, Portugal

## 1.    INTRODUCTION

Adhesion and cytotoxicity are important mechanisms in *Escherichia coli* uropathogenicity, both in man and animals. There are few comparative studies regarding urovirulence in human and animal *E. coli* strains[1,2].

In this study 90 human, 35 dog and 5 cat *E. coli* strains were evaluated by a multiplex polymerase chain reaction, for the presence of adhesin-encoding operons (*pap*, *sfa/foc*, *afa*), hemolysin operon (*hly*), cytotoxic necrotizing factor 1 (*cnf 1*) and aerobactin (*aer*) genes.

## 2.    VIRULENCE FACTORS DETECTION

Simultaneous genotypic detection of urovirulence factors allows rapid strain characterization and can also act as an epidemiological marker [3,4]. Futhermore, existence of multiple virulence determinants in a single *E. coli* strain could be revealing of a pathogenicity island and hence reinforce its uropathogenic character [5,6].

*Genes and Proteins Underlying Microbial Urinary Tract Virulence*
Edited by L. Emödy *et al.*, Kluwer Academic/Plenum Publishers, 2000

305

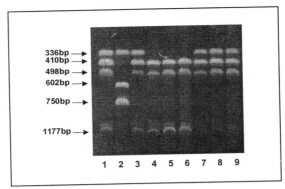

*Figure 1.* Analysis of multiplex PCR products – lane 1, *Escherichia coli* J96 (*pap* 336bp,*sfa* 410bp, *cnf* 498bp, *hly* 1177bp); lane 2, *Escherichia coli* KS52 (*pap* 336bp, *aer* 602bp, *afa* 750bp); lanes 3 to 9, clinical strains.

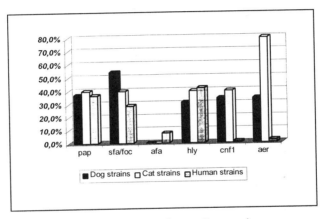

*Figure 2.* Virulence factors frequencies.

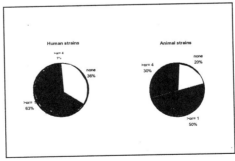

*Figure 3.* Number of virulence determinants *per* strain.

## 3.     VIRULENCE FACTORS FREQUENCIES

In human strains only 58/90 (64,4%) had at least one virulence factor; the frequencies detected were: 33/90 *pap* (36,7%), 26/90 *sfa/foc* (28,9%), 7/90 *afa* (7,8%), 38/90 *hly* (42,2%), 1/90 *cnf1* (1,1%) and 2/90 *aer* (2,2%).

The majority [32/40 (80%)] of animal uropathogenic *E. coli* encoded for one or more factors. Twelve of the fourty studied strains (40%) carried simultaneously 4 virulence determinants. The frequencies detected were for canine strains: 13/35 *pap* (37,1%), 19/35 *sfa/foc* (54,3%), 0 *afa* (0%), 11/35 *hly* (31,4%), 12/35 *cnf1* (34,3%), 12/35 *aer* (34,3%); and for feline strains 2/5 *pap* (40,1%), 2/5 *sfa/foc* (40%), 0 *afa* (0%), 2/5 *hly* (40%), 2/5 *cnf1* (40%), 4/5 *aer* (80%).

Detection of adhesin encoded operons was different between animal and human strains. Adhesin-encoding *afa* operon was not detected in animal strains; *sfa* operon was more frequent than *pap* operon in animals; conversely human strains presented more Pap than Sfa fimbrae.

In what concerns cytotoxins, hemolysin gene detection was important both in animal and human *E.coli,* but *cnf1* and aerobactin genes were detected more frequently in animal strains.

## 4.     CONCLUSION

Genotypic differences regarding virulence factors between human and animal *E.coli* strains were observed in this work. They consisted mainly on the frequencies and type of adhesin encoded operons detected, which may reveal uropathogenic *E.coli* adaptation to different host cell receptors. Low detection of the *cnf1* gene in human hemolytic *E.coli* strains suggests the possibility that, in these strains, other cytotoxins may be involved in the pathogenesis of urinary tract infection.

Simultaneous presence of 4 or more virulence factors was more important in animal (12/40), than in human (1/90) *E.coli* strains. This may be due to the fact that these animal strains caused primary urinary tract infection (11/40). Simultaneous carriage of virulence determinants by these strains may occur in fundamental gene blocks, previously designated as "pathogenicity-associated-islands". This hypothesis is under investigation.

## ACKNOWLEDGMENTS

This study was financially supported by Centro de Investigação Interdisciplinar em Sanidade Animal (CIISA).

# REFERENCES

1. Low, D., Braten, B.A., Ling, G.V., Johnson, D.L., and Ruby, A.L., 1988, Isolation and comparison of *Escherichia coli* strains from canine and human patients with urinary tract infection. *Infect. Immun.*, **56**: 2601-2609.
2. Yuri, K., Nakata, K., Katae, H., Yamamoto, S., and Hasegawa, A., 1998, Distribution of uropathogenic virulence factors among *Escherichia coli* strains isolated from dogs and cats. .J. *Vet. Sci.* **60**: 287-290.
3. Le Bouguenec, C., Archambaud, M., and Labigne, A., 1992, Rapid and specific detection of the pap, afa and sfa adhesin-encoded operons in uropathogenic *Escherichia coli* strains by polymerase chain reaction. *J. Clin.Microbiol.* **30**:1189-1193.
4. Yamamoto, C., Terai, A., Yuri, K., Korazano,, H., Takeda, Y., and Yoshida, O., 1995, Detection of virulence factors in *Escherichia coli* by multiplex polymerase chain reaction. *FEMS Immunol. Med. Microbiol.*, **12**: 85-90.
5. Kao, J.-S., Stucker, D.M., Warren, J.W., and Mobley, H.L.T., 1997, Pathogenicity island sequences of pyelonephritogenic *Escherichia coli* CFT073 are associated with virulent uropathogenic strains. *Infect. Immun.* **65**: 2812-2820.
6. Guyer, D., Kao, J.-S., and Mobley, H.L.T., 1998, Genomic analysis of a pathogenicity island in uropathogenic *Escherichia coli* CFT073: distribution of homologous sequences among isolates from patients with pyelonephritis, cystitis and catheter-associated bacteriuria and from fecal samples. *Infect. Immun.* **66**: 4411-4417.

# ASYMPTOMATIC BACTERIURIA CAN BE CONSIDERED A DIABETIC COMPLICATION IN WOMEN WITH DIABETES MELLITUS

[1]Suzanne E. Geerlings*, [2]Ronald P. Stolk , [3]Marielle J.L. Camps, [4]Paetrick M. Netten, [5]Joost B.L. Hoekstra, [4]Paul K. Bouter, [3]Bert Braveboer, [7]Theo J. Collet, [6]Arjen R. Jansz, and [1]Andy M. Hoepelman

[1]*Dept. Med., Div. Infect Dis. & AIDS*, [2]*Julius Center for Patient Oriented Research, Univ. Hospital Utrecht*, [3]*Dept. Med., Catharinahospital, Eindhoven*, [4]*Dept. Med., Bosch Medicentrum's Hertogenbosch*, [5]*Dept. Med., Diakonessenhuis, Utrecht*, [6]*Lab. Microbiol., St. Josephhospital, Veldhoven*, [7]*Dept. Med, Univ. Hospital Utrecht, The Netherlands*

## 1.     INTRODUCTION

Patients with diabetes mellitus (DM) have an increased risk for infections.[1,2] The urinary tract is the most important site of these infections.[3,4] Many urinary tract infections (UTI) are asymptomatic and it is not known whether symptomatic UTI are preceded by asymptomatic bacteriuria (ASB). In contrast to men, a higher prevalence of ASB has been found in women with DM compared to women without DM.[4,5,6,7] However, others could not confirm this finding.[8,9] Because more complications of UTI are seen in diabetic patients compared to nondiabetic patients[10] and renal involvement, even without the presence of symptoms (subclinical pyelonephritis), is common,[11,12] it is important to investigate the association between ASB and symptomatic UTI in women with DM. Various risk factors for ASB in diabetic women have been suggested.[5,7,13,14,15,16] However, most studies only included a small number of patients from one hospital, often without distinguishing between DM type 1 and 2.

*Genes and Proteins Underlying Microbial Urinary Tract Virulence*
Edited by L. Emődy  *et al.*, Kluwer Academic/Plenum Publishers, 2000

The aim of the present multi-center study was to determine the prevalence of ASB as well as the risk factors for ASB in a large number of women both with type 1 and type 2 diabetes.

## 2.    METHODS

### 2.1    Patients' Enrolment and Evaluation

The patients were recruited in the diabetes outpatient clinics of the University Hospital Utrecht (tertiary care hospital), four non-university hospitals (Diakonessenhuis Utrecht, Bosch Medicentrum 's Hertogenbosch, Catharinahospital Eindhoven) and the offices of seven general practitioners in The Netherlands. Women were included with either DM type 1 or DM type 2, age between 18-75 years. All patients were asked to collect two consecutive midstream urine specimens during a 2-4 month period. Exclusion criteria were: Pregnancy, recent hospitalization or surgery (< 4 months), known urinary tract abnormalities, symptoms of a UTI or the use of antimicrobial drugs in the previous 14 days. Finally 636 women entered the study group. During the first visit of the study all patients were interviewed and the medical history was obtained from the hospital files using a standardized questionnaire, which included: Age, type and duration of DM, medication, secondary complications of the DM (retinopathy, macrovascular diseases, peripheral neuropathy), pregnancies or urinary tract surgery in the previous years, number of urinary tract infections in the last year, recent sexual intercourse (<1 week), contraceptive method, menopausal status and use of (local) estrogens. Blood pressure, weight and height (Body Mass Index, BMI) were recorded. The following laboratory values were obtained: Serum hemoglobin A1c (HbA1c), serum creatinine, blood group, microalbuminuria, glucosuria, leucocyturia and urinary pH. In addition, in 106 patients the bladder residue in ml after micturition was measured by a bladderscan and in 40 patients the Ewing test was performed to assess cardiovascular autonomic neuropathy.

To investigate the prevalence of ASB in nondiabetics, females visiting the eye and trauma outpatient clinic and not having DM, were asked to collect two consecutive midstream urine specimens. Exclusion criteria were the same as for the diabetic females. Hundred fifty-three women were included (mean age 47.8 year, standard deviation 16.4 year).

## 2.2    Urine

One or two midstream urine specimens were collected for evaluation of bacteriuria with an interval of 2-4 months. Urine culture was performed according to the standard procedures. Asymptomatic bacteriuria was defined as the presence of at least $10^5$cfu/ml of one or two microorganisms in a culture of a clean voided midstream urine isolated from an individual without symptoms of a urinary tract infection or fever.[17] Glycosuria, leucocyturia and urinary pH values were determined by a dipslide method (Combur-Test, Boehringer Mannheim, Almere, The Netherlands).

## 2.3    Statistical Analysis

The t-test, Mann Whitney U-test and logistic regression analysis were used. The p-values and odds ratios (OR) of all variables, except the duration of DM, were adjusted for age.

## 3.    RESULTS

## 3.1    Study Population

One non-contaminated midstream urine specimen was collected in 636 women. In 412 of these women a second non-contaminated urine specimen with the same result was collected after 2-4 months. Of the total study group (n=636) (DM type 1 and DM type 2 grouped together) 163 (26%) women had ASB. In the nondiabetic control group (153 patients) 9 patients (6%) had a positive urine culture result. The prevalence of ASB was significantly higher in the diabetic patients than in the control group (*p*<0.001.) Fifty-three women with DM type 1 (whole group: n=258) had ASB (prevalence 21%). One hundred and ten women with DM type 2 (whole group: n=378) had ASB (prevalence 29%).

## 3.2    Risk Factors For Asb

In Table 1, 2 and 3 we show the significant risk factors of the women, who collected at least one noncontaminated urine specimen.

In both DM type 1 and DM type 2 patients the HbA1c level did not influence the risk for ASB. The presence of cardiovascular autonomic dysfunction or a post-voiding bladder residue did not increase the chance of developing ASB.

*Table 1* Risk factors for women with DM type 1 and DM type 2 (grouped together) for having asymptomatic bacteriuria (ASB)

| Risk factors for all women with DM n=636 | ASB- n=473 (74%) | ASB+ n=163 (26%) | OR | p-value |
|---|---|---|---|---|
| Age | 50.3 (15.2) | 56.6 (14.5) | | <0.001 |
| Duration DM (years) | 13.1 (10.9) | 14.9 (11.5) | | 0.07 |
| Retinopathy | 119 (26%) | 57 (36%) | 1.5 | 0.01 |
| Macroalbuminuria (n=428) | 18 (6%) | 18 (16%) | 3.1 | 0.002 |
| BMI | 27.8 (6.1) | 26.8 (4.8) | 0.95 | 0.004 |
| Number of UTI previous year | 83 (18%) | 43 (26%) | 1.9 | 0.01 |
| HbA1c (%) | 8.5 (1.6) | 8.6 (2.1) | | 0.6 |

Number (n) of patients is given when concerning variable is not measured in all patients. Values are given as means (with standard deviations SD) or numbers (with percentages %). All odds ratios (OR) and p-values are adjusted for age.

*Table 2.* Risk factors for women with DM type 1 for having asymptomatic bacteriuria (ASB)

| Risk factors for women with DM type 1 N=258 | ASB- n=205(79%) | ASB+ n=53(21%) | OR | p-value |
|---|---|---|---|---|
| Age | 40.3 (13.5) | 43.1 (13.1) | | 0.2 |
| Duration DM (years) | 17.9 (12.9) | 22.4 (12.1) | | 0.02 |
| Peripheral neuropathy (n=245) | 44 (23%) | 20 (40%) | 2.2 | 0.03 |
| Macroalbuminuria | 8 (5%) | 7 (16%) | 3.6 | 0.02 |
| HbA1c (%) | 8.5 (1.5) | 8.8 (2.9) | | 0.3 |

Legends: see Table 1.

*Table 3.* Risk factors for women with DM type 2 for having asymptomatic bacteriuria (ASB).

| Risk factors for women with DM type 2 N=378 | ASB- n=268 (71%) | ASB+ n=110 (29%) | OR | p-value |
|---|---|---|---|---|
| Age | 58.0 (11.7) | 63.0 (10.0) | | <0.001 |
| Age =45 year | 240 (90%) | 105 (96%) | 2.4 | 0.07 |
| Age =50 year | 212 (79%) | 97 (88%) | 2.0 | 0.04 |
| Duration DM (years) | 9.3 (7.1) | 11.3 (9.1) | | 0.05 |
| Macroalbuminuria (n=231) | 10 (6%) | 11 (15%) | 2.9 | 0.03 |
| BMI | 29.9 (6.2) | 28.3 (4.8) | 0.96 | 0.04 |
| UTI previous year | 48 (18%) | 30 (27%) | 1.9 | 0.02 |
| HbA1c (%) | 8.6 (1.7) | 8.5 (1.6) | | 0.7 |

Legends: see Table 1.

## 4.    CONCLUSION

1. Women with DM have an increased prevalence of ASB compared with women without DM.

2. Risk factors for ASB for all women with DM are: age, duration of DM, retinopathy, macroalbuminuria, a lower BMI and a symptomatic UTI in the previous year.

3. Risk factors for ASB for women with DM type 1 are: duration of DM, peripheral neuropathy and macroalbuminuria.

4. Risk factors for ASB for women with DM type 2 are: age, duration of DM, macroalbuminuria, a lower BMI and a symptomatic UTI in the previous year.

5. Poor regulation of DM or postvoiding bladder residue are no risk factors for ASB in women with DM.

## REFERENCES

1. Pozzilli, P., and Leslie, R.D.G., 1994, Infections and diabetes: Mechanisms and prospects for prevention. *Diabetic Medicine* **11**: 935-941.
2. Carton, J.A., Maradona, J.A., Nuno, F.J., Fernandez-Alvarez, R,, Perez-Gonzalez, F., and Asensi, V., 1992, Diabetes mellitus and bacteraemia: A comparative study between diabetic and non-diabetic patients. *E.J.M.* **1**: 281-287.

3. MacFarlane, I.A., Brown, R.M., Smyth, R.W., Burdon, D.W., and Fitzgerald, M.G., 1986, Bacteraemia in diabetics. *J. Infect.* **12:** 213-219.

4. Wheat, L.J., 1980, Infection and diabetes mellitus. *Diabetes Care* **3:** 187-197.

5. Schmitt, J.K., Fawcett, C.J., and Gullickson, G., 1986, Asymptomatic bacteriuria and hemoglobin A1. *Diabetes Care* **9:** 518-520.

6. Vejlsgaard, R., 1966 Studies on urinary infection in diabetics. I. Bacteriuria in patients with diabetes mellitus and in control subjects. *Acta Med Scand* **179:** 173-182.

7. Osterby Hansen, R., 1964, Bacteriuria in diabetic and non-diabetic out-patients. *Acta Med. Scand.* **176:** 721-730.

8. Brauner, A., Flodin, U., Hylander, B., and Ostenson, C.G., 1993, Bacteriuria, bacterial virulence and host factors in diabetic patients. *Diabet. Med.* **10:** 550-554.

9. Pometta, D., Rees, S.B., Younger, D., and Kass, E.H., 1967, Asymptomatic bacteriuria in diabetes mellitus. *N. Engl. J. Med.* **276:** 1118-1121.

10. Patterson, J.E., and Andriole, V.T., 1997, Bacterial urinary tract infections in diabetes. *Infect. Dis. Clin. North. Am.* **11:** 735-750.

11. Forland, M., and Thomas, V.L., 1985, The treatment of urinary tract infections in women with diabetes mellitus. *Diabetes Care* **8:** 499-506.

12. Forland, M., Thomas, V., and Shelokov, A., 1977, Urinary tract infections in patients with diabetes mellitus. Studies on antibody coating of bacteria. *JAMA* **238:** 1924-1926.

13. Zhanel, G.G., Nicolle, L.E., and Harding, G.K.M., 1995, Manitoba Diabetic Urinary Infection Study Group: Prevalence of asymptomatic bacteriuria and associated host factors in women with diabetes mellitus. *Clin. Infect. Dis.* **21:** 316-322.

14. Perez Luque, E.L., de la Luz Villalpando. M., and Malacara, J.M., 1992, Association of sexual activity and bacteriuria in women with non-insulin-dependent diabetes mellitus. *J. Diabetes Complications* **6:** 254-257.

15. Sawers, J.S., Todd, W.A., Kellett, H.A., Miles, R.S., Allan, P.L., Ewing, D.J., and Clarke, B.F., 1986, Bacteriuria and autonomic nerve function in diabetic women. *Diabetes Care* **9:** 460-464.

16. Vejlsgaard, R., 1966, Studies on urinary infection in diabetics. II Significant bacteriuria in relation to long-term diabetic manifestations. *Acta Med. Scand.* **179:** 183-188.

17. Members of the Medical Research Council Bacteriuria Committee, 1979, Recommended terminology of urinary tract infection. *.Br. Med. J.* **2:** 717-719.

# DETERMINATION OF GENETIC DIVERSITY OF *PROTEUS PENNERI* STRAINS USING REP-PCR

Marcin Kowalczyk and Zygmunt Sidorczyk
*Department of General Microbiology, Institute of Microbiology and Immunology, University of Łódź, Banacha 12/16, 90-237 Łódź, Poland*

## 1.     INTRODUCTION

*Proteus penneri* bacteria, formerly known as "indol negative" *Proteus vulgaris* or "*Proteus vulgaris* biogroup 1"[1] have been isolated from a variety of clinical sources, such as urine, blood, stools, abdominal wounds, burns and bronchial exudates. These bacteria could also play a role in urinary tract infections and primary diseases: *meningitidis, osteomielitis*[2], recently described urosepsis[3] and acute *pyelonephritis*[4]. Natural habitat of *Proteus penneri* rods is unknown and their etiological role in infectious processes has not been fully established so far. Potential virulence factors, like urease, IgA proteases, fimbriae, hemagglutinins and hemolysins of *Proteus penneri* have been described[5,6]. Also the swarming growth phenomenon is the most characteristic feature which distinguishes *Proteus* bacteria from other members of *Enterobacteriaceae* family[5].

The aim of this study was to apply the technique known as rep-PCR to the analysis of *Proteus* genomic DNA in order to differentiate the individual strains within the species *P. penneri* and particularly the various species in the genus *Proteus*. The rep-PCR method uses primers complementary to endogenous repetitive elements of DNA in the PCR of bacterial, genomic DNA. PCR amplification of such genomic DNA leads to products having different molecular masses (bp), presumably reflecting the distance and position of endogenous repeating sequences. This DNA fingerprint appears

*Genes and Proteins Underlying Microbial Urinary Tract Virulence*
Edited by L. Emödy *et al.*, Kluwer Academic/Plenum Publishers, 2000

315

to be strain specific and may be useful in the identification of particular strains[7,8,9].

## 2.    MATERIALS AND METHOD

**Bacterial strains** – all strains were from the collection of our Department.

**DNA preparation** – the extractions of DNA were made according to the instructions of the manufacturer.

**PCR conditions** – BOX A1R primer[9] had the following sequence: 5' – CTACGGCAAGGCGACGCTGACG – 3'. Thermal cycling conditions included: an initial denaturation step at 95°C for 7 min, followed by elongation in 32 cycles at 65°C for 225 sec, then again a denaturation step at 90°C for 30 sec, followed by annealing of primer at 50°C for 60 sec and final extension of DNA at 65°C for 16 min.

**Electrophoresis** - 5µl samples of amplified DNA were run in a 1,2 % agarose gel together with molecular weight markers in TAE buffer.

**Computer analysis** - The approximate length of corresponding DNA fragments and distances between the bands on the gel were calculated using the computer programme *Sigma Gel^{TM} 1995, Gel Analysis Software, Jandel Scientific, USA.*

## 3.    RESULTS AND DISCUSSION

In this work, genetic differentiation of a collection of 68 *Proteus penneri* strains being unique in the world was tested. The following repetitive sequences were used: ERIC 1R/ERIC 2, REP1R-Dt/REP2-Dt, REP2-I/REP1R-I and BOX A1R. On the basis of the tentative experiments (not included in this article), only one primer - **BOX A1R** supplied the most complex fingerprint patterns with the largest number of bands, and therefore this primer was chosen for further analysis of *Proteus penneri* genomic DNA.

In the next step of this work all *Proteus penneri* strains were examined in PCR reaction with earlier selected primer (Fig 1.).

- **Photo 1** shows that DNA of *P. penneri* strains 4-6 and 9-13 are similar to each other while strains 1 and 3 that are different from the others.
- On **photo 2** one can observe many different profiles of DNA in *Proteus penneri* strains but it is also obvious that there are bands being present in all strains.

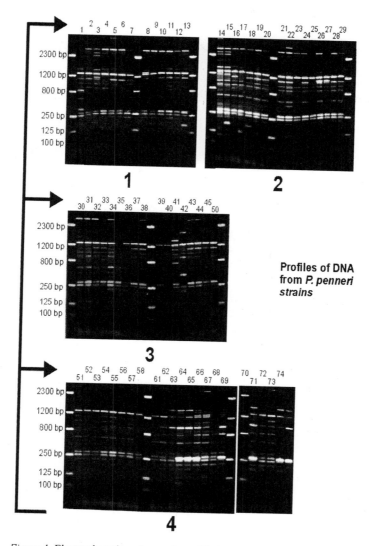

*Figure 1.* Electrophoretic patterns of amplified DNA from *P. penneri* strains.

- **Photo 3** shows some strains with a large number of bands (strains: 30-34, 41 and 42) and four other strains (35, 36, 39 and 40) with a very small number of bands.
- On **photo 4** one can notice several strains presenting with very intensive bands (64-66, 69, 70, 73 and 74) and also strains giving a larger number of bands than others (66, 67 and 72).

At that step of investigations it was obvious, that for the analysis of such a great variation of genetic profiles of *Proteus penneri* strains the use of a computer programme was necessary. Therefore computer analysis of the gel electrophoretic profiles of amplified DNA was performed (Fig 2).

Analysis of the dendrogram has shown that the strains can be divided into two major groups containing six clusters of DNA from *Proteus penneri* strains at the level of similarity between 40-60%. Only 2 pairs of *Proteus penneri* strains: 19 and 20, 39 and 40 showed identical DNA fingerprint pattern.

- **- group I consisted of 18 isolates**
- **- group II included 50 isolates**

## 4.    CONCLUSION

The results of our study have shown that REP-like repetitive DNA elements are present in the genome of *Proteus* strains and the rep-PCR technique is useful for generating DNA fingerprints of *Proteus penneri* strains. Beside evident differences in DNA band patterns of the strains there were bands specific for all of the *Proteus penneri* isolates. Analysis of these results showed a large degree of genetic heterogenity among these bacteria.

Furthermore, a PCR fingerprint technique was used in this study in order to characterise clinical *Proteus penneri* strains and to determine the applicability of this technique for identification and comparison of *Proteus* strains from clinical and other biological materials, for diagnostic and epidemiological purposes.

Additionally, because phenotypic expression of virulence determinants of bacterial strains may be affected by storage and culture conditions, such genotyping techniques may be also used as an additional tool for differentiation of strains from patients with different clinical disorders.

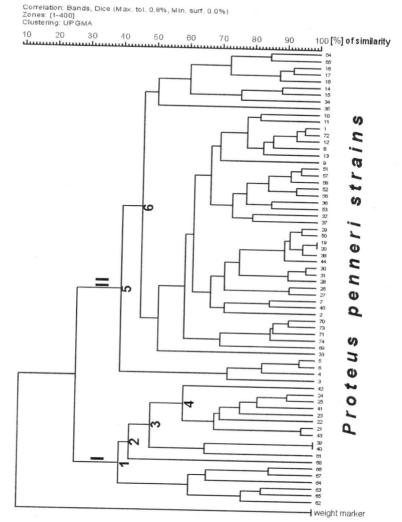

*Figure 2.* Dendrogram of *P. penneri* DNA fingerprints after polymerase chain reaction of repetitive extragenic palindromic sequences (rep-PCR).

## ACKNOWLEDGEMENTS

This work was supported by a grant 6 P04A 059 14 of the Sciences Research Committee (KBN), Poland.

## REFERENCES

1. Hickman F. W., Steigerwalt, A.G.,J. J. Farmer III, J.J., and Brenner, D.J., 1982, Identification of *Proteus penneri species nova*, formerly known as *Proteus vulgaris* indole negative or as *Proteus vulgaris* biogrup 1. *J. Clin. Microbiol.* **15**: 1097-1102.

2. Penner, J.L., 1991, The genera *Proteus, Providencia* and *Morganella*, In *The Procaryotes* (A. Ballows, H. G. Trüper, H. Dworkin, W. Harder and K. H. Schleifer, eds), Springer - Verlag, Berlin, PP.2849-2862.

3. Latuszyński, D. K., Schoch, P., Quadir, M.T., and Cunha, B.A., 1998, *Proteus penneri* urosepsis in a patient with diabetes mellitus. Heart & Lung **27**: 146-148.

4. Craig, J., 1997,Acute *pyelonephritis* in a child caused by *Proteus penneri*. *Australian & New Zealand Journal of Medicin* 1997, **27**: 347-348.

5. Różalski A., Sidorczyk, Z., and Kotełko, K., 1997, Potential virulence factors of *Proteus* bacilli. *Microbiol. Mol. Biol. Rev.* **61**: 65-89.

6. Zych K., Świerzko, A., and Sidorczyk, Z., 1992, Serological characterisation of *Proteus penneri species novum*. Arch. Immun. Ther. Exp. **40**: 89-92.

7. Versalovic J., Koeuth, T., and Lupski, J.R., 1991, Distribution of repetitive DNA sequences in eubacteria and application to fingerprinting of bacterial genomes. *Nucl. Acids Res.* **24**: 6823-6831.

8. Versalovic J., Schneider, M., de Bruijn, F.J., and Lupski, J.R., 1994, Genomic fingerprinting of bacteria using repetitive sequence - based polymerase chain reaction. *Meth. Mol. Cell. Biol.* **5**: 25-40.

9. Versalovic, J., Kapur, V., Koeuth, T., Mazurek, G.H., Wittham, T.S., Muser, J.M., and Lupski, J.R., 1995, DNA fingerprinting of pathogenic bacteria by fluorophore-enhanced repetitive sequence-based polymerase chain reaction. *Arch. Path. Lab. Med.* **119**: 23-29.

# USE OF RANDOMLY AMPLIFIED POLYMORPHIC DNA (RAPD) ANALYSIS FOR IDENTIFICATION OF *PROTEUS PENNERI*

[1]Iwona Kwil, [2]Jarosław Dziadek, [1]Dorota Babicka, [2]Aleksandra Cierniewska-Cieślak and [1]Antoni Różalski
*[1]Department of Immunobiology of Bacteria, University of Łódź, 12/16 Banacha Street, Łódź, Poland;[2]Microbiology and Virology Centre of The Polish Academy of Sciences, 106 Lodowa Street, Łódź, Poland*

## 1. INTRODUCTION

The genus *Proteus* consists of four species: *P. vulgaris*, *P. mirabilis*, *P. penneri* and *P. myxofaciens*. *P. penneri* was formerly known as *P. vulgaris* biogrup 1 and was later proposed as the novel species on the basis of DNA-DNA relatedness found among *P. vulgaris* biogrups[1]. *P. mirabilis*, *P.vulgaris* and *P. penneri* strains are widely distributed in the natural environment, were they play an important role in decomposing organic matter of the animal origin. They are also present in the intestines of humans and domestic animals. *Proteus* bacilli are opportunistic pathogens which are able to cause under favourable conditions several types of infections of which urinary tract infections (UTI) are the most important ones.

Different methods have been used to identify and type *Proteus* bacteria including biochemical tests, serotyping, the Dienes types, susceptibility to phage lysis, analysis of cell proteins, rybotyping, AP-PCR and rep-PCR[2,3,4].

### 1.1 Aim of the Study

The aim of our study was to apply a technique of randomly amplified polymorphic DNA (RAPD) PCR to distinguish between *P. penneri* and *P.*

*Genes and Proteins Underlying Microbial Urinary Tract Virulence*
Edited by L. Emődy *et al.*, Kluwer Academic/Plenum Publishers, 2000

*vulgaris*, *P. mirabilis* and strains of other bacterial species of *Enterobacteriaceae* family.


## 2.    MATERIALS AND METHODS

### 2.1    Bacterial Strains

A total of 162 strains were studied including *P. penneri* 69 strains, *P. vulgaris* 32 strains, *P. mirabilis* 19 strains, *E. coli* 12 strains, *K. pneumoniae* 4 strains, *E. cloaceae* 5 strains, *M. morganii* 3 strains, *Acinetobacter* sp. 3 strains, *S. marcescens* 3 strains, *S. enteritidis* 2 strains, *S. aureus* 2 strains, the other genus of bacteria: *K. pneumoniae*, *C. freundii*, *E. aerogenes*, *S. typhimurium*, *S. agona*, *P. stuartii*, *Y. enterocolitica*, *P. aeruginosa*-1 strain of each. *P. vulgaris* and *P. mirabilis* strains were from the Czech National Collection of Type Cultures (Institute of Epidemiology and Microbiology, Prague). *P. penneri* strains and others strains used in this study come from Institute of Microbiology and Immunology, University of Łódz.

### 2.2    Culturing, DNA Preparation and PCR-Assay

Bacterial strains were cultured on Luria-Broth and genomic DNA was obtained by employing two methods:1) The Genomic Prep Plus Kit and 2) the method described by Jacobs[5]. The oligonucleotid sequences of the primers used for RAPD PCR are presented below:

1 - 5′ TAT CCC CAT CTA TAG CCA GTT C 3′,
2 - 5′ TTG GCA CTA GGG CGG TGC TAT C 3′,

The used primers were designed on the basis of the inner fragment of *hpmA* gene of *Proteus mirabilis* coding for cell-bound hemolysin[6] but the condition of the termocycle allowed amplification of random products. The amplification cycle consisted of an initial 7 min denaturation at 95°C followed by 35 cycles of 5 min at 92°C, 1 min at 39°C and 4.25 min at 65°C. The PCR products were separated by electrophoresis in 7% polyacrylamide gel in TAE buffer[7].


## 3.    RESULTS

The PCR pattern obtained using *P. penneri* total DNA contained four main products 750, 500, 250, 150 bp in length, respectively (Fig 1). The amplification assay was performed for 69 *P. penneri* clinical isolates. In every case, the amplification patterns contained each of the four *P. penneri* specific bands described above.

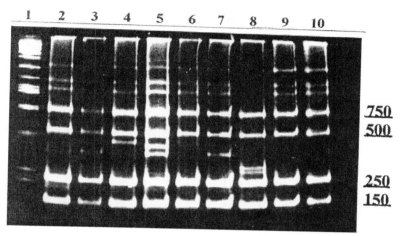

*Figure 1.* Analysis of amplification products of chromosomal DNA from *P. penneri strains;* **Lane 1**, size marker; **lane 2**, *P. penneri* 70; **lane 3**, *P. penneri* 26; **lane 4**, *P. penneri* 71; **lane 5**, *P. penneri* 66; **lane 6**, *P. penneri* 62; **lane 7**, *P. penneri* 25;**lane 8**, *P. penneri* 15; **lane 9**, *P. pennri* 12; **lane 10**, *P. penneri* 4.

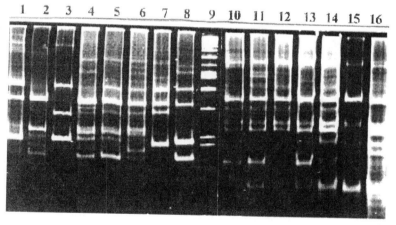

*Figure 2.* Analysis of amplification products of chromosomal DNA from *P. vulgaris* and *P. mirabilis* strains; **Lane 1**, *P. vulgaris* 30/57; **lane 2**, *P. vulgaris* 73/57; **lane 3**, *P. vulgaris* 49990; **lane 4**, *P. vulgaris* 9/57; **lane 5**, P. vulgaris 3/57; **lane 6**, P. vulgaris 71/57; **lane 7**, P. vulgaris 70/57; **lane 8**, *P. pennri* 22; **lane 9**, size marker; **lane 10**, *P. mirabilis* 69/57; **lane 11**, *P. mirabilis* 53/57; **lane 12**, *P. mirabilis* 20/57; **lane 13**, *P. mirabilis* 68/57; **lane 14**, *P. mirabilis* 19/57; **lane 15**, *P. mirabilis* 51/57; **lane 16**, *P. mirabilis* 29906.

The PCR patterns obtained for *P. vulgaris*, *P. mirabilis* (Fig 2) and other Gram-negative bacteria from *Enterobacteriaceae* family (data not shown) were not similar to the specific one of *P. penneri*, however single mentioned above products could be observed.

## 4. CONCLUSIONS

The RAPD assay applied in our study confirmed the taxonomic position of *P. penneri* bacteria. The low annaealing temperature and the 22-oligonucleoide primers used in our study resulted in PCR patterns highly specific for *P. penneri* species. The analysis of a number of *Proteus* clinical isolates as well as other Gram-negative bacteria showed that *P. penneri* strains composed a clonally related group which can be distinguished from other bacteria including *P. mirabilis* and *P. vulgaris*. Moreover, the RAPD assay performed by us could be useful in one step PCR based identification of *P. penneri* strains.

## ACKNOWLEDGMENTS

This work was supported by grant 4 P05A 140 14 of Sciences Research Committee (KBN) Poland

## REFERENCES

1. Hickman, F. W., Steigerwalt, J., Farmer III, J. J., Brenner, D. J., 1982, Identification of *Proteus penneri* sp. nov., formerly known as *Proteus vulgaris* biogroup 1. *J. Clin. Microbiol.* **15**: 1092-1102.
2. Różalski, A., Sidorczyk, Z., and Kotełko, K., 1997, Potential virulence factors of *Proteus* bacilli. *Microbiol. Mol. Biol. Rev.* **61**: 65-89.
3. Kowalczyk, M., Serwecińska, L., and Sidorczyk, Z., 1998, DNA fingerprinting of *Proteus penneri* by rep-PCR. In *Conference on Molecular Biology in Diagnostics of Infectious Diseases and Biotechnology*, Warsaw Agricultural Univ. Publishers, Poland, pp.70-76.
4. Serwecińska, L., Cieślikowski, T., Pytlos, M., Jaworski, A., and Kaca, W., 1998, Genomic fingerprinting of *Proteus* species using repetitive sequence based PCR (rep-PCR). *Acta Microbiol. Polon.* **47**: 313-319.
5. Jacobs, W. R. Jr., Kalpana, G. V., Cirillo, J. D., Pascopella, L., Snapper, S. B., Udani, R. A., Jones, W., Barletta, R. G., Bloom, B. R., 1991, Genetic systems for *Mycobacteria*. *Meth. Enzymol.* 204: 537-555.
6. Uphoff, T. S., Welch, R. A., 1990, Nucleotide sequencing of the *Proteus mirabilis* calcium independent hemolysin genes (*hpmA* and *hpmB*) reveals sequence similarity with *Serratia marcescens* hemolysin genes (*shlA* and *shlB*). *J. Bacteriol.* **172**: 1206-1216.
7. Sambrook, J., Fritsch, E. F., Maniatis, T., 1989, Molecular Cloning, Cold Spring Harbor Laboratory Press.

# OVERVIEW ON THE CLINICAL STUDIES WITH UROSTIM IMMUNOSTIMULATOR AGAINST UROGENITAL INFECTIONS

Plamen Nenkov

*Department of Applied Immunology and Biotechnology, National Center of Infectious and Parasitic Diseases, 26 Yanko Sakazov Blvd. Sofia 1504, Bulgaria*

## 1.     INTRODUCTION

Urinary tract infections (UTI) are among the most widely spread bacterial infections in humans. Chronic or recurrent UTI often cause serious therapeutic problems in clinical practice. Antibiotics and chemotherapeutics used for treatment are often ineffective and may even be immunosuppressive after continuous application. Their extensive use resulted in the selection and distribution of polyresistant bacterial strains and the rising number of immunodeficient patients leads to the involvement of a great variety of Gram-negative and Gram-positive species from the genera *Escherichia, Proteus, Klebsiella, Pseudomonas, Enterococcus faecalis, Staphylococcus epidermidis* etc. in urinary tract diseases.

The polybacterial preparation Urostim was developed in the form of tablets for oral immunoprophylaxis and immunotherapy of chronic and recurrent urinary tract infections. Urostim consists of killed bacterial cells and their lysates of four microbial species: *E.coli* expressing type 1 and P pili, Rc mutant of *E. coli, K .pneumoniae, P. mirabilis* and *E. faecalis*.

The oral application of Urostim stimulated phagocytosis, humoral immunity and functional activity of lymphocytes in experimental animal models and also protected animals against systemic and local infections caused by homologous and heterologous Gram-negative bacteria.

*Genes and Proteins Underlying Microbial Urinary Tract Virulence*
Edited by L. Emődy *et al.*, Kluwer Academic/Plenum Publishers, 2000

Urostim has been licensed and distributed in Bulgaria since 1992.

## 2.     AIM OF THE WORK

This work summarises the results of studies on the effectiveness of Urostim applied on children and adults for immunotherapy and immunoprophylaxis of infections of the urogenital tract in seven different clinics in Bulgaria.

## 3.     MATERIALS AND METHODS

The assessment of the therapeutic effect of Urostim was performed on 320 patients selected on the basis of the following criteria:
-    chronic or recurrent  kidney and/or other urinary tract infections;
-    relapsing androgenological infections

Infections were caused by different bacterial species: *E.coli*, *P.mirabilis*, *K.pneumoniae*, *E. faecalis*, *C. trachomatis* etc.

Urostim was applied as a 1-tablet dosage daily before breakfast for 3 months. In some cases when necessary antibiotics were applied during Urostim administration.

## 4.     RESULTS

*Table 1.* UROSTIM treatment of patients with recurrent non-obstructive UTI - bacteriuria, clinical symptoms, antibacterial treatment and leucocyturia

|                          | Before Treatment | After treatment with UROSTIM | | |
| --- | --- | --- | --- | --- |
|                          |    | 3 months<br>28 patients | 6 months<br>26 patients | 12 months<br>17 patients |
| Bacteriuria              | 28 | 39,28% | 34,61% | 35,29% |
| Clinical symptoms        | 27 | 10,71% | 7,69%  | 0%     |
| Antibacterial treatment  | 24 | 14,28% | 7,69%  | 5,88%  |
| Leucocyturia             | 12 | 7,14%  | 3,84%  | 17,64% |

(In cooperation with Kiroytcheva et al ., Clinic of Nephrology, Medical University, Sofia)

*Table 2.* Mean values of S-IgA (mg/I) in urine of patients treated with UROSTIM

| Patients | Before treatment | After treatment | | |
|---|---|---|---|---|
| | | 3 months | 6 months | 12 months |
| Total 28 | 4,94±2,97 | 6,18±3,42 | 6,15±2,73 | 5,03±2,28 |
| Low levels 5 | 1,61±0,29 | 4,49±1,29 | 5,62±1,75 | 7,50±3,0 |

(In cooperation with Kiroytcheva et al., Clinic of Nephrology, Medical University, Sofia )

*Table 3.* Results of 3 months treatment with UROSTIM of children with pyelonephritis and vesico-ureteral reflux

| Patients treated with Urostim | Patients not treated with Urostim |
|---|---|
| 2[R] / 33[T] | 24/25 |
| 6% reinfected | 96% reinfected |
| R – Reinfected  T – Total | |

(In cooperation with Anadolijska, Clinic of Pediatrics, Medical University, Sofia, )

*Table 4.* Effect of 3 months UROSTIM treatment of patients with uroinfections not influenced by 2 courses of antibacterial treatment in the last 6 months

| | Before treatment | | After treatment | |
|---|---|---|---|---|
| Bacteriuria | 18 | 100% | 10/18 | 56% |
| Clinical symptoms | 18 | 100% | 1/18 | 5,5% |
| Antibacterial treatment | 18 | 100% | 11/18 | 61,1% |

(In cooperation with Pencheva et al., National Institute for Urgent Medicine, Sofia)

*Table 5.* Treatment of patients in acute phase of recurrent or chronic diseases with UROSTIM

| Diagnosis | Results after treatment | Positive effect |
|---|---|---|
| Hyperthrophy of prostate gland and cystopyelitis | 5[P]/8[T] | 62,5% |
| Chronic calculosis pyelonephritis | 7/12 | 58,3% |
| Acute cystopyelitis after treansuretral rejection of tumor bladder adenom, structure | 7/11 | 66,6% |
| P- Positive effect; T –Total | | |

(In cooperation with Panchev et al., Clinic of Urology, Medical University, Sofia )

*Table 6.* Microbiological finding in ejaculate of androgenological patients before and after treatment with UROSTIM

| Treated with Urostim | Isolated bacteria | Before treatment with Urostim | After treatment with Urostim | % Positive results |
|---|---|---|---|---|
| Chronic | *E.coli* | 12 | 2 | 83,4% |
| prostatitis | *Enterococcus* | 6 | 2 | |
| 30 patients | *Proteus* | 4 | - | |
| | *Staphylococcus* | 4 | - | |
| | *Streptococcus* | 4 | 1 | |
| Chronic | *E. coli* | 6 | 2 | 80% |
| exacerbate | *Enterococcus* | 2 | - | |
| urethritis | *Staphylococcus* | 9 | - | |
| 20 patients | *Streptococcus* | 3 | 2 | |
| Chronic | *E.coli* | 6 | - | 100% |
| prostatitis and | *Enterococcus* | 3 | - | |
| urethritis | *Proteus* | 2 | - | |
| 20 patients | *Klebsiella* | 1 | - | |
| | *Staphylococcus* | 3 | - | |
| | *Streptococcus* | 3 | - | |
| | *Ch.trachomatis* | 20 | - | |
| Chronic | *E.coli* | 11 | 5 | 60% |
| prostatitis and | *Enterococcus* | 2 | 1 | |
| urethritis | *Staphylococcus* | 6 | 2 | |
| 20 patients without Urostim | *Streptococcus* | 4 | 1 | |

(In cooperation with J. Uzunova et al., Faculty of Medicine, Medical University, Sofia)

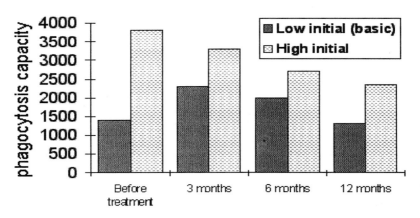

*Figure1.* Changes of phagocytosis capacity after Urostim treatment
(In cooperation with Kiroytcheva et al., Clinic of Nephrology, Medical University, Sofia)

## 5. CONCLUSION

The results obtained characterize Urostim as an effective immunostimulator in the immunotherapy of chronic and recurrent infections of the urogenital tract. Patients with UTI had relapses only in 35% 12 months after treatment with U and the number of relapses was significantly lower than in the control group. In patients with low basic levels of S-IgA these levels were increased after treatment with Urostim. U prevented the re-infection of children with vesico-ureteral reflux. Patients not positively influenced by antibacterial treatment in the last 6 months were free from bacteriuria in 46% after treatment with U. U was effective in immunotherapy of prostatitis and urethritis. Positive influence of U on the phagocytosis capacity in patients with low basic values was also observed.

# PORCINE POSTWEANING DIARRHEA ISOLATES OF ESCHERICHIA COLI WITH UROPATHOGENIC CHARACTERS

[1]István Tóth, [2]Eric Oswald, [3]Jacques Mainil, [4]Mohamed Awad-Masalmeh and [1]Béla Nagy

[1]*Veterinary Medical Research Institute of Hungarian Academy of Sciences, Budapest, Hungary* [2]*Microbiol. Mol. INRA-ENVT, Toulouse, France:* [3]*Chaire Bactériologie, Facult. Med. Vétérinaire, Univ. Liége, Belgium:* [4]*II. Medical Klinik, Univ. Veterinary Sciences, Vienna, Austria*

## 1.    INTRODUCTION

Diarrhoea of just weaned pigs is often a multifactorial disease in which enterotoxic *Escherichia coli* (ETEC) is thought to be the main factor in most cases. Verotoxic *E. coli* (VTEC) can also complicate postweaning diarrhea or may cause oedema disease of weaned pigs. Both porcine postweaning ETEC and VTEC strains strains are known to carry fimbrial adhesins F18[1]. It is however possible that *Escherichia coli* strains with no classical enterotoxic or verotoxic character could also be involved in this multifactorial disease.

## 2.    INITIAL COMMENTS

Our aim was to investigate whether cytotoxic necrotic factors (CNF) or cytolethal dystending toxin (CDT) could also be among the dominant *E. coli* in the porcine small intestine in case of severe diarrhea after weaning.

*Genes and Proteins Underlying Microbial Urinary Tract Virulence*
Edited by L. Emödy *et al.*, Kluwer Academic/Plenum Publishers, 2000

331

Furthermore it was questioned whether enteric CNF+ and/or CDT+ *E. coli* (NTEC) from that age group of pigs could have fimbriae (P or S) or afimbrial adhesins (AFA), characteristic to uropathogenic *E. coli*[2,3].

## 3.      RESULTS

*E. coli* bacteria representing 100 cases of porcine postweaning diarrhea (small intestinal isolates), and 10 other *E. coli* strains from extraintestinal organs or tissues of pigs (5 urogenital and 5 abscess isolates) were PCR tested for genes of necro- and cytotoxins (CNF and CDT)[4,5]. All CNF[+] and selected CNF[-] strains were also tested for fimbrial (P and S) and afimbrial (AFA) adhesins[3,6] known to be responsible for urinary tract virulence in man. Necro- and cytotoxic activity of selected CNF+ strains was also controlled by rabbit skin test[7] and by HeLa cell assay[8]. We have detected 12 enteric NTEC isolates as CNF1[+] and one being also positive for a recently described toxin CDT.

All NTEC possessed the genes for P or S fimbriae or both, but were negative for AFA. One strain also contained the genes for CDT and produced F18 fimbriae (Table 1).

*Table 1.* P- and S fimbrial genes in CNF producing porcine postweaning enteric *E. coli* strains

| NETEC strains | CNF1 | CDT | P-fimbria | S-fimbria | AFA |
|---|---|---|---|---|---|
| 12 | 12/12 | 1/12 | 12/12 | 9/12 | 0/12 |
| non-NETEC strains | | | | | |
| 10 | 0/10 | 0/10 | 0/10 | 0/10 | 0/10 |

On the other hand, none of 10 non-necrotoxic, non-enterotoxic enteric isolates possessed such adhesin genes (Table 2). Out of 10 extraintestinal *E. coli*, only 3 had one or more of the following urinary tract virulence characters: one (from abscess) proved to have CNF1 and P plus S fimbriae and further two strains were either P- or S fimbriated (Table 2). None of the last two possessed necrotoxin genes (Table 2).

*Table 2.* P and S fimbria genes in extraintestinal clinical *E. coli* isolates of adult swine

| Shelf Nr. | CNF1 | P-fimbria | S-fimbria | Clinical background |
|---|---|---|---|---|
| 376 | - | - | + | uterus |
| 422 | - | + | - | liver abscess. |
| 414 | + | + | + | pelvic abscess. |

## 4. CONCLUSION

Our studies confirm earlier findings of Dozois et al. 1997[8], and de Brito et al.1999[9] about the occurence of necrotoxic and P or S fimbriated *E. coli* among enteric and extraintestinal isolates from suckling pigs, and provide additional evidence for similar properties of *E. coli* in diarrheal weaned pigs.

It was suggested that porcine enteric *E. coli* population may contain strains carrying pathogenicity islands more characteristic to human uropathogenic *E. coli*. The pathogenetic significance of such strains for weaned pigs remains to be investigated.

## ACKNOWLEDGEMENT

Support of OMFB-EU-98-D10-115, FAIR3-CT96-1335, OTKA T026150, Ministry of Health T-10 186/96 and of OECD (Paris, France) as well as personal contribution of Márta Tóth-Szekrényi and of Péter-Zsolt Fekete is gratefully acknowledged.

## REFERENCES

1. Rippinger, P., Bertschinger, H.U., Imberechts, H., Nagy, B., Sorg, I., Stamm, M., Wild, P., and Witting W., 1995, Designation F18ab and F18ac for the related fimbrial types F107, 213P and 8813 of *Escherichia coli* isolated from porcine postweaning diarrhoea from oedema disease. *Vet. Microbiol.* **45**: 281-295.
2. Hacker, J., 1990, Genetic determinants coding for fimbriae and adhesins of extraintestinal *Escherichia coli*. *Curr. Topics Microbiol. Immunol.* **151**: 1-27.
3. Le Bougenec, C., and Bertin, Y., 1999, AFA and F17 adhesins produced by pathogenic *Escherichia coli* strains in domestic animals. *Vet. Res.* **30**: 317-342.
4. Blanco, M., Blanco, J.E., Mora, A., and Blanco, J., 1998, Distribution and characterization of faecal necrotoxigenic *Escherichia coli* CNF1+ and CNF2+ isolated from healthy cows and calves. *Vet. Microbiol.* **59**: 183-192.
5. Oswald, E., personal communication
6. Le Bouguenec, C., Archaumband, M., and Labigne, A., 1992, Rapid and specific detection of *pap, afa*, and *sfa* adhesin-encoding operons in uropathogenic *Escherichia coli* strains by polimerase chain reaction. *J Clin Microbiol.* **30**: 1189-1193.
7. Caprioli, A., Falbo, V., Roda, L.G., Ruggeri, F.M., and Zona, C., 1983, Partial purificatiobn and characterization of an Escherichia coli toxic factor that induces morphological cell alterations. *Infect. Immun.* **39**: 1300-1306.
8. Dozois, C.M., Clement, S., Desautels, C., Oswald, E., and Fairbrother, J.M., 1997., Expression of P, S, and F1C adhesins by cytotoxic necrotizing factor 1-producing Escherichia coli from septicemic and diarrheic pigs. *FEMS Microbiol. Lett.* **152**: 307-312.
9. De Brito, B.G., Leite, D.S, Linhares, R.E, and Viditto, M.C., 1999, Virulence-associated factors of uropathogenic *Escherichia coli* strains isolated from pigs. *Vet. Microbiol.* **65**: 123-132.

# VIRULENCE MARKERS OF HUMAN UROPATHOGENIC *ESCHERICHIA COLI* STRAINS ISOLATED IN HUNGARY

[1]István Tóth,[2]Eric Oswald,[3]Béla Szabó,[4]István Barcs and [5]Levente Emődy
[1]*Veterinary Medical Research Institute of Hungarian Academy of Sciences, Budapest, Hungary;* [2]*Microbiol. Mol. INRA-ENVT, Toulouse, France;* [3]*Medical University School of Debrecen, Debrecen;* [4]*Central Military Hospital, Budapest;* [5]*Medical University School of Pécs, Pécs, Hungary*

## 1.    INTRODUCTION

Uropathogenic E. coli (UPEC) strains acquire traits that distinguish them from commensal and diarrheagenic *E. coli* strains. Characteristically, UPEC strains produce haemolysin and cytotoxic necrotizing factor type 1 (CNF1), P fimbriae, aerobactin, exhibit serum resistance, and are encapsulated[1]. Clustered sets of virulence genes, termed pathogenicity island (PAI) was first described in an UPEC strain by Hacker and colleagues[2,3,4].

## 2.    INITIAL COMMENTS

Our aim was to monitor the presence of CNF- and CDT (Cytolethal Distending Toxins) genes in *E. coli* strains isolated from patients with urinary tract infections in Hungary, and to test the strains for haemolysin production.

Additionally, we wanted to monitor the presence of urovirulence adhesin genes encoding pyelonephritis associated pili (*pap*), S fimbriae (*sfa*) and afimbrial adhesin (*afa*) among toxigenic strains.

*Genes and Proteins Underlying Microbial Urinary Tract Virulence*
Edited by L. Emődy *et al.*, Kluwer Academic/Plenum Publishers, 2000

## 3.     RESULTS

Altogether 202  *E. coli* strains were   isolated and identified by standard bacteriological procedures in three different Hungarian hospitals.  190 *E. coli* strains were isolated from urine specimens of patients with urinary tract infections.  Eight strains were isolated from wound infections, two strains were cultivated from bile and 1-1 strain originated from a haemoculture and vaginal infection (extraintestinal strains).

### 3.1     CNF, CDT and Haemolysin Production

CNF-specific sequences were detected by multiplex PCR using previously described CNF1 and CNF2- specific primer pairs[5]. Forty-two (22.1 %) UPEC strains produced CNF1. CDT-specific sequences were detected from 15 (7.9 %) UPEC strains by PCR using universal primers[6]. Twelve out of the 15 CDT strains produced CNF1, and 3 CDT producing strains did not produce CNF. None of the extraintestinal strains contained either CNF or CDT genes.

Eighty strains (42.1 %) of the UPEC strains produced haemolysin. Only 4 out 12 (33.3 %) extraintestinal strains produced haemolysin. Much higher incidence was detected among CNF1- and CDT producing strains: 41 strains produced haemolysin, only 2 CNF$^+$ and 2 CDT$^+$ strains did not produce haemolysin.

### 3.2     Detection of P-, S Fmbriae Specific Genes

All the 42 CNF1$^+$ strains and three CDT$^+$ only strains were tested for the *pap*-, *sfa*-, and *afa*-related sequences encoding P,S and AFA adhesins by multiplex PCR[7].   P- and S fimbriae genes were detected with high frequency: 86.7 % (39/45) of the toxigenic strains coded S fimbriae, 71.1 % (32/45) P fimbriae and none of the strains coded for AFA.

### 3.3     Virulence Marker Patterns

Forty-four strains possessed more than one virulence markers, and one strain produced CDT only. The virulence genes were clustered and gave seven virulence marker patterns. Most frequently, in 16.3 % (31/190) of UPEC strains *cnf1* gene was associated with Hly, *pap* and *sfa* and had the same virulence marker pattern as the prototypic uropathogenic strain J96[3,8]. In 10 out of these J96-like strains CDT was associated to the characteristic virulence marker cluster encoded by PAIs. Six strains produced CNF1, haemolysin and S fimbriae. Three strains produced CNF and haemolysin, two strains produced CNF and CDT and possessed S fimbria gene. In one strain CDT and haemolysin and in another one CDT and P fimbria genes were present.

# 4. CONCLUSION

As high as 21.1% of the UPEC strains isolated in Hungary produced CNF1. Most of the CNF1 strains had additional virulence markers.

Our results suggest that J96-like strains (*cnf1*, *hly*, *pa*p, *sfa*) are spread in Hungarian human population.

Interestingly one third of these strains produced CDT, indicating that CDT could be considered as a potential new virulence factor in urinary tract infections caused by *E. coli*.

# ACKNOWLEDGEMENT

Support of OMFB-EU-98-D10-115, FAIR3-CT96-1335, OTKA T026150, Ministry of HealthT-10 186/96 and of OECD (Paris, France) as well as personal contribution of Márta Tóth-Szekrényi and of Péter-Zsolt Fekete is gratefully acknowledged.

# REFERENCES

1.. Johnson, J.R., 1991, Virulence factors in *Escherichia coli* urinary tract infections. *Clin. Microbiol. Rev.* **4:** 80-128.
2. Hacker,J., Bender, L., Ott, M., Wingender, J., Lund, B., Marre, R., and Goebel, W., 1990, Deletions of chromosomal regions coding for fimbriae and hemolysin occur *in vitro* and *in vivo* in various *Escherichia coli* isolates. *Microb. Pathog.* **8:** 213-225.
3. Blum, G., Ott, M., Lischewski, A., Ritter, A., Imrich, H., Tschape, H., and Hacker, J., 1994, Excision of large DNA region termed pathogenicity islands from tRNA-specific loci in in the chromosome of an *Escherichia coli* wild-type pathogen. *Infect. Immun.* **62:** 606-614.
4. Hacker, J., Blum-Oehler, G., Mühldorfer, I., and Tschape, H., 1997, Pathogenicity islands of virulent bacteria: structure, function and impact on microbial evolution. *Mol. Microbiol.* **23:** 1089-1097.
5. Blanco, M, Blanco. J.E., Mora, A., and Blanco, J., 1998, Distribution and characterization of fecal necrotoxigenic *Escherichia coli* CNF1+ and CNF2+ isolated from healthy cows and calves. *Vet. Microbiol..* **59:** 183-192.
6. Oswald, E., personal communication
7. Le Bouguenec, C., Archaumband, M., and Labigne, A., 1992, Rapid and specific detection of *pap, afa,* and *sfa* adhesin-encoding operons in uropathogenic *Escherichia coli* strains by polimerase chain reaction. *J. Clin. Microbiol.* **30:** 1189-1193.

8. Blum, G., Falbo, V., Caprioli, A., and Hacker, J., 1995, Gene clusters encoding the cytotoxic necrotizing factor type 1, Prs-fimbriae and hemolysin from the pathogenicity island II of uropathogenic *Escherichia coli* strain J96. *FEMS Microbiol. Lett.* **126:**189-196.

# NEW SEROGROUPS OF THE GENUS *PROTEUS* CONSISTING OF PROTEUS *PENNERI STRAINS* ONLY

*Determination of some LPS epitopes responsible for specificity*

[1]Krystyna Zych, [1]Marcin Kowalczyk, [2]Yuriy A. Knirel, and [1]Zygmunt Sidorczyk

[1]*Department of General Microbiology, Universty of Lodz, Banacha 12/16, 90-237 Lodz, Poland;*
[2]*ND Zelinsky Institute of Organic Chemistry, Russian Academy of Sciences, Moscow, Russian Federation*

## 1.     INTRODUCTION

Gram-negative rods from the genus *Proteus* are important opportunistic pathogens causing urinary tract infection (UTI). Their serological classification based on specificity of somatic O-antigens (lipopolysaccharides, LPS) contains 60 O-serogroups and includes two species only: *P. mirabilis* and *P. vulgaris*[1,2]. The third species – *P. penneri* has not been classified yet. Chemical, immunochemical and serological studies have been undertaken aiming to understand the immunospecificity of *P. penneri* LPS and its potential role in the pathogenicity of the bacteria on the molecular level.

In this work serological classification of *P. penneri* strains is described and cross reactivity of various *P. penneri* strains is discussed in a view of the chemical structures of the O-antigens.

*Genes and Proteins Underlying Microbial Urinary Tract Virulence*
Edited by L. Emődy *et al.*, Kluwer Academic/Plenum Publishers, 2000

## 2.    METHODS

Structures of O-specific polysaccharides from *P. penneri* strains were studied by means of sugar and methylation analyses and different variants of NMR spectroscopy[4]. Serological investigations were performed with use of enzyme immunoabsorbent assay (EIA), passive immunohemolysis and its inhibition tests, absorption and Western Blot analysis[5]; also a set of polyclonal *P. penneri* O-antisera and LPSs from complete collection of *Proteus* strains: 68 (*Pp*), 37 (*Pm*) and 28 (*Pv*) were used[3].

## 3.    RESULTS AND DISCUSSION

In this work a first set of 8 *P. penneri* O-antisera was tested with lipopolysaccharides from 68 of *P. penneri*, 37 of *P. mirabilis* and 28 of *P. vulgaris* strains.

Serological analysis of more than 1000 tested systems (8 *P. penneri* antisera and 133 *Proteus* lipopolysaccharides) have shown the following four cross-reacting groups of strains.

*Table 1.* Cross-reactivity of *P. penneri* LPSs with *P. penneri* 52 O- antiserum

| LPS from *P. penneri* strains | Enzyme immunosorbent assay | Passive immunohemolysis test | Minimal dose of LPS in inhibition of passive Immuno-hemolysis in the homologous test system |
|---|---|---|---|
| | reciprocal titer | | ng |
| 21 | 25600 | 25600 | 2 |
| 33 | 25600 | 51200 | 1 |
| 43 | 12800 | 25600 | 2 |
| 50 | 25600 | 25600 | 1 |
| 51 | 12800 | 25600 | 2 |
| 52 | *51200* | *25600* | *2* |
| 53 | 25600 | 51200 | 1 |
| 54 | 25600 | 51200 | 1 |
| 55 | 25600 | 25600 | 1 |
| 57 | 25600 | 25600 | 2 |
| 58 | 51200 | 25600 | 1 |
| 66 | 25600 | 25600 | 2 |
| 67 | 25600 | 51200 | 2 |
| 68 | 25600 | 25600 | 2 |
| 69 | 25600 | 25600 | 2 |
| 72 | 25600 | 25600 | 2 |

Data for the homologous LPS are italicized.

1. The first group contained 16 of *Proteus penneri* strains cross reacting with *P. penneri* 52 O-antiserum (Table 1.)

*P. penneri* 52 O-antiserum was highly reactive with all the 15 LPSs in all the applied tests. The heterologous reactions with this antiserum were identical or very similar to the homologous reaction.

Absorption of the *P. penneri* 52 antiserum with alkali-treated LPSs from each strain of this group completely removes both homologous and cross-reacting antibodies. These results are confirmed by Western blots, where specific antibodies against *P. penneri* 52 recognised tested O-antigens from all the cross-reactive strains.

Structural analysis of O-specific polysaccharides from selected strains (*P. penneri* 21, 53 and 67) has shown that they have the same structures as that of *P. penneri* 52[3].

Therefore, on the basis of the obtained data it was concluded that all the investigated *P. penneri* strains (21, 33, 43, 50-55, 57, 58, 66-69 and 72) belong to the same, new serological group *Proteus* O61.

2. The next group of eight *P. penneri* strains cross-reacted with *P. penneri* 41 O-antiserum (Table 2.)

On the basis of serological studies with tested LPSs, it can be concluded that *P. penneri* strains: 41, 56, 61, 64, 65, 70 and 74 belong to the same, new *Proteus* O62 serogroup consisting of *P. penneri* strains only. Structural identity of the O-specific polysaccharides of *Proteus* O62 serogroup was demonstrated after the investigation of three randomly selected LPSs from *P. penneri* strains 41, 65 and 74[4].

*Table 2.* Cross-reactivity of *P. penneri* LPSs with *P. penneri* 41 O- antiserum

| LPS from *P. penneri* Strains | Enzyme Immuno-Sorbent Assay | Passive immuno-Hemolysis test | Minimal dose of LPS in inhibition of passive immunohemolysis in the homologous test system |
|---|---|---|---|
| | reciprocal titer | | ng |
| *41* | *102400* | *51200* | *1* |
| 56 | 102400 | 51200 | 1 |
| 61 | 102400 | 51200 | 2 |
| 64 | 102400 | 51200 | 1 |
| 65 | 102400 | 51200 | 1 |
| 70 | 102400 | 51200 | 1 |
| 73 | 102400 | 25600 | 1 |
| 74 | 102400 | 51200 | 1 |

Data for the homologous LPS are italicized.

3. The next two strains reacted with *P. penneri* 26 O-antiserum (Table 3).

*Table 3.* Cross-reactivity of *Proteus* LPSs with *P. penneri* 26 O-antiserum

| LPS from Strains | Enzyme immuno-sorbent assay | Passive immuno-hemolysis test | Minimal dose of LPS in inhibition of passive Immunohemolysis in the Homologous test system |
|---|---|---|---|
| | reciprocal titer | | ng |
| *P. penneri* 26 | 12800 | 25600 | 4 |
| *P. vulgaris* OX2 | 8000 | 1600 | 3000 |

Cross-reactions of *P. vulgaris* LPS OX2 were much weaker. Absorption of the antiserum with this antigen (Table 4.) left some fraction of antibodies reacting with homologous LPS.

*Table 4.* Passive immunohemolysis data after absorption of *P. penneri* 26 O-antiserum with alkali-treated LPS (LPS-OH)

| Antiserum absorbed with LPS-OH | Reciprocal titer for P. penneri 26 antiserum reactivity with LPS-OH from: | |
|---|---|---|
| | P. penneri 26 | P. vulgaris OX2 |
| Control | 25600 | 1600 |
| P. penneri 26 | <100 | <100 |
| P. vulgaris OX2 | 3200 | <100 |

After comparison of serological results with the chemical structure of both O-antigens[6, 7] it was evident that cross-reaction was associated with the presence of the common trisaccharide fragment:

$\alpha$-D-Glc$p$NAc-(1→3)-$\alpha$-L-Qui$p$NAc-(1→3)-$\alpha$-D-Glc$p$NAc

Thus, *P. penneri* 26 strain is the only representative of the next, new *Proteus* O70 serogruop.

4. The last group of *P. penneri* strains reacted with their homologous O-antisera only. They did not show any cross-reactions and each represented a new, separate *Proteus* serogroup (Table 5.).

*Table 5.* New *Proteus* serogroups represented by a single *P. penneri* strain each

| Number of group | *P. penneri* strain | *Proteus* O serogroup | References (structures of O-antigens) |
|---|---|---|---|
| 8 | 22 | O63 | [8] |
| 9 | 34 | O65 | [9] |
| 10 | 2 | O66 | [10] |
| 11 | 25 | O69 | [11] |
| 12 | 42 | O71 | [12] |

*Table 6.* Proposed new *Proteus* serogroups

| No of group | Proposed *Proteus* serogroup | *P. penneri* strain representing this serogroup | References |
|---|---|---|---|
| 1 | O61 | 21, 33, 43, 50, 51, 52, 53, 54, 55, 57, 58, 66, 67, 68, 69 and 72 | 3 |
| 2 | O62 | 41, 56, 61, 64, 65, 70, 73 and 74 | 4 |
| 3 | O70 | 26 | 6 |
| 4 | O63 | 22 | 8 |
| 5 | O65 | 34 | 9 |
| 6 | O66 | 2 | 10 |
| 7 | O69 | 25 | 11 |
| 8 | O71 | 42 | 12 |

# 4.    CONCLUSION

On the basis of serological investigations of 133 *Proteus* strains and structural analysis of *P. penneri* O-polysaccharides the following new *Proteus* serogroups have been proposed (Table 6.).

# ACKNOWLEDGMENTS

This work from our laboratory was supported by grants 6 PO4A 007 14 and 6 PO4A 059 14 of the Sciences Research Committee (KBN, Poland).

# REFERENCES

1.  Larsson, P., 1984, Serology of *Proteus mirabilis* and *Proteus vulgaris. Methods Microbiol.* **14:** 187-214.
2.  Penner, J.L. and Hennessy, C., 1980, Separate O-grouping schemes for serotyping clinical isolates of *Proteus mirabilis* and *Proteus vulgaris. J. Clin. Invest.* **12:** 77-82.
3.  Sidorczyk, Z., Zych, K., Świerzko, A., Vinogradov, E.V. and Knirel, Y.A., 1996, The structure of the O-specific polysaccharide of *Proteus penneri* 52. *Eur. J. Biochem.* **240:** 245-251.
4.  Zych, K., Knirel, Y.A., Paramonov, N.A., Vinogradov, E.V., Arbatsky, N.P., Senchenkova, S.N., Shashkov, A.S. and Sidorczyk Z., 1998, Structure of the O-specific polysaccharide of *Proteus penneri* strain 41 from a new proposed serogroup O62. *FEMS Immunol. Med. Microbiol.* **21:** 1-9.
5.  Sidorczyk, Z., Świerzko, A., Knirel, Y.A., Vinogradov, E.V., Chernyak, A.Y., Kononov, L.O., Cedzyⁿski, M., Różalski, A., Kaca, W., Shashkov, A.S. and Kochetkov, N.K., 1995, Structure and epitope specificity of the O-specific polysaccharide of *Proteus penneri* 12 (ATCC 33519) containing amide of D-galacturonic acid with threonine. *Eur. J. Biochem.* **230:** 713-721.

6. Shashkov, A.S., Arbatsky, N.P., Widmalm, G., Knirel, Y.A., Zych, K. and Sidorczyk, Z., 1998, Structure and cross-reactivity of the O-specific polysaccharide of *Proteus penneri* strain 26, another neutral *Proteus* O-antigen containing 2-acetamido-2,6-dideoxy-L-glucose (*N*-acetyl-L-quinovosamine). *Eur. J. Bochem.* **253**: 730-733.

7. Ziółkowski, A., Shashkov, A.S., Świerzko, A., Senchenkova, S.N., Tukach, F.V., Cedzyński, M., Amano, K.-I., Kaca, W., and Knirel, Y.A., 1997, Structures of the O-antigens of Proteus bacilli belonging to OX group (serogroups O1-O3) used in Weil-Felix test. FEBS Lett., **411**: 221-224.

8. Arbatsky, N.P., Shashkov, A.S., Mamyan, S.S., Knirel, Y.A., Zych, K. and Sidorczyk, Z., 1998, Structure of the O-specific polysaccharide of a serologically separate *Proteus penneri* strain 22. *Carbohydr. Res.* **310**: 85-90.

9. Toukach, F.V., Arbatsky, N.P., Shashkov, A.S., Knirel, Y.A., Zych, K. and Sidorczyk, Z., 1998, Structure of a neutral O-specific polysaccharide of *Proteus penneri* 34. *Carbohydr. Res.* **312**: 97-101.

10. Shashkov, A.S., Arbatsky, N.P., Toukach, F.V., Knirel, Y.A., Moll, H., Zähringer, U., Zych, K. and Sidorczyk, Z., 1999, Structure of the O-specific polysaccharide of a serologically separate strain of *Proteus penneri* 2 from a new proposed serogroup O66. *Eur. J. Biochem.* **261**: 392-397.

11. Shashkov, A.S., Arbatsky, N.P., Widmalm, G., Knirel, Y.A., Zych, K. and Sidorczyk, Z., 1998, Structure and cross-reactivity of the O-specific polysaccharide of *Proteus penneri* strain 26, another neutral *Proteus* O-antigen containing 2-acetamido-2,6-dideoxy-L-glucose (*N*-acetyl-L-quinovosamine). *Eur. J. Bochem.* **253**: 730-733.

12. Knirel, Y.A., Shashkov, A.S., Vinogradov, E.V., Świerzko, A. and Sidorczyk, Z., 1995, The structure of the O-specific polysaccharide chain of *Proteus penneri* strain 42 lipopolysaccharide. *Carbohydr. Res.*, **275**: 201-206.

# THE ROLE OF *CHLAMYDIA TRACHOMATIS* IN ASYMPTOMATIC AND SYMPTOMATIC UROGENITAL INFECTIONS

Judith Deák and Elisabeth Nagy
*Department of Clinical Microbiology, Albert Szent-Györgyi Medical University, Somogyi Béla tér 1. 6725 Szeged, Hungary*

## 1.     INTRODUCTION

*Chlamydia trachomatis* (*C. trachomatis*) is the most frequent etiological agent involved in sexually transmittable bacterial infections. WHO estimates suggest that the annual number of newly acquired *C. trachomatis* infections worldwide is close to 90 million[1]. The asymptomatic and symptomatic infections display varying distributions in different countries in Europe[2] (Table 1). Screening for *C. trachomatis* infections is extremely widespread in Sweden, and concerns not only risk groups. Clinical and laboratory examinations and antibiotic treatment are promoted by the Swedish state. The number of new cases of *C. trachomatis* infections in Sweden in 1994 was 14 thousand[3]. An eradication programme has been elaborated with a view to decreasing pelvic inflammatory diseases[4]. There is insufficient information concerning the prevalence and incidence of chlamydia and the type of laboratory examinations in Russia, but the number of infections increased between 1993 and 1997: 169 834 new cases were registered in 1997, 3.1 times the number in 1993[5]. In the majority of European countries the incidence and prevalence of *C. trachomatis* have decreased.

The recent statistical data for Hungary are presented in Table 2. Within a given country, the prevalence and incidence of infections depend on different factors. Diagnostic and directed examinations were performed in small Hungarian populations at the beginning of 1990. Later, screening programmes

*Genes and Proteins Underlying Microbial Urinary Tract Virulence*
Edited by L. Emödy *et al.*, Kluwer Academic/Plenum Publishers, 2000

345

were elaborated for examinations of different risk groups, and in 1995 a screening program was introduced in a search for asymptomatic risk groups[6].

The diagnosis of *C. trachomatis* is based on detection of the bacterium. Amplified methods are the new gold standards of the diagnostics, e.g. LCR, PCR and TMA. Serological diagnosis may be useful in cases of PID, ectopic pregnancy, periappendicitis, perihepatitis and SARA.

*Table 1.* Incidence/prevalence of *Chlamydia trachomatis* in some European countries (1994-95)

| Country | Year | % | Asymptomatic Infections | Symptomatic Infections |
|---|---|---|---|---|
| Austria | 1995 | 7.2 | Pregnant women | |
| Bulgaria | 1995 | 6.1 | Females | |
| Denmark | 1995 | 4.8 | | Males and females |
| England | 1995 | 3-12 | | Males and females |
| France | 1993-95 | 6-11 | | Males and females |
| Greece | 1995 | 4-7 | Females | |
| The Netherlands | 1994 | 5.1-12.3 | | Females |
| Croatia | 1995 | 17.1 | | Males and females |
| Hungary | 1995 | 14.5 | | Males and females |
| Germany (East region) | 1995 | 4.7-6.5 | Females | |
| Germany (West region) | 1995 | 2.7 | Females | |
| Norway | 1995 | 4.4 | Females | |
| Switzerland | 1994 | 4.6 | | Males and females |

Table 2. Prevalence of *Chlamydia trachomatis* infection in Hungary (1993-98)

| Year | No | Positive | % |
|---|---|---|---|
| 1993 | 4 636 | 433 | 9.3 |
| 1994 | 8 913 | 1 515 | 17.0 |
| 1995 | 9 633 | 1 401 | 14.5 |
| 1996 | 13 981 | 1 495 | 10.7 |
| 1997 | 9 596 | 615 | 6.4 |
| 1998 | 9 405 | 547 | 5.8 |

## 2.    METHODS

Commercial data relating to the methods used in the eight examination procedures applied are as follows:

Amplicor *C. trachomatis* PCR Detection Kit, Roche Diagnostics System
*C. trachomatis* specific PCR, primer pair (INT, Corallsville, IA, USA)[7]

*C. trachomatis* Transcription Mediated Amplification (TMA) Amplified Gene Probe 2, USA

PACE 2 *C. trachomatis* Gen-Probe, USA

LCR, LCx *C. trachomatis* Assay, Abbott, USA

SYVA MikroTrac *C. trachomatis* direct Specimen IF test, SYVA-Behring Diagnostics Inc.

DAKO IDEA chlamydia EIA test, DAKO A/S

Sanofi Diagnostics Pasteur, Chlamydia Microplate ELISA

# 3.     RESULTS

## 3.1     First Study

Between 1994 and 1996, 7 495 asymptomatic pregnant women were screened with the PACE 2 Gen-Probe method in geographically different clinics and hospitals of Hungary. The overall average incidence of *C. trachomatis* cases was 5.7%. The data from different centers ranged between 1.6 and 9.8%. The incidence of *C. trachomatis* in Szeged was 3.6% (Table 3). In recent years, the prevalence of infections has exhibited an overall slow decrease, both in Hungary and in Szeged.

*Table 3.* Prevalence of *Chlamydia trachomatis* infection in asymptomatic pregnant women (1994-96)

| Centre | N | Positive | % |
|---|---|---|---|
| Budapest I | 364 | 28 | 7.7 |
| Budapest II | 715 | 20 | 2.8 |
| Debrecen | 472 | 6 | 1.3 |
| Miskolc | 2 327 | 227 | 9.8 |
| Nyíregyháza | 1 703 | 92 | 5.4 |
| Szombathely | 757 | 12 | 1.6 |
| Szeged | 1 157 | 42 | 3.6 |
| Total | 7 495 | 427 | 5.7 |

## 3.2     Second Study

*C. trachomatis* was examined in 50 patients by means of 7 different methods simultaneously [ELISA (2 methods), IF, PCR (2 methods), LCR and TMA]. The patients were otherwise asymptomatic for genital infection and presented with infertility. *C. trachomatis* was detected in 3 cases (6%) with the amplified methods: PCR (Roche and laboratory-developed PCR), LCR and TMA. The IF method was not adequately specific or sensitive, and one of the ELISA methods gave negative results in all cases (Table 4) [8].

*Table 4.* Detection of *Chlamydia trachomatis* in ejaculatum samples from asymptomatic males in Hungary in 1997

| Methods | Results | | |
|---|---|---|---|
| | Positive | Borderline | Negative |
| PCR | 3 | 0 | 47 |
| PCR (laboratory-developed) | 3 | 0 | 47 |
| LCR | 3 | 0 | 47 |
| TMA | 3 | 0 | 47 |
| Direct IF | 2 | 10 | 38 |
| EIA I | 1 | 1 | 48 |
| EIA II | 0 | 0 | 50 |

## 3.3     Third Study

In January 1998, an amplified method, LCR, was instituted as diagnostic method in our laboratory. Cervical, urethral, vaginal and conjunctival swab, urine and semen samples were examined by LCR from gynecological, urological, venerological and ophthalmological patients.

The overall average incidence of *C. trachomatis* infections was 1.9%. The incidence of pathogens in gynecological patients was 1.2%, in urological patients it was 6.8%, in the couples participating in the in vitro fertilization programme it was 1.2% (females) and 0.96% (males), and in the ophthalmological cases it was 4.3% (Table 5).

*Table 5.* Diagnostic chlamydial examinations of symptomatic males and females in Szeged in 1998

| Samples | N | Positive | % |
|---|---|---|---|
| Cervix | 425 | 5 | 1.2 |
| Semen | 313 | 3 | 0.96 |
| Urethra | 117 | 8 | 6.8 |
| Urine | 83 | 1 | 1.2 |
| Conjunctiva | 23 | 1 | 4.3 |
| Total | 961 | 18 | 1.9 |

## 4.     CONCLUSION

In the first screening study, a high prevalence of *C. trachomatis* was detected with a non-amplified PACE 2 Gen-Probe method. Before this screening programme there had been no similar chlamydia screening programme in Hungary. After the evaluation of these results, the number of *C.*

*trachomatis* laboratory examinations increased and the incidence of positive cases decreased.

In the second study, the incidence of positive cases conformed with the European literature data. The importance of the method of sampling is emphasized if the bactericidal effect of the semen is to be minimized. The molecular biological methods are recommended for the detection of *C. trachomatis*[9, 10, 11].

In the third study, diagnostic chlamydia examinations were performed in Szeged, where the earlier prevalence in asymptomatic women was 3.6%. One of the most sensitive methods, LCR, was used for the diagnosis of *C. trachomatis.*

Which factors have played a role in the decreasing rate of infections? The *C. trachomatis* diagnostic methods were introduced first in Hungary, in Szeged, in 1985. Doxycycline is one of the most widely used antobiotics in Hungary, and is suitable among others for the treatment of *C. trachomatis* infections. However, can we unambiguosly explain this apparent decreasing tendency as a true decrease in the number of *C. trachomatis* infections? Have most of the clinical samples from symptomatic patients been sent to microbiological laboratories for chlamydia detection in recent years[12]? Have the 14-18-year-old males and females, the most important group at risk of chlamydial infections been screened[13, 14, 15]?

The CDC has suggested the introduction of national programmes for the eradication of *C. trachomatis* infections. A national health education programme involving the sexual health of students $\geq 12$ years old would be very important in Hungary. Teenager outpatient clinics have been founded in different hospitals in Hungary for 14-18-year-old girls, where contraception advice, and programmes for the prevention and diagnostics of STDs have been introduced. This possibility is separate from adult attendance both in time and in place. There have as yet been no similar clinics for teenager males. The screening and treatment of the *C. trachomatis*-positive population below 20 years of age would have a great epidemiological effect[16]. The use of sensitive and specific microbiological methods and the treatment of sexual partners can form an effective part of eradication programmes.

## ACKNOWLEDGMENTS

The authors express their thanks to those colleagues who participated in the three chlamydial studies.

## REFERENCES

1. Gerbase, A.C., Rowley, J.T., Mertens, T.E., 1998, Global epidemiology of sexually transmitted diseases. *Lancet* **351** (suppl III): 2-4.

2. Nyári, T., 1998, PhD Thesis, *The frequency and the role of Chlamydia trachomatis infection in premature labour – multicenter epidemiological study in Hungary.* Albert Szent-Györgyi Medical University, Szeged.

3. Kallings, I., 1996, Genital chlamydial infections in Sweden. In *Proceedings Third Meeting of the European Society for Chlamydia Research,* (A Stary, ed.), Societa Editrice Esculapio, Bologna, 3. p. 401.

4. Kamwendo, F., Forslin, L., Bodin, L. Danielsson, D., 1998, Programmes to reduce pelvic inflammatory disease – the Swedish experience. *Lancet* **351** (suppl III): 25-28.

5. Gromyko, A., 1998, Joint efforts are required to control HIV and STD epidemics in Eastern Europe. *Official J. Hung. STD Soc.,* **2:** 227-232.

6. Deák, J., Veréb, I., Nagy, E. Mészáros, Gy., Kovács, L., Nyári, T., Berbik, I., 1997, Prevalence of Chlamydia trachomatis infection in a low-risk population in Hungary. *Sex. Transm. Dis.* **24:** 38-542.

7. Brule, van den C.J.A., Hemrika, J.D., Walboomers, M.M.J., Raaphorst, P., van Amstel, N., Bleker, P.O., Meijer, M.L.J.C., 1993, Detection of Chlamydia trachomatis in semen of artificial insemination donors by the polymerase chain reaction. *Fertil. Steril.* **59:** 1098-1104.

8. Corradi, Gy., Deák, J., Budai, I., Nagy, B., 1999, Comparison of molecular biological and conventional methods for detection of Chlamydia trachomatis in semen. *Hum. Reprod.* **14:** 141.

9. Corradi, Gy., Konkoly, T.M., Pánovics, J., Molnár, Gy., Bodó, Á., Frang, D., 1995, Is seminal fluid a suitable specimen for detecting chlamydial infection in men? *Acta Microbiol. Immunol. Hung.* **42:** 389-394.

10. Yoshida, K., Kobayashi, N., Negishi, T., 1994, Chlamydia trachomatis infection in the semen of asymptomatic infertile men: Detection of the antigen by in situ hybridization. *Urol. Int.* **53:** 217-221.

11. Weidner, W..M.W., 1997, Diagnostic workup and therapeutical management of the prostatitis syndrome. *Eur. Urol. Today* **7:** 4-5.

12. Dean, D., Suchland R.J., Stamm, W.E., 1998, Apparent long-term persistence of Chlamydia trachomatis cervical infections – analysis by OMP1 genotyping. In *Chlamydial infections* (Stephens, R.S., Byrne, G.I., Christiansen, G. et al., eds.), San Francisco, pp. 31-34.

13. Gaydos, C.A., Crotchfelt, K.A., Howell, M.R., Kralian, P., Hauptman, P., Quinn, T.C., 1998, Molecular amplification assays to detect chlamydial infections in urine specimens from high school female students and to monitor the persistence of chlamydial DNA after therapy. *J. Infect. Dis.* **177:** 417-24.

14. Gaydos, C.A., Howell, M.R., Quinn, T.C., Gaydos, J.C., McKee, K.T. Jr., 1998, Use of ligase chain reaction with urine versus cervical culture for detection of Chlamydia trachomatis in an asymptomatic military population of pregnant and nonpregnant females attending Papanicolaou smear clinics. *J. Clin. Microbiol.* **36:** 1300-4.

15. Burstein, G., Waterfield, G., Hauptman, P., Joffe, A., Quinn, T., Gaydos, C., 1998, High prevalence of Chlamydia trachomatis and Neisseria gonorrhoeae documented in middle school students by urine based DNA screening. In *Chlamydial infections* (Stephens, R.S., Byrne, G.I., Christiansen, G. et al., eds.), San Francisco, pp. 11-14.

16. Katz, B.P., Fortenberry, D., Orr, D., 1998, Factors affecting chlamydial persistence or recurrence one and three months after treatment. In *Chlamydial infections* (Stephens, R.S., Byrne, G.I., Christiansen, G. et al., eds.), San Francisco, pp. 35-38.

# LIST OF CONTRIBUTORS

| | |
|---|---|
| Abraham, Soman N. | Duke University, Durham, NC, USA |
| Akbulut, Didem | Department of Microbiology, University of Istanbul, Istanbul Faculty of Medicine, Turkey |
| Anğ, Özdem | Department of Microbiology, University of Istanbul, Istanbul Faculty of Medicine, Turkey |
| Anğ-Küçüker, Mine | Department of Microbiology, University of Istanbul, Istanbul Faculty of Medicine, Turkey |
| Auckenthaler, Raymond | Hôpital Cantonal Universitaire, Geneva, Switzerland |
| Awad-Masalmeh, Mohamed | University Clinic, Veterinary University, Vienna, Austria |
| Babicka, Dorota | Department of Immunology of Bacteria, Institute of Microbiology and Immunology, University of Łodz, Poland |
| Balsalobre, Carlos | Department of Microbiology, Umeå University, Umeå, Sweden |
| Barcs, István | Central Military Hospital, Budapest, Hungary |
| Bartodziejska, Beata | Department of Immunology of Bacteria, Institute of Microbiology and Immunology, University of Łodz, Poland |
| Bergsten, Göran | Institute of Laboratory Medicine, Department of MÍG, Lund University, Lund, Sweden |
| Blum-Oehler, Gabriela | Institut für Molekulare Infektionsbiologie, Universität Würzburg, Würzburg, Germany |

351

Boquet, Patrice                 INSERM, Unit 452, Faculty of Medicine, Nice, France

Bouter, Paul K.                 Department of Medicine, Bosch Medicentrum's
                                Hertogenbosch, The Netherlands

Braun, Michael                  Mikrobiologie/Membranphysiologie, Universität
                                Tübingen, Tübingen, Germany

Braun, Volkmar                  Mikrobiologie/Membranphysiologie, Universität
                                Tübingen, Tübingen, Germany

Braveboer, Bert                 Department of Medicine, Catharina Hospital, Eindhoven,
                                The Netherlands

Brouwer, Ellen C.               Eijkman-Winkler Institute, University Hospital, Untecht
                                University, Utrecht, The Netherlands

Büyükbaba-Boral,                Department of Microbiology, University of Istanbul,
                                Istanbul Faculty of Medicine, Özden, Turkey

Camps, Marielle J.L.            Department of Medicine, Catharina Hospital, Eindhoven,
                                The Netherlands

Carrascal, Montserrat           Espectrometria de Massas Estructural y Biologica,
                                Departamento Bioanalitica IIBB, IDIBARS, CSIC,
                                Barcelona, Spain

Cho Seunghak                    Institut für Molekulare Infektionsbiologie, Universität
                                Würzburg, Würzburg, Germany

Cierniewska-Cieslak             Department of Immunology of Bacteria, Institute of
Aleksandra                      Microbiology and Immunology, University of Łodz,
                                Poland

Collet, Theo J.                 Department of Medicine, University Hospital Utrecht,
                                The Netherlands

Correia, José D.                CIISA, Facultade de Medicina Veterinaria, Universidade
                                Técnica de Lisboa, Portugal

Cotterill, Claire               Department of Veterinary Pathology, Royal (Dick)
                                School of Veterinary Studies, University of Edinburgh,
                                Edinburgh, UK

Cramton, Sarah E.               Universität Tübingen, Mikrobielle Genetik, Tübingen,
                                Germany

| | |
|---|---|
| Cuenca, Sonja | Max von Pettenkofer-Institut, LMU München, München, Germany |
| Daryab, Neda | Institut für Molekulare Infetionsbiologie, Universität Würzburg, Würzburg, Germany |
| Deák, Judith | Department of Clinical Microbiology, Albert Szent-Györgyi Medical University, Szeged, Hungary |
| Dietirch, Katja | Institut für Molekulare Infektionsbiologie, Universität Würzburg, Würzburg, Germany |
| Dobrindt, Ulrich | Institut für Molekulare Infektionsbiologie, Universität Würzburg, Würzburg, Germany |
| Dziadek, Jarosław | Department of Immunology of Bacteria, Institute of Microbiology and Immunology, University of Łodz, Poland |
| Emődy, Levente | Department of Medical Microbiology and Immunology, University Medical School, Pécs, Hungary |
| Féria, Constança P. | CIISA, Facultade de Medicina Veterinaria, Universidade Técnika de Lisboa, Portugal |
| Forsman-Semb, Kristina | AstraZeneka, Molecular Biology, Mölndal, Sweden |
| Fischer, Daniela | Max von Pettenkofer-Institut, LMU München, München, Germany |
| Frendéus, Björn | Institute of Laboratory Medicine, Department of MIG, Lund University, Lund, Sweden |
| Fünfstück, Reinhard | Department of Internal Medicine, University of Jena, Germany |
| Gaastra, Wim | Veterinary Faculty, Utrecht University, Utrecht, The Netherlands |
| Gally, David L. | Department of Veterinary Pathology, Royal (Dick) School of Veterinary Studies, University of Edinburgh, Edinburgh, UK |
| Geerlings, Suzanne E. | Department of Medicine, Division of Infectious Diseases AIDS, Utrecht University, Utrecht, The Netherlands |
| Georgellis, Dimitris | Microbiology and Tumorbiology Centre, Karolinska Institute, Stockholm, Sweden |

| | |
|---|---|
| Godaly, Gabriela | Institute of Laboratory Medicine, Department of MIG, Lund University, Lund, Sweden |
| Gonçalves, José | CIISA, Facultade de Medicina Veterinaria, Universitade Técnica de Lisboa, Portugal |
| Goebel, Werner | Lehrstuhl für Mikrobiologie, Universiät Würzburg, Würzburg, Germany |
| Göransson Mikael | Department of Microbiology, Umeå University, Umeå, Sweden |
| Götz, Friedrich | Universität Tübingen, Mikrobielle Genetik, Tübingen, Germany |
| Hacker, Jörg | Institut für Molekulare Infektionsbiologie, Universität Würzburg, Würzburg, Germany |
| Hang, Long | Institute of Laboratory Medicine, Department of MIG, Lund University, Lund, Sweden |
| Hasty, David L. | University of Tennesee and VAMC, Memphis, TN, USA |
| Hedlund, Maria | Institute of Laboratory Medicine, Department of MIG, Lund University, Lund, Sweden |
| Heesemann, Jürgen | Max von Pettenkofer-Institut, LMU München, München, Germany |
| Heilmann, Christine | Universität Tübingen, Mikrobielle Genetik, Tübingen, Germany |
| Hengge-Aronis, Regine | Department of Biology-Microbiology, Freie Universität Berlin, Berlin, Germany |
| Hess, Petra | Institut für Molekulare Infektionsbiologie, Universität Würzburg, Würzburg, Germany |
| Hoekstra, Joost B.L. | Department of Medicine, Diakonessenhuis, Utrecht, The Netherlands |
| Hoepelman, Andy M. | Department of Medicine, Division of Infectious Diseases and AIDS, and Eijkman-Winkler Institute, University Hospital, Utrecht University, Utrecht, The Netherlands |
| Holden, Nicola | Department of Veterinary Pathology, Royal (Dick) School of Veterinary Studies, University of Edinburgh, Edinburgh, UK |

| | |
|---|---|
| Hormaeche, Carlos E. | Department of Microbiology and Immunology, The Medical School, Newcastle University, Newcastle upon Tyne, UK |
| Jacobi, Christoph A. | Max von Pettenkofer-Institut, LMU München, München, Germany |
| Jacobson, Niels | Department of Internal Medicine, University of Jena, Germany |
| Janke, Britta | Institut für Molekulare Infektionsbiologie, Universität Würzburg, Würzburg, Germany |
| Jansz, Arjen R. | Laboratory of Microbiology, St. Josephhospital, Veldhoven, The Netherlands |
| Jass, Jana | Department of Microbiology, Umeå University, Umeå, Sweden |
| Johansson Jörgen | Department of Microbiology, Umeå University, Umeå, Sweden |
| Juárez, Antonio | Departament de Microbiologia, Universitat de Barcelona, Barcelona, Spain |
| Karch, Helge | Institut für Hygiene und Mikrobiologie, Universität Würzburg, Würzburg, Germany |
| Karpman, Diana | Institute of Laboratory Medicine, Department of MIG, Lund University, Lund, Sweden |
| Keegan, Sally J. | Department of Microbiology and Immunology, The Medical School, Newcastle University, Newcastle upon Tyne, UK |
| Khan, A. Salam | Institut für Molekulare Infektionsbiologie, Universität Würzburg, Würzburg, Germany |
| Kilár, Ferenc | Central Research Laboratory, University Medical School, Pécs, Hungary |
| Killmann, Helmut | Mikrobiologie/Membranphysiologie, Universität Tübingen, Tübingen, Germany |
| Klemm, Per | Department of Microbiology, Technical University of Denmark, Lyngby, Denmark |

Knirel, Yury A.            N.D. Zelinsky Institute of Organic Chemistry, Russian
                           Academy of Sciences, Moscow, Russian Federation

Kocsis, Béla              Department of Medical Microbiology and Immunology,
                           University Medical School, Pécs, Hungary

Korhonen, Timo K.         Division of General Microbiology, Department of
                           Biosciences, Helsinki University, Helsinki, Finland.

Kowalczyk, Marcin         Department of General Microbiology, University of Łodz,
                           Poland

Köhler, Gerwald           Zentrum für Infektionsforschung, Universität Würzburg,
                           Würzburg, Germany

Kretschmar, Marianne      Zentrum für Infektionsforschung, Universität Würzburg,
                           Würzburg, Germany

Kustos, Ildikó            Department of Medical Microbiology and Immunology,
                           University Medical School, Pécs, Hungary

Küçükbasmaci, Ömer        Experimental Medical Research Institute, University of
                           Istanbul, Turkey

Kwil, Iwona               Department of Imunology of Bacteria, Institute of
                           Microbiology and Immunology, University of Łodz,
                           Poland

Laurila, Minni            Division of General Microbiology, Department of
                           Biosciences, Helsinki University, Helsinki, Finland

Lång, Hannu               Division of General Microbiology, Department of
                           Biosciences, Helsinki University, Helsinki, Finland

Lorenz, Udo               Department of Surgery, Universität Würzburg, Würzburg,
                           Germany

Lößner, Isabel            Institut für Molekulare Infektionsbiologie, Universität
                           Würzburg, Würzburg, Germany

Machado, Jorge            Centro de Bacteriologica, Instituto Nacional de Saúde,
                           Portugal

Madrid, Cristina          Departament de Microbiologia, Universitat de Barcelona,
                           Barcelona, Spain

Mainil, Jacques           Chaire Bactériologie, Faculté Medicine Veterinaire,
                           Université Liege, Belgique

| | |
|---|---|
| Mäki, Minna | Division of General Microbiology, Department of Biosciences, Helsinki University, Helsinki, Finland |
| Mellefors, Öjar | Microbiology and Tumorbiology Centre, Karolinska Institute, Stockholm, Sweden |
| Michaelis, Kai | Institut für Molekulare Infektionsbiologie, Universität Würzburg, Würzburg, Germany |
| Miquelay, Elisabet | Departament de Microbiologia, Universitat de Barcelona, Barcelona, Spain |
| Morschhäuser, Joachim | Zentrum für Infektionsforschung, Universität Würzburg, Würzburg, Germany |
| Muscholl-Silberhorn, Albrech | Universität Regensburg, Institut für Mikrobiologie NWF III, Regensburg, Germany |
| Nagy, Erzsébet | Department of Clinical Microbiology, Albert Szent-Györgyi Medical University, Szeged, Hungary |
| Nagy, Gábor | Institut für Molekulare Infektionsbiologie, Universität Würzburg, Würzburg, Germany |
| Naureckiene Saule | Department of Microbiology, Umeå University, Umeå, Sweden |
| Nenkov, Plamen | National Center of Infectious and Parasitic Diseases, Sofia, Bulgaria |
| Netten, Paetrick M. | Department of Medicine, Bosch Medicentrum's Hertogenbosch, The Netherlands |
| Nichterlein, Thomas | Institut für Mikrobiologie, Universität Heidelberg, Germany |
| Nieto, José M. | Department de Microbiologia, Universitat de Barcelona, Barcelona, Spain |
| Normark, Staffan J. | Microbiology and Tumorbiology Centre, Karolinska Institute, Stockholm, Sweden |
| Oelschlaeger, Tobias A. | Institut für Molekulare Infektionsbiologie, Universität Würzburg, Würzburg, Germany |
| Ofek, Itzhak | Tel Aviv University, Tel Aviv, Israel |

Ohlsen, Knut — Institut für Molekulare Infektionsbiologie, Universität Würzburg, Würzburg, Germany

Oswald, Eric — Microbiologie Moléculaire INRA-ENVT, Toulouse, France

Otto, Gisela — Institute of Laboratory Medicine, Department of MIG, Lund University, Lund, Sweden

Pajor, László — Department of Urology, Albert Szent-Györgyi Medical University, Szeged, Hungary

Pál, Tibor — Department of Medical Microbiology and Immunology, University Medical School, Pécs, Hungary

Pátri, Eszter — Department of Medical Microbiology and Immunology, University Medical School, Pécs, Hungary

Pearson Jeffery P. — Department of Physiology, The Medical School, Newcastle University, Newcastle upon Tyne, UK

Perepelov, Andrei V. — N.D. Zelinsky Institute of Organic Chemistry, Russian Academy of Sciences, Moscow, Russian Federation

Pernestig, Anna-Karin — Microbiology and Tumorbiology Centre, Karolinska Institute, Stockholm, Sweden

Piechaczek, Katherine — Institut für Molekulare Infektionsbiologie, Universität Würzburg, Würzburg, Germany

Pouttu, Riita — Division of General Microbiology, Department of Biosciences, Helsinki University, Helsinki, Finland

Prenafeta, Antoni — Departament de Microbiologia, Universitat de Barcelona, Barcelona, Spain

Puustinen Terhi — Division of General Microbiology, Department of Biosciences, Helsinki University, Helsinki, Finland

Rachid, Shwan — Institut für Molekulare Infektionsbiologie, Universität Würzburg, Würzburg, Germany

Rantakari, Anssi — Division of General Microbiology, Department of Biosciences, Helsinki University, Helsinki, Finland

Reisenauer, Anita — Institut für Molekulare Infektionsbiologie, Universität Würzburg, Würzburg, Germany

| | |
|---|---|
| Roberts, Ian, S. | School of Biological Sciences, University of Manchester, Manchester, UK |
| Rozalski, Antoni | Department of Immunology of Bacteria, Institute of Microbiology and Immunology, University of Łodz, Poland |
| Rozdzinski, Eva | Universitätsklinik Ulm, Abteilung für Medizinische Mikrobiologie und Hygiene, Ulm, Germany |
| Samuelsson, Patrik | Institite of Laboratory Medicine, Department of MIG, Lund University, Lund, Sweden |
| Schubert, Sören | Max von Pettekofer-Institut, LMU München, München, Germany |
| Sharon, Nathan | Weizmann Institute of Science, Tel Aviv, Israel |
| Sidorczyk, Zygmunt | Department of General Microbiology, University of Łodz, Poland |
| Sondén, Berit | Department of Microbiology, Umeå University, Umeå, Sweden |
| Sorsa, Johanna L. | Max von Pettenkofer-Institut, LMU München, München, Germany |
| Staib, Peter | Zentrum für Infektionsforschung, Universität Würzburg, Würzburg, Germany |
| Stein, Günter | Department of Internal Medicine, University of Jena, Germany |
| Stolk, Ronald P. | Julius Center for Patient Oriented Research, University Hospital, Utrecht, The Netherlands |
| Svanborg, Catharina | Institute of Laboratory Medicine, Department of MIG, Lund University, Lund, Sweden |
| Svennson, Majlis | Institute of Laboratory Medicine, Deparment of MIG, Lund University, Lund, Sweden |
| Szabó, Béla | Department of Microbiology, University Medical School, Debrecen, Hungary |
| Szabó, Edina | Department of Medical Microbiology and Immunology, University Medical School, Pécs, Hungary |

| | |
|---|---|
| Szőke, Ildikó | Department of Clinical Microbiology, Albert Szent-Györgyi Medical University, Szeged, Hungary |
| Tekin, Mehmet | Experimental Medical Research Institute, University of Istanbul, Turkey |
| Thiede, Arnulf | Department of Surgery, Universität Würzburg, Würzburg, Germany |
| Torzewska, Agnieszka | Deaprtment of Immunology of Bacteria, Institute of Microbiology and Immunology, University of Łodz, Poland |
| Tóth, István | Veterinary Medical Research Institute of the Hunagarian Academy of Sciences, Budapest, Hungary |
| Tóth, Vilmos | Department of Stomatology, University Medical School, Pécs, Hungary |
| Toukach, Filip V. | N.D. Zelinsky Institute of Organic Chemistry, Russian Academy of Sciences, Moscow, Russian Federation |
| Török, László | Department of Urology, Albert Szent-Györgyi Medical University, Szeged, Hungary |
| Uhlin, Bernt Eric | Department of Microbiology, Umeå University, Umeå, Sweden |
| Urbonaviciene, Jurate | Department of Microbiology, Umeå University, Umeå, Sweden |
| van Kessel, Kok P.M. | Eijkman-Winkler Institute, University Hospital, Utrecht University, Utrecht, The Netherlands |
| Vidal, Rui | Facultade de Farmácia de Lisboa, Portugal |
| Virkola, Ritva | Division of General Microbiology, Department of Biosciences, Helsinki University, Helsinki, Finland |
| Wirth, Reinhard | Universität Regensburg, Institut für Mikrobiologie NWF III, Regensburg, Germany |
| Wullt, Björn | Institute of Laboratory Medicine, Department of MIG, Lund University, Lund, Sweden |
| Wykrota, Marianna | Department of Immunology of Bacteria, Institute of Microbiology and Immunology, University of Łodz, Poland |

Xia, Yan      Department of Microbiology, Umeå University, Umeå, Sweden

Ziebuhr, Wilma      Institut für Molekulare Infektionsbiologie, Universität Würzburg, Würzburg, Germany

Zych, Krystyna      Department of General Microbiology, University of Łodz, Poland

# INDEX

## DATE DUE